SKIN CANCER OVERVIEW

Edited by **Yaguang Xi**

Skin Cancer Overview
Edited by Yaguang Xi

Published by InTech
Janeza Trdine 9, 51000 Rijeka, Croatia

Publishing Process Manager Tajana Jevtic

Technical Editor Teodora Smiljanic

Cover Designer InTech Design Team

Additional hard copies can be obtained from orders@intechopen.com

Skin Cancer Overview, Edited by Yaguang Xi
p. cm.
ISBN 978-953-307-746-8

For EU product safety concerns:
IN TECH d.o.o., Prolaz Marije Krucifikse Kozulić 3, 51000 Rijeka, Croatia,
info@intechopen.com or visit our website at intechopen.com.

Meet the editor

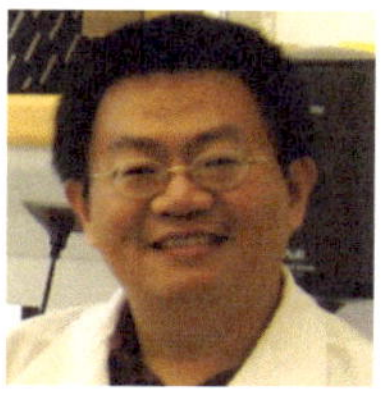

Dr. Yaguang Xi is an Assistant Professor at the Mitchell Cancer Institute, University of South Alabama in Mobile, Alabama, United States. Before coming to the United States, Dr. Xi earned his MD and PhD in China and was trained as a postdoctoral fellow at the International Agency for Research on Cancer (IARC) in Lyon, France. Dr. Xi won the Scholar-In-Training Award for the American Association for Cancer Research (AACR), and the Merit Award from the American Society of Clinical Oncology (ASCO). He is an author of publications in Cell Death and Differentiation, Oncogene, Clinical Cancer Research, Carcinogenesis, RNA, Molecular Cancer Therapeutics, Bioinformatics, PLoS ONE, and more. Dr. Xi is a member of Editorial Boards of Thoracic Cancer, TheScientificWorldJOURNAL, and Micro RNA. He was also invited to be a reviewer for a number of journals and research grant foundations.

Contents

Preface

Skin cancer is one of the most common types of tumors in Western countries. In the United States only, more than one million people are diagnosed with skin cancer each year. Although the absolute number of skin cancer patients is increasing, the death is inversely decreasing, due to the early detection and treatment. Basal cell carcinoma (BCC), squamous cell carcinoma (SCC), and melanoma are three major types of skin cancer. BCC and SCC rarely have metastasis; over 95 percent BCC and SCC patients can be cured. Melanoma only accounts for a small percentage of skin cancer, but it causes 75 percent death of this disease. In this book, we invited a number of experts to present their latest accomplishments on skin cancer research. Although the topics are varied, the authors did great work to help readers better understand skin cancer and learn the knowledge to prevent this disease.

There are three sections in this book, starting with etiology. Ultraviolet (UV) light exposure is overwhelmingly believed to be the most frequent cause of skin cancer. In this section, the association between UV and photodermatoses, as well as skin cancer is discussed. Desmosomal cadherins are important molecules in tumor cell adhesion and invasion, and their important roles in BCC are also presented in details.

In the diagnosis and treatment section, a few new methodologies are described. As known, the outcome of malignant melanoma greatly depends on the thickness of the tumor at the time of treatment. Accurate determination of melanoma lateral and depth of margins using non-invasive imaging technologies is of importance when making sound decisions for treatment and evaluating a five year survival rate. A novel method named differential scanning calorimetry is capable of predicting metastasis of melanoma patients by monitoring the temperature changes of plasma. Electronic miniature X-ray brachytherapy is introduced as a new technology to treat non-melanoms skin cancer.

Although its potential has not yet been fully realized, chemoprevention, in terms of using chemical agents that naturally occur in foods, or are administered as pharmaceuticals to retard or reverse the process of carcinogenesis and progression of cancer, has been recognized to benefit individuals with precancerous lesions or genetic susceptibilities to cancer. In the prevention section, two chapters summarized the most recognized dietary phytochemicals and their potential application in skin cancer.

This book would not have been possible without the contributions of all authors and the support from the publisher. Especially, I will convey my sincere appreciation to Ms. Tajana Jevtic, who has always been available and supportive of me to accomplish this project.

Yaguang Xi, M.D., Ph.D.
Assistant Professor of Oncologic Sciences,
University of South Alabama,
USA

Part 1

Etiology

1

Photodermatoses and Skin Cancer

Serena Lembo, Nicola Balato, Annunziata Raimondo,
Martina Mattii, Anna Balato and Giuseppe Monfrecola
Department of Dermatology – University of Naples Federico II
Italy

1. Introduction

Photodermatoses are a group of skin diseases caused or exacerbated by light. Their classification is traditionally based on the cause of the disorder and on the pathology of cutaneous response. **Polymorphic light eruption (PLE)** is the commonest photosensitive disorder affecting up to 20% of the population, characterized by an intermittent eruption of non scarring pruritic erythematous papules, vesicles or plaques that develop on ultraviolet (UV) radiation (UVR)-exposed skin (Stratigos et al., 2002). The course of the disease is mainly chronic. The disease is multifactorial: a genetic susceptibility has been identified as well as environmental components. The spectrum of radiation that induces PLE is most commonly UVA and/or UVB wavelengths and, rarely, visible light. Epstein first hypothesized, over 60 years ago, that PLE was an immune-mediated disease. He postulated that PLE was a delayed-type hypersensitivity reaction (DTHR) to UVR induced cutaneous antigens (Epstein, 1986). Only during the past 20 years have studies emerged that support this theory. It is hypothesized that the DTHR associated with PLE is secondary to a partial failure of UVR-induced immunosuppression in patients with PLE. Multiple studies highlighted the greater role of Langerhans cells (LCs) in the sensitization phase and therefore suggested that LC dysfunction may be the underlying cause of PLE. In fact, in patients with PLE, LCs persist in the epidermis after intermittent UVB exposure whereas, in normal subjects, LCs disappear from the epidermis. In contrast, neutrophil infiltration in the skin after UVB exposure is significantly decreased in patients with PLE. Less neutrophilic infiltration may lead to impaired local production of cytokines such as interleukin (IL)-4 and IL-10. Altering the local skin milieu after UVR exposure eventually leads to activation of the skin immune response instead of suppression (Cooper et al., 1992). These observations would lead one to suppose that failure of immunosuppression following UVR exposure might give an advantage with regard to recognition of UV-induced tumour antigens and more effective elimination of such antigenic cells by the immune system. UVR-induced **skin cancer (SC)** is the most prevalent form of human neoplasm. It is well known that UVB (280–320 nm) and UVA (320-400 nm) radiation can induce DNA damage leading to melanoma or non melanoma SC by provoking mutations and immunosuppressive effects. The molecular changes induced by UV generate multiple consequent or concomitant mechanisms: DNA damage with thymidine dimer formation, urocanic acid (UCA) isomerization from trans-UCA to cis-UCA, depletion of some protective cytokines such as IL-1, IL-12 and interferon-γ (IFN-γ), or the increase of tumour necrosis factor-α (TNF-α), IL-6, IL-10 and IL-15, resulting in the immunosuppressed skin milieu that permits and maintains the proliferation of mutated cellular clones (Kamiya, 2003). It would seem that the skin performs a 'balancing act' between adequate elimination of early cancerous cells and suppression of abnormal reactions against UV-exposed cells that may suffer transient aberrations. PLE appears to be associated with an 'imbalance' between UV-induced proinflammatory and UV-induced suppressive immunoreaction. From previous experiences, a reduced incidence of SC has been shown in patients with PLE compared with gender- and age-matched controls (Lembo et al., 2008). In support of the findings of this study, other studies indicated that either LC subtypes or tumour-derived cytokines play a crucial role in UV-induced skin tumours, determining LC depletion, attraction and immunoprotective function. Whereas there is considerable circumstantial evidence that disruption in the density and function of these cells, during the early stages of UVR-induced carcinogenesis, may be important for enabling developing neoplasms to escape immune destruction, the role of the large number of these cells found infiltrating developed skin tumours, remains unclear. Our aim was to provide an overview of UVR effects, photodermatoses and skin cancer, their epidemiology, incidence and the relationship of UVR-induced imbalance between immunosuppression or immunoactivation in PLE with relative skin cancer risk

2. Ultraviolet radiation

Sunlight is a continuous spectrum of electromagnetic radiation that is divided into three major spectrums of wavelength: ultraviolet, visible and infrared. The UV range is the most significant spectrum of sunlight that causes photoaging and skin cancer. UVR is subdivided into: ultraviolet A [UVA (320–400 nm)], ultraviolet B [UVB (280–320 nm)] and ultraviolet C [UVC (100–280 nm)]. UVA represent the 90–99% of the solar UVR energy that reaches the earth's surface; it is not filtered by the stratospheric ozone layer in the atmosphere and has long wavelength and low energy so it can penetrate deeper into the skin. Once considered harmless, but now believed to be harmful, in case of excessive and long-term exposure, causes skin aging and induces immediate and persistent pigmentation (tanning). In the recent years a carcinogenic role for UVA has also been proved. Only approximately 1–10% of UVB reaches the earth's surface because it is filtered by the stratospheric ozone layer in the atmosphere; it has short wavelength and high energy so it can penetrate the upper layers of the epidermis. UVB is responsible for sunburns, tanning, wrinkling, photoaging and skin cancer. UVC is filtered by the stratospheric ozone layer in the atmosphere before reaching earth; the major artificial sources are germicidal lamps. UVC burns the skin and causes skin cancer. Ultraviolet radiation that reaches the earth's surface can increase or decrease based on a variety of factors. One factor is the ozone layer, which forms a thin shield in the stratospheric atmosphere, protecting life on earth from the sun's UV rays; this layer absorbs all UVC radiation, most UVB radiation and very little UVA radiation. Since the mid 1980s, scientists began to be concerned that the ozone layer was being depleted. The reason for thinning of the stratospheric ozone is resulting from the release of ozone-depleting substances and chemicals (chlorofluorocarbons) that are released from industry and motor vehicle into the atmosphere. An approximate 1% decrease in ozone levels corresponds to a 1–2% increase in the mortality caused by melanoma (World Health Organization, 2009). Likewise, a 10% decrease in the ozone levels will cause 300,000 new non-melanoma and 4500 new melanoma skin cancer cases moreover, multiple factors such as time of the day, time of the year, latitude and altitude, determine UVR levels reaching earth's surface.

Depletion of the ozone layer results in increased UVR, (especially UVB) reaching the earth's surface. UVB is directly absorbed by DNA and causes structural DNA damage. UVA causes indirect DNA damage through the formation of reactive oxygen species, which create breaks in DNA. These events lead to mutations and then to skin cancer (Brenner et al., 2008). The sun exerts its highest peak between 10 AM to 4 PM. During this time, the sun's rays have the least distance to travel through the atmosphere and UVB levels are at their highest. In the early morning and late afternoon, the sun's rays pass through the atmosphere at an angle and their intensity is greatly reduced. The sun's angle varies with the seasons, causing the intensity of UV rays to change. UV intensity tends to be the highest during the summer season. Environmental factors that increase the amount of UVR exposure to humans include latitudes closer to the equator. At higher latitudes the sun is lower in the sky, so UV rays must travel a greater distance through ozone-rich portions of the atmosphere and in turn, less UVR is emitted. Hence, living closer to the equator increases UV exposure, thus increasing the incidence of skin cancers. For every 1000 meters increase in elevation, the UVR intensity increases by 10–12%. UV levels also depend on cloud cover; thus, there are lower UV levels at higher cloud cover densities. In the summer, the sun is higher in the sky, and less ultraviolet radiation is absorbed during its passage through the atmosphere. Fog, haze, clouds and pollutants can reduce ultraviolet levels by 10–90%. Snow, sand and metal can reflect up to 90% of ultraviolet radiation. Sea water can reflect up to 15%, whereas little reflection occurs on still water (e.g., a pool). Shade alone reduces solar UVR by 50–95%. The amount of protection varies considerably between different shades settings, with a beach umbrella showing the least and dense foliage the most protection. The best technique for reducing ultraviolet exposure is to avoid the sun, especially in the middle of the day (Lautenschlager et al., 2007) . There is accumulating evidence that UVR in physiological doses exerts multiple effects on the immune system: such as inducing immune system but suppressing the adaptive one. Both effects may be beneficial, protecting from microbial infections on the one hand and toning down allergic and autoimmune reactions on the other hand; but these effects on the immune system are also responsible of the dangerous effects of UVR such as photodermatoses and skin cancer.

2.1 UVR effects

Solar UVR makes up just 5% of the electromagnetic spectrum that reaches the earth's surface. Three spectral regions have been designated based on their biological effects. Terrestrial UVR consists of 3- 6% UVB and 94- 97% UVA. Negligible amounts of UVC reach the earth's surface due to the filtering capacity of the ozone layer (Diffey, 2002). UVR is a potent environmental carcinogen and is largely responsible for the development of the most common cancer worldwide: skin cancer. The steady increases in melanoma and non-melanoma skin cancer cases, contrast with the recent downward incidence for all other cancers (excluding lung cancer in women). The increases in skin cancer are largely attributed to recreational sun exposure (including tanning beds) practiced by the population. Concern that further increases in skin cancer incidence may result due to ozone depletion, may be tempered by positive global efforts to reduce ozone-depleting substances in the atmosphere (Jemal et al., 2007). The genetic mechanisms by which UVR transforms and promotes various skin cancers have been under intense investigation for decades, and much progress has been made in identifying genes that contribute to the oncogenic process in the development of melanoma, squamous cell carcinoma (SSC) and basal cell carcinoma

(BCC). However, in addition to generating genetic mutations, UVR actively suppresses the normal processes of immune surveillance responsible for eliminating mutant cells, and permits tumor growth. UVR is highly mutagenic but is only partially absorbed by the outer stratum corneum of the epidermis Depending on melanin content UVR can penetrate into the deeper layers of the epidermis, where induces DNA damage and apoptosis in epidermal cells, including those in the germinative basal layer. The cellular decision, to initiate either the cellular repair processes or undergo apoptosis, has evolved to balance the acute need to maintain skin barrier function with the long-term risk of retaining precancerous cells. Langerhans cells are positioned suprabasally, where they may sense UV damage directly, or indirectly through recognition of apoptotic vesicles and soluble mediators derived from surrounding keratinocytes. Apoptotic bodies will contain UV-induced altered proteins (enzymes, proteins that regulate cells proliferation and apoptosis process) that may be presented to the immune system as foreign. The observation that UVR induces immune tolerance to skin-associated antigens suggests that this photodamage response has evolved to preserve the skin barrier by protecting it from autoimmune attack. LC involvement in this process is not clear and controversial. In order to ameliorate the world-wide burden of UVR related pathologies such as sunburn, aging, autoimmunity, immune suppression and skin cancer, it is imperative that we gain a better understanding of the mechanisms of UVA and UVB induced photodamage and how they relate to the molecular and immunologic nature of photodamage responses.

2.1.1 The link between UV-induced inflammation and carcinogenesis

UV augments blood flow and infiltration by blood leukocytes, such as macrophages and neutrophils into the skin, observed clinically as inflammation. Increased production of NO and prostaglandins contribute to these events. UVR-induced lipid peroxidation increases production of prostaglandins (PG), including PGE2, which, in turn, cause inflammation in the skin. PGE-2 is produced from arachidonic acid by the inducible form of cyclooxygenase (COX), COX-2. This is thought to be due to UV increasing phospholipase activity, thus enhancing arachidonic acid availability for PG production. Dietary supplementation with fish oils has been shown to reduce UV-induced inflammation in humans, probably due to a reduction in UV-induced PGE-2 production. Other UV-induced mediators, such as tumour necrosis factor and interleukin 1 also contribute to UV-induced inflammation. The inflammatory cells, infiltrating UV exposed skin, produce ROS that further drive damage to lipids, proteins and DNA. Thus, UV-induced oxidative damage to lipids, and activation of NO synthase (Warren, 1994) initiates a cascade of events resulting in inflammation, which causes further reactive oxygen stress in the skin. As ROS produced by inflammatory cells is linked to gene mutations, it seems to be a reasonable hypothesis that UV-induced inflammation results in genetic damage, which contributes to photocarcinogenesis. There is a large amount of literature supporting a role for inflammation in driving tumour progression, and anti-inflammatory drugs have been shown to reduce the incidence of cancer (Balkwill & Mantovani, 2001). A number of animal models have shown that inhibition of COX-2 helps prevent skin cancer: Celecoxib, a COX-2 inhibitor, decreases macrophages and neutrophils infiltration into skin tumours; Indomethacin, which inhibits both COX-1 and 2, reduces photocarcinogenesis in mice. The cancer protective effect of COX-2 inhibition may be due to prevention of inflammation: it has been suggested, in fact, that this may enhance apoptosis of UV damaged keratinocytes as PGE2 signalling is required for growth of skin tumour cells (Thompson et al., 2001). UV-induced infiltration of the skin by granulocytes and macrophages has been shown to enhance the growth of a UV-induced regressor skin tumour. UV-induced regressor skin tumours grow for about 1–2 weeks after transplantation into syngeneic mice before being rejected by the immune system, so that they decrease in size after this time. In these studies, a single inflammatory dose of UVR caused infiltration of the skin by CD11b+, Gr-1+, CD45+, MHC Class II+ cells, which were likely to be macrophages and or granulocytes (Thompson et al., 2001). Time courses demonstrated an enhancement of tumour growth only when these cells were present at high numbers in the skin: therefore UV-induced inflammatory cells promoted skin tumour growth. Other studies have shown that UV radiation induces infiltration of neutrophils and macrophages into the skin of mice and humans. As UV-induced inflammatory cells produce hydrogen peroxide and NO, it is likely that ROS produced by these inflammatory cells contribute to skin tumour development at least in part by enhancing gene mutation, but they may also suppress immunity. Moreover, it has also been suggested that inflammatory cytokine induction of iNOS results in increased NO production which inhibits DNA repair, thus promoting carcinogenesis. Both of these are likely to contribute to skin cancer formation.

2.1.2 UV-induced oxidative damage and gene mutation

There is little direct evidence for oxidative damage to DNA making a substantial contribution to photocarcinogenesis.

The formation of micronuclei is an indication of chromosomal rearrangement or genetic instability. UVA-induced micronucleus formation in cultured HaCaT cells was reduced by treatment with catalase, suggesting a role for hydrogen peroxide in this form of UVA-induced genetic damage (Phillipson et al., 2002). UVB absorbed by two adjacent cytosine (C) residues in DNA causes the formation of cyclobutane pyrimidine dimers (CPD), which result in GC to AT mutations. These only occur in response to UVB and can be regarded as fingerprints for UVB; UVA-induced CPD formation is orders of magnitude less frequent. In contrast, UVA indirectly induces the fingerprint mutations AT to CG at high frequency, but these rarely result from UVB or other mutagens. Reactive oxygen and nitrogen species can cause many different types of gene mutations, but guanine is the most sensitive of the DNA bases to oxidation, as it has the lowest oxidation potential. Hence, G to T, G to C and G to A mutations at sites other than dipyrimidines are frequently caused by ROS (Kamiya, 2003). However, ROS cannot be assigned to be the mutagen as confidently in these cases as UVB and UVA can be identified when the fingerprints mentioned above are observed. UVA itself can cause oxidation of guanine indirectly via ROS production, or the ROS can come from other sources such as inflammatory cells. However, in combination with UVA-induced fingerprints to account for the role of UVA, mutations at guanine sites can give an indication of the likely extent to which DNA is mutated in response to ROS from sources other than UVA, such as inflammatory cells. In a recent study, different regions of about 20 keratinocytes from human solar keratosis (SK) and SCC were microdissected to analyse the p53 gene for mutations. Using the criteria described above, the mutations could be grouped into those most likely caused by ROS, UVB or UVA. When the cause of the mutations could not be unambiguously identified they were grouped as "other", but some of these could have been due to ROS, UVB or UVA. About one-third of the mutations in SK were caused by sunlight with an equal number resulting from UVA and UVB. ROS caused a slightly larger number of mutations than UV, showing that ROS make a significant contribution to the mutational burden in these benign pre-malignant lesions. When comparing SK to SCC, it was found that SCC contained an increase in mutational burden of 14 ROS, 5 other, 4 UVB, but 0 UVA-induced mutations (Agar et al., 2004). Thus, ROS appear to be responsible for the majority of the increase in mutations as SK progress into SCC. UV does not appear to be the major mutagen driving SK progression towards SCC, as there was little difference in UVB and UVA fingerprints between these lesions. Therefore, the increase in ROS induced mutations probably did not result from UVA-induced ROS. This data appear to indicate that the mixture of UVA and UVB in sunlight is largely responsible for the mutations that lead to SK, but the main factor that then drives these benign lesions to progress to malignancy is ROS. The cause of a large number of the mutations could not be identified, and therefore some caution is required in interpreting this data. These mutations could have been caused by UVB, UVA or ROS, but were not identifiable as such, or they may have resulted from a yet unknown event. It has been reported that patients with SK have reduced plasma antioxidant defence (Vural et al., 1999), which may contribute to oxidation induced gene damage in SK. Most SK do not develop into SCC and often spontaneously regress. However, an inflammatory response, developing for unknown reasons in a small subset of SK appears to be associated with progression towards malignant SCC. The major mutagen driving SK progression to SCC appears to be ROS, rather than sunlight, suggesting that reactive oxygen and nitrogen species from inflammatory cells is responsible for progression of SK into SCC. While UVA can cause gene mutations indirectly, via reactive oxygen mediated processes, the absence of a large increase in UVB-induced gene mutations as SK progress towards SCC suggests that little of the ROS-mediated damage driving progression of SK to SCC arose from sunlight.

2.1.3 UV-induced immunosuppression

Ultraviolet radiation not only causes DNA damage but also is a potent immunosuppressive agent. This was demonstrated in a series of elegant experiments carried out by Kripke (Fisher & Kripke, 1977). In syngeneic mice, UVR-induced skin cancers were transplanted into mice which were either irradiated with UVB or not irradiated. In those mice irradiated with UVB the tumours continued to grow, whereas those not irradiated were able to reject the transplanted tumours. The induced immunosuppression was also transferable by lymphocytes from irradiated mice (unable to reject the tumours) injected into non irradiated mice. It is known that UVR-induced immunosuppression is a complex process (Figure 1). ***UVR action*** spectrum for induction of CPDs is now known to be identical to that of Tumour necrosis factor alpha which in turn is induced by Interleukin-1. Direct immunosuppression locally in the skin comes about when UVB directly impacts on Langerhans cells. LCs: dendritic cells critical for the presention of antigens to the immune system, very sensitive even to UVR minimal dose. In a series of human experiments, solar simulated radiation whether, given as a single minimal erythema dose, or over ten times the time period, but with irradiance at 10% of the dose, or over 10 days at one tenth of MED, the outcome was the same: LCs numbers were depleted (Figure 1). The ability to do this appears to be genetic, and, in those individuals who fail to deplete LCs when initially exposed to antigen in the setting of UV exposure, PLE occurs. This ability to resist UV-induced depletion appears to be protective against skin cancer development. This hypothesis is supported by an epidemiological study of the prevalence of polymorphic light eruption in those who have skin cancer, despite apparently equivalent UVR exposure, the prevalence of PLE appeared reduced (Lembo et al., 2008). Kripke's experiments in mice suggest that SCCs are highly antigenic, thus mechanisms whereby antigen is recognised are relevant in the process of preventing UVR initiated skin cancers (Timares et al., 2008). Mutated cells carrying highly relevant p53 mutations are well described. Such clones of mutated cells are found in chronically UVR exposed skin. If the immune system is functioning, such mutant cells may be policed by antigen presenting cells and T memory cells and progression to skin cancers can be stopped. CPD are linked with the suppression of T memory cells thus UVR reduces immune surveillance by this mechanism. Therefore when immune regulation is perturbed, such as with ongoing sun-exposure, chronic lymphatic leukaemia or with long term systemic immuno-suppression, failure of immune regulation leads to progression of these clones to actinic keratoses and frankly invasive squamous cell carcinomas. Nucleotide excision repair is a very important protective response against skin cancer. Pyrimidine dimer formation in DNA initiates the tanning response in UV-irradiated mice. DNA repair results in fragments of DNA being excised from the DNA molecule, these tiny oligomers have been shown to directly cause immunoprotective effects when applied to the skin (Arad et al., 2006). A further UVR immunosuppressive effect is the isomerisation of a chemical component of the stratum corneum.: urocanic acid normally exists in its trans-isoform but with irradiation by UVB is transformed to its cis-isomer which is a powerful systemic immunosuppressant (Figure 1). The action spectrum for the induction of this process appears to be in the UVB range. There is evidence to suggest that cis-urocanic acid's ability to suppress contact hypersensitivity is mediated via TNF-α (McLoone et al., 2005). UV-irradiated urocanic acid is also able to suppress delayed hypersensitivity reactions to herpes simplex in mice (Ross et al., 1986). The complexity of UV-induced immunosuppression is compounded by the ability of UVR to modulate four main families of growth factors: epidermal growth factor receptor (EGFR), platelet-derived growth factor receptor (PDGFR), fibroblast growth factor receptor (FGFR), and insulin receptor (IR), and in addition primary cytokines each of which has immunosuppressive effects. Apart from TNF-α, the interleukin family have wide ranging effects often interdependent. UV induces IL-1, IL-6, IL-10 amongst others. IL-10 is considered very important as a mediator of systemic immunosuppression (Ghoreihi & Dutz, 2006): tolerance induction by immunisation through UVR irradiated skin is transferable through CD4+CD25+ T regulatory cells and is dependant on IL-10 produced by the host. The mechanisms underlying UVR-induced tolerance therefore are complex and constantly being refined. UVR also induces platelet-derived growth factor (PDGF) thought to be pivotal both in UVB-induced immunosuppression and also the immunosuppression induced by PUVA. UVB activates receptors for the primary cytokines interleukin-1 and tumor necrosis factor-α and the death receptor Fas. UV also induces melanin stimulating hormone (MSH) locally, from keratinocytes; such paracrine secretion plays a critical role in local cell regulation from an immunosuppressive and proinflammatory point of view. The receptor for pigment regulation within melanocytes: melanocortin receptor (MCR) is also regulated by UVR (Figure 1). While increasing doses of UVB were found to cause increasing levels of immunosuppression, only a narrow range of UVA or solar-simulated UV suppressed the immune system. Doses of about 1.8 J/cm2 solar-simulated UV (0.5 minimum erythema dose [MED]) delivered for three consecutive days, but not twice this dose-suppressed immunity to an antigen delivered to un-irradiated skin (induction of systemic immunosuppression). The ***UVA component*** of this, 1.68 J/cm2, was also immunosuppressive, but twice this dose was not. It appears that while this low dose of UVA damages the immune system, higher doses can actually protect the immune system from UVB effects . UVA has also been reported to be as effective as solar-simulated UV at suppressing the reactivation of secondary immunity in mice (Moyal & Fourtanier, 2001). It, therefore, appears that different doses of UVA can affect immunity in quite different ways, presumably because UVA has complex dose effects on unknown molecular events. Doses of UVA within the range used some studies have been shown to produce ROS in human skin, and these ROS can be inhibited with reactive oxygen quenchers (Ou-Yanh, 2004). As increasing doses of UVA cause higher levels of ROS in the skin. It is likely that ROS are involved in UVA-induced immunosuppression. High dose UVA, which reverses UVB-induced immunosuppression has been shown to mediate this effect via production of the antioxidant heme oxygenase enzyme. Thus, it seems probable that low doses of UVA initiate ROS production, which suppress skin immunity. In contrast, higher does of UVA stimulate production of protective antioxidant enzymes, thus reversing the suppressive effects of ROS and UVB. There has been some experimentation that supports the above hypothesis that UVA causes immunosuppression via a ROS-dependent mechanism, but considerably more work is required to definitively answer this issue and determine the steps involved. Other mediators may also be involved in UVA modulation of immunity, such as PGE2. It has been suggested that a cascade of events, initiated by UV-induced PGE2 production in the skin, in turn induces production of IL-4 and IL-10, which cause systemic immunosuppression (Figure 1). As increase PGE2 is a downstream event of lipids oxidative damage, the important role of UV-induced oxidative damage in photoimmunosuppression is highlighted. PGE2 has also been implicated in immunosuppression during chemical carcinogenesis in the skin (Andrews et al., 1991). More recently it has been shown that oxidized lipids, such as phosphatidylcholine, are recognized by the platelet activating factor receptor able to trigger immunosuppression (Walterscheid et al., 2002). The practical and visible consequences of these immunological perturbations are those of carcinogenesis, photoallergic reactions and infections. ***Latent viral infection*** can be triggered or enhanced by UVR. The action spectrum for induction or activation of Herpes Simplex and/or Varicella Zoster virus seems to be in the UVB range. A new viral infection linked with UVR is the recently described ***Merkel cell polyoma virus*** (Paulson et al., 2009) and ***Human papilloma virus (HPV)***. HPV is ubiquitous in human skin, it is thought that the skin is colonised shortly after birth. More than 100 different virus subtypes are described and divided into mucosal and non-mucosal types. Different subtypes are associated with different clinical pictures. Up to recently, it was assumed that cutaneous sub-types did not interfere with apoptosis, as is the case for high risk subtypes, in which the E6 protein functions as a block in the apoptotic pathway interfering with the tumour suppressor gene p53. The consequence for those carrying high risk mucosal HPV may be anogenital squamous cell carcinoma. The role of human papilloma virus in carcinogenesis is well established in cervical cancer, in which persistent carriage of high risk viral types 16, 18, 31 and 33 are incontrovertibly implicated in cancer pathogenesis. In keratinised skin, until recently, the story was less clear other than in the rare syndrome epidermodysplasia verruciformis (EV), where medium risk oncogenic type 5, 7 and 12 HPV interact with UVR to induce cancer. High risk HPV types 16 and 18 on keratinised skin are found rarely in periungual warts. Something important is supposed to occur in transitional areas: keratinised skin-mucosal epithelium or keratinised skin-nail. HPV favours anogenital areas, lips nose and also UV-irradiated skin. Plane warts are almost inevitably found on the dorsum of the hands and the face, sites of maximal UV dose. Immunosuppression caused by UVR in irradiated areas leads to skin exquisitely suited to the proliferation of HPV; with the defences down, immune surveillance at a minimum, it is no surprise therefore that warts or dysplastic lesions, depending on HPV type, will flourish in these circumstances (O' Connor, 2001). Recently mechanistic evidence has emerged implicating medium risk HPV in the aetiology of non-melanoma skin cancer, particularly squamous cell carcinomas, specially in immunosuppressed individuals. Mutated cells normally are shifted to the apoptotic pathway, but HPV has the ability to abrogate the proapoptotic BAK signalling via the E6 protein, leading to damaged cell survival (Leverrier et al., 2007). One of the difficulties when discussing immunosuppression is the absence of a good and standardized measure of immunosuppression. Most studies have measured effects of UVR on abrogating delayed hypersensitivity responses. In the context of contact dermatitis the immunosuppression-immunosurveillance state can be clinically evident through patch testing before and after UVR exposure. There is no good marker which reliably determines immunosuppression: the only epidemiological marker is circulating CD4 count.

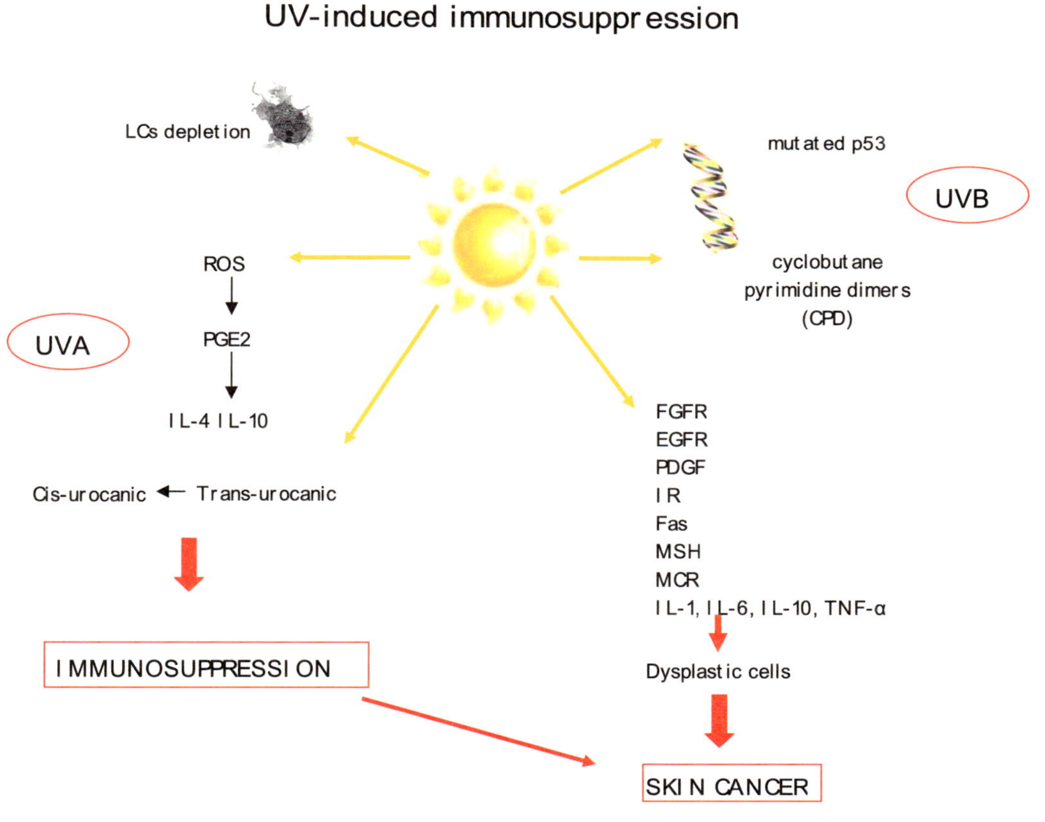

Fig. 1. UV-induced immunosuppression.

3. Photosensitive disorders

Photosensitive disorders occur when human skin reacts abnormally to UVR or visible light (Murphy et al., 2001). Normal human skin produces a range of responses designed to protect man from adverse effects of UVR. The normal response is determined by skin colour, which is in part genetically determined, and skin thickness, which is influenced by adaptive responses to UVR (Murphy et al., 1991). The presence, extent and thickness of hair determine photoprotection. Age, pigment adaptation, body site and also antiinflammatory agents influence responsiveness to UVR. Classification of the photodermatoses traditionally is based on the cause of the disorder, where known, and on the pathology of cutaneous response (Table 1). Observation of the clinical patterns of skin reactivity and the timing of the response helps the investigator to classify disorders as many photodermatoses are of unknown cause. Photosensitive disorders may be broadly classified as primarily UVR induced such disorders include the idiopathic (some of which may perhaps now be better described as autoimmune) photodermatoses: Polymorphic light eruption, Juvenile spring eruption, Actinic prurigo (AP), Solar urticaria (SU), Hydroa vacciniforme, Chronic actinic dermatitis (CAD), Brachioradial pruritus, Actinic folliculitis. Phototoxic diseases are caused by external agents either systemic, or topically applied, which predictably lower the threshold for abnormal UVR responses. Photoallergic disorders occur idiosyncratically and may not be predicted, they are less common than phototoxic reactions and are determined by either delayed hypersensitivity responses or, more rarely, immediate hypersensitive reactions IgE mediated. Diseases that are characteristically *photosensitive,* but with other manifestations, include: xeroderma pigmentosum (XP), trichothiodystrophy (TTD), the Rothmund-Thompson syndrome and the cutaneous porphyries. *Photoaggravated* diseases are numerous: Lupus erythematosus (LE), Dermatomyositis, Psoriasis, Rosacea, Lichen Planus, Autoimmune bullous disease; these disorders occur independently of environmental UVR exposure, but may be worsened by exposure to UV. History and physical examination are most important aspects in the diagnosis of the photodermatoses. Most photodermatoses are manifest by cutaneous response to the sun at a lower dose to that which might be expected. The responses may be summarized either as inappropriate redness of the skin occurring immediately or as a delayed response. Immediate erythema occurring minutes after UVR exposure may be caused by SU, drugs, chemicals such as tar or creosote. Erythropoietic protoporphyria or rarely porphyria cutanea tarda may exhibit immediate erythema and urticaria, these latter responses are observed during formal testing with UVR and visible light more than with ambient daylight. Immediate erythema may, rarely be caused by contact allergens such as sunscreens. The morphology of responses is very variable and polymorphic: maculopapular eruptions occurring after UV are, most frequently, expression of PLE. However, similar reactions may also occur with LE, AP, erythema multiforme and drug eruptions. *Urticaria* case occurs in response to UV in SU, rarely as a response to drugs and in case of porphyria (erythropoietic protopophyria (EPP). *Eczema,* as a late reaction to UVR, occurs in CAD, in photosensitive atopic eczema and in AIDS where patients at a young age may develop photosensitive eczema (Wong & Khoo, 2003). In drug-induced photosensitivity, eczema also may be the consequence of agents such as thiazides. *Lichenoid responses* also may occur in response to many drugs including thiazides (Johnston, 2002). *Bullous reaction* to UVR and visible light can represent the clinical picture of Hydroa vacciniforme (HV), a rare childhood disorder, mainly induced by UVA. Umbilicated blisters occur on the face and other exposed areas. Blistering, most frequently on the backs of the hands, can be seen also in cutaneous porphyrias. Drugs such as frusemide, nalidixic acid and amino-quinolones do not infrequently produce blistering in sunlight. Pseudo-porphyria is also recognized as a reaction to numerous agents. This disorder may occur not only with drugs, but also to sunbed over-exposure, and in those who sunbathe excessively with poor sun protection, with excessive UVA exposure. Endogenous porphyrins may be the relevant chromophore in the absence of a relevant drug (Murphy, 1989). *Telangiectasia* may be the endpoint of photosensitivity in some situations. ACE inhibitors lead to photodistributed telangiectasia in patients, especially in renal transplant patients. *Phototoxic burning* represents an immediate discomfort of the skin on exposure to UVR or visible light in the absence of visible signs. This may also occur with drugs, topical agents such as tar or porphyria, especially in patient attended with EPP, or in treatment with photodynamic therapy (PDT) using amino-laevulinic acid or its esters that are metabolized to protoporphyrin IX. Phototoxic burning with PDT is particularly a problem with renal transplant patients where interactions may occur with the many photoactive drugs being taken. *Hyperpigmentation* also occurs as a response to photosensitivity, this may represent post-inflammatory hyperpigmentation, or interaction of UV/visible light with hormonally induced pigmentation as in melasma. In dark skin, photosensitivity may be primarily observable as hyperpigmentation. All dermatologists will be aware of the ability of PUVA to pigment skin. Lichen planus may be photoaggravated; clinically this may look like hyperpigmentation, but histology shows a lichenoid infiltrate. *Hypopigmentation* may be seen in CAD, and this seems to be post-inflammatory hypopigmentation. In some patients, as post-inflammatory reaction because of the Koebner phenomenon, vitiligo occurs. Vitiligo is made worse by sun exposure in some patients. Prurigo lesions, in the absence of obvious primary lesions are seen in AP, excoriations are maximally seen in UV-exposed areas but sun-protected sites also may be affected possibly as autosensitization. *Photo-onycholysis* may occur as an idiopathic phenomenon, but may be caused by some drugs, particularly tetracyclines, psoralens or it may occur in porphyria. It is infrequent because of the protective nature of the nail itself: thick keratin is very photoprotective. *Photorecall* reactions may also occur. Perhaps, 5-fluorouracil given systemically is the most frequent cause of this reaction. Patients undergoing chemotherapy with this agent may develop florid redness and burning and even erosion of photodamaged skin even though they may not have been outdoors for weeks. Presumably the reaction is similar to that of topical Efudix that selectively kills cells with the most UV-induced damage. *Pruritus* may be the sole manifestation of photosensitivity. Immediate pruritus suggests SU, and it rarely occurs in the absence of erythema and urticaria. *Pruritus* occurring within hours with the same time course as PLE has been described sine eruptione. Itching can occur 1–2 weeks after sunburn probably representing the reaction of sensitive skin to desquamation, soothed by emollients. *Dysaesthesia* occurring after intense UV exposure may persist for weeks; threshold responses are normal, and brachioradial pruritus appears to be neuralgia secondary to UVR damage to the skin. Many disorders develop *photoadaptation*; thus, the patient and clinician may be misled by the fact that the face is unaffected, but sites only occasionally exposed to the sun are worst affected. Photodermatoses may occasionally be highly localized and the nature of the disorder can be elucidated only by testing. Formal testing is essential to make a definite diagnosis of CAD. In the absence of abnormal tests, the diagnosis cannot be made. Most patients have abnormal threshold responses to UVR with the same action spectrum as the human erythema spectrum, suggesting that the chromophore for CAD is DNA. A minority of patients exhibit UVA photosensitivity, but this is more commonly the pattern of drug-induced photosensitivity and thus drugs should be excluded in such cases. PLE and juvenile spring eruption usually exhibit normal light tests; 30% of PLE patients demonstrate abnormal responses, either to UVB, UVA or both, and very rarely PLE may be induced by visible light. AP is more often UVA-induced with about 70% of patients showing abnormal reactions. HV is also usually UVA sensitive. SU patients usually produce immediate responses with erythema and urticaria to the eliciting wavelengths. The action spectrum of SU is usually UVA, often UVB and visible light. In individual patients, the action spectrum may broaden, and in some patients, the disorder may spontaneously clear (Beattie, 2001). A solar simulator is a xenon arc lamp fitted with filters such that the output of the lamp reproduces terrestrial sunlight. The intensity of the lamp is much higher so photodermatoses may be reproduced in the laboratory, confirming diagnosis and proving photosensitivity if a patient has normal monochromator tests. Depending on the population tested, 100% of patients with CAD have abnormal responses. Seventy per cent of patients with PLE have reproducible PLE as do AP and HV. SU is almost always reproduced, but occasional patients only react to natural sunlight. Different schedules are used to provoke photodermatoses (van de Pas et al., 2004). Large areas of 4x4 cm^2 or more, need to be used, on body sites where the rash normally occurs. Thirty per cent of patients react with one exposure, repeating the irradiation twice more increases the yield to 70%. This is useful to prove a rash is UV-induced in the absence of other pointers. All patients with exposed surface eczema should be patch and photopatch tested. Photoallergic contact dermatitis is uncommon (Darvay et al., 2001). Review of the relevant allergens for photopatch testing shows that virtually all positive photopatch tests in recent years are because of sunscreen ingredients. Previous photoallergens such as 6-methyl coumarin, musk ambrette and related molecules have been discontinued by the perfume industry in Europe because of previous relatively frequent sensitization. Tetrachlorosalicylanilide also is no longer encountered; thus, it is no longer relevant to test with these agents. Testing perfume ingredients, plant materials and drugs such as promethazine, chlorpromazine and non steroidal anti-inflammatory drugs leads to such a number of false-positive phototoxic reactions that it is better to omit these agents. In the rare true allergic reaction it is important to use a low concentration of the allergen and administer no more than 5 J/cm2 UVA or even 1–2 J/cm2. The crescendo pattern of test reaction, with most intense picture observed the second reading, compared with the first, distinguishes allergy from phototoxic reactions that fade after the time of the first reading. Some patients may need testing to their own products, but if a new agent is being assessed, it is essential to test a control panel of 20 subjects to this agent to exclude false-positive results. Investigation of the photodermatoses offers a considerable amount of information not otherwise available. Some patients are surprisingly photosensitive when formally tested. Clinical impressions may be completely overturned. Formal testing conclusively proves the diagnosis of photosensitivity if the tests are abnormal. Photosensitive individuals may, however, have normal light tests. Photoprovocation using a solar simulator is helpful to demonstrate that the disorder is UV-induced.

Idiopathic photodermatoses	Photoallergic contact dermatitis/photoxic contact sensitivity Drug induced (photoxic/photoallergic)	Genophotodermatoses	Photoaggravated disease	Disease aggravated or precipitated by UVR-induced immunosuppression
Polymorphic light eruption	Antibiotics	Xeroderma pigmentosum	Lupus erythematosus	Herpes simplex infection
Juvenile spring eruption	Diuretics	Trichothiodystrophy	Dermatomyositis	Viral exanthemata
Actinic prurigo	Antipsychotics	Bloom's syndrome	Eczema	Plane wart
Solar urticaria	Sedatives	Cutaneous porphyries	Psoriasis	Skin cancers
Hydroa vacciniforme	Antihypertensive agents	Kindler-Weary syndrome	Rosacea	
Chronic actinic dermatitis	Non-steroid anti-inflammatory drugs	Smith-Lemli-Opitz syndrome	Lichen planus	
Brachioradial pruritus	Antidiabetic-agents		Autoimmune bullous diseases	
Actinic folliculitis	Lipid-lowering agents		Vitiligo	
	Protease inhibitors		Vitamin B6, niacin deficiency	

Table 1. Classification of photodermatoses

3.1 Polymorphous light eruption

Polymorphic light eruption (PLE) is the most common of the idiopathic photodermatoses. It is an acquired disorder characterized by an intermittent, transient, delayed response, 30 minutes to several hours after UV light exposure. The cutaneous response has been described as nonscarring, pruritic, erythematous papules, vesicles, or plaques on light-exposed skin. Other presentations include vesiculobullous, hemorrhagic, erythema multiforme-like, and strophulus-like (insect bite) appearances. In the absence of additional UV exposure, the eruptions resolve in hours to as long as 2 weeks, leaving completely normal skin. PLE is the most common photosensitivity. It affects females two to three times more often than males and onset is typically in the first three decades of life. The incidence is estimated at 10% in the United States, 21% in Sweden, 15% in the United Kingdom, and 5% in Australia. All racial skin types have been documented as being affected in the medical literature, however, it most commonly occurs in fair-skinned individuals of Fitzpatrick skin types I–IV. PLE has been widely reported, but it occurs most frequently in temperate climates and is least prevalent in subtropical and tropical areas. Episodes of PLE usually occur in the spring and occasionally in the fall. Patients are usually less susceptible during the summer and winter. This prevalence during the spring and fall, as well as the predilection for temperate climates, may be explained by the greater proportion of UVA to UVB light in these settings. It is possible that the higher proportion of UVB to UVA during the summer months may inadvertently reduce UVA exposure because of earlier sunburning and, therefore, reduce susceptibility through a UVB-induced alteration in immunologic reactivity. Although classified as an acquired idiopathic photodermatoses, familial clustering is suggestive of a genetic etiology. A recent study examined 119 monozygotic twin pairs and 301 dizygotic twin pairs, revealing an incidence of 21% among the monozygotic twins and 18% in dizygotic twins. The study also demonstrated that PLE was present in one or more first-degree relatives (excluding the co-twin) in 12% of affected twin pairs compared with 4% of relatives in unaffected twin pairs, thus providing statistically significant evidence of familial clustering ($p< 0.0001$) (Milliard et al., 2000). Ultimately a combination of genetic and environmental factors is probably responsible for expression of PLE. PLE has been considered, for long as a possible, delayed-type hypersensitivity (DTH) response to an endogenous, cutaneous UV-induced antigen, because of the hours or days delay between sun exposure and manifestation of symptoms, and the histological appearance of lesional skin. Firm evidence, however, has been lacking and the responsible allergen has not been identified. UV irradiation may convert a potential precursor in the skin to an antigen that causes a DTH reaction, resulting in the clinical appearance of the disease. The nature of this hypothetical precursor or antigen, however, remains obscure. More recently, timed biopsies following irradiation with artificial light sources, with doses below the MED, have shown perivascular infiltrates of mainly CD41 T lymphocytes within a few hours and CD81 cells within days; an increased number of dermal and epidermal Langerhans cells and dermal macrophages has also been observed, suggesting the DTH pattern seen in allergic contact dermatitis and the tuberculin reactions. In addition, E-selectin, vascular cell adhesion molecule-1 (VCAM-1) and intercellular adhesion molecule-1 (ICAM-1), identified on keratinocytes above areas of dermal leukocyte infiltration, are also expressed as in other DTH responses. UV-induced immunosuppression is a consistent finding in normal skin and it was hypothesized that this process may protect the skin from UV-induced photoallergens. Thus, susceptibility of individuals to PLE could arise from a failure of normal UV-induced immunosuppression. Kolgen et al. reported that the skin of PLE patients was less susceptible to UVB-induced migration of CD11 Langerhans cells. Following a six MED dose of UVB, there was a significant failure of LC to migrate from the epidermis of PLE as compared with normal subjects. They also found a significant reduction in UVB-induced infiltration by CD11b1 macrophage-like cells in PLE compared with healthy skin, which was considered to represent an important finding in view of the prominent role of these cells in the secretion of the immunosuppressive cytokine IL-10. It was thus postulated that the pathologic defect underlying PLE might be a failure of normal photoimmunosuppression. If this is the case, the balance of UV-induced suppression and UV-induced provocation would be altered, allowing sunlight exposure to provoke PLE eruption. More recently, Kolgen et al. assessed whether there are abnormalities of UV-induced secretion of TNF-α and interleukin-1b, cytokines known to be important in affecting LC migration. Secondly, they examined the effects of UV on secretion of T-helper cell type 2 (TH2) cytokines IL-4 and IL-10, which mediate immunosuppression. They concluded that the reduced expression of TNF-α, IL-4, and IL-10 in the UVB irradiated skin of patients with PLE appears largely attributable to a lack of neutrophils and it is indicative of reduced Langerhans cell migration and reduced TH2 skewing. Impairment of these mechanisms essential for UVB-induced immunosuppression may be important in the pathogenesis of PLE (Kolgen, 2004). Palmer and Friedmann performed functional studies examining DTH responses in PLE and concluded that induction of sensitization by 2,4-dinitrochlorobenzene (DNCB) is less suppressed by UV in patients with PLE compared with healthy controls. Beyond this, van de Pas et al. recently showed a reduction in UV-induced suppression of DTH response to DNCB in PLE, such that these patients are less easily sensitized to DNCB than in healthy subjects. Also Schornagel et al. suggested a role for neutrophils in the pathogenesis of PLE, by showing a relative reduction in UVB-induced infiltration with neutrophils. It is conceivable that abnormalities in both neutrophil and mononuclear cell activity could be implicated in the pathogenesis of PLE. However, the most recent findings on the effect of solar-simulated radiation on the elicitation phase of contact hypersensitivity revealed no significant difference between controls and patients with PLE. These results contrasted with previous findings of the same group that had indicated a resistance to UV-induced suppression of sensitization to DNCB in PLE. This difference may reflect the greater importance of Langerhans cells in the sensitization phase, and is consistent with the hypothesis that PLE arises from impaired suppression of Langerhans cell activation or migration (Palmer, 2005). The reason for the occurrence of PLE appears likely to be genetic with a significant environmental component, with 70% of the population perhaps having a tendency to the condition but not all expressing it because of poor penetrance. However, the culprit gene has not been identified yet. This genetically determined factor, which leads to the putative immune recognition of an autologous cutaneous antigen generated by UV radiation in PLE, but not normal subjects, although the antigen is presumably expressed in all individuals. The inducing UV absorbers and antigens in PLE have not been characterized; tough has been suggested a form of heatshock protein. A variety of such antigens within and between patients, however, seems more likely. In addition, the induction of lesions by a UVA sun bed in the non-tanning sacral pressure area further suggests that the UV–chromophore interaction in at least some patients may be oxygen independent. Determination of the action spectrum of PLE by experimental reproduction of skin lesions using artificial radiation sources has led to conflicting results. A lack of response, often to adequate doses of artificially produced UV radiation, by patients who react readily to just suberythemogenic doses of natural sunlight may be attributed to a number of variables. These include the size of the UV irradiation site and its location, the irradiation of small, normally unaffected areas perhaps not eliciting sufficient immunologic stimulus to activate the response, but also to the UV spectrum, irradiation dose, dose rate, and degree of cutaneous immunologic tolerance, which may be increased by any recent prior exposure. Moreover, there is a lack of universally accepted, standardized phototest protocols under revision of board of experts. The complex interrelationships between factors such as these, have clearly contributed significantly to the conflicting nature of reports concerning the most effective wavelengths for PLE induction. In most series, UVA has been more effective than UVB. Thus, in one of these studies, following exposures of buttock skin to UVA or UVB daily for 4–8 days, the action spectrum was in the UVA range in 56%, UVB in 17%, and both in 27%. In another study 68% of reaction were triggered by UVA, 8% by UVB, and 10% by both wavelengths. This apparent diversity in action spectrum of PLE is possibly the result of different UV-provoked inducing antigens, and perhaps also of different cutaneous levels for these antigens. Variation in the proportions of UVA and UVB present in terrestrial sunlight may also explain certain clinical characteristics of PLE. Thus, the greater proportion of UVA to UVB in temperate climate zones, and during the spring and fall months, might be expected to contribute to a higher incidence of PLE in temperate, rather than tropical regions, with greater susceptibility to the condition in spring and occasionally autumn, rather than summer in most patients. Moreover, the higher proportion of UVB to UVA in summer sunlight also probably inhibits PLE development through a predominantly UVB-induced cutaneous immunosuppressive mechanism. Older generation sunscreens without substantial UVA protection, encouraged to stay much longer in the sun, thereby receiving a much higher UVA dose than without UVB protection, did not provide adequate protection against provocation of PLE. Clinical features of PLE are characterized by lesions that, generally, develop symmetrically and affect only some sun-exposed areas of the skin, often those that are normally covered in winter, such as the V area of the chest, the external aspects of the arms and forearms and lower anterior aspect of the neck. Occasionally, the face can be involved. Symptoms are worse in spring and early summer. The eruption typically begins each spring or early summer, on sunny vacations, or after recreational tanning use, often moderating with continuing exposure. Also outdoor activities in winter may induce the rash, and it may also occur by exposure through window glass (Hampton, 2004), which is penetrated by UVA such as light cotton clothing. The eruption develops after minutes to hours or sometimes days of sun exposure and lasts for one to several days or occasionally weeks, particularly with continuing exposure. Skin eruption, however, often fades or ceases as summer or the vacation proceeds ('hardening process'). A PLE severity index (PLESI) has been proposed to produce a simple, valid, and reproducible method to assess the severity of the disease (Palmer, 2004). In the absence of further exposure, lesions gradually subside completely, without scarring over a few days, occasionally over a week or two. In a given patient, the eruption tends always to affect the same skin sites. Associated systemic symptoms are quite rare: chills, headache, fever, and nausea have been reported but may have been the consequence of accompanying sunburn.This condition may last life-long but gradually improves over years in many patients: over 7 years, 64 of a series of 114 patients (57%) reported steadily diminishing sun sensitivity, including 12 (11%) that totally cleared. PLE has many morphologic variants, as indicated by the name. Lesions vary widely between patients, but are generally pruritic, grouped, erythematous or skin-colored papules of varying size, not infrequently coalescing into large, smooth or rough-surfaced plaques, sometimes resembling subacute cutaneous lupus erythematosus. Vesicles, bullae, and papulovesicles, as well as confluent edematous swelling (particularly of the face), are also possible, while rarely erythema or pruritus alone (PLE sine eruptione) may occur. Insect bite-like, and erythema multiforme-like variants have also been described. A particular variant in African Americans occurs as 'pinpoint' variant. In addition, the helices of the ears may be primarily affected often with vesicles, particularly in boys. This form of PLE was previously termed 'juvenile spring eruption'. The papular form, of either large or small separate or confluent lesions, generally tending to be in clusters, is the most common, followed by the papulovesicular and plaque variants; the others are rare. The eczematous form probably does not exist, representing rather chronic actinic dermatitis instead. A final morphologic variant, a small papular form generally sparing the face and occurring after several days of exposure on vacations has been designated as benign summer light eruption in Europe. Hematoxylin and eosin staining of PLE reveals superficial and deep dermal inflammatory cell infiltrate. While the infiltrate is predominantly perivascular, there is sometimes a heavy interstitial infiltrate of lymphocytes in the upper dermis, in those variants characterized by prominent subepidermal edema. The upper dermis frequently exhibits edema, particularly in plaque-like lesions. Epidermal changes, if present, are variable and range from mild spongiosis to acanthosis. A study performed to explore the immunohistopathology of photoinduced cutaneous lesions in LE patients revealed some important differences between these lesions and the cutaneous lesions seen in PLE patients. Of 22 person enrolled in this study, 16 patients had LE and 6 PLE. The study explored both cellular infiltrate and deposition of immunoreactants in the epidermis and dermis of lesions. The biopsies that were taken from two patient groups were examined for multiple classes of cellular infiltrates using standardized markers. The biopsies were screened for CD3+, CD4+, CD8+, M718+, CD15+, CD1+, CD22+ cells, and lue7 cellular marker. Specific attention was paid to the perivascular and dermoepidermal interface. Summation of the cellular populations from these samples revealed two significant differences. The first observation noted was the high prevalence of M718 cells at the dermoepidermal interface in LE patients, suggestive of active migration of M718+ monocytes toward the epidermis. The other significant difference was the increased CD1+ cell population seen throughout the entire dermis of PLE patients. The findings seen in the biopsies agree with past studies conducted on PLE patients. Current data suggests that this increased population of CD1+ cells represents the epidermal Langerhans cell population that is migrating toward the area's lymph nodes to present their antigen and elicit a type IV immune reaction. To examine if there were any significant findings related to immunoreactant deposition, the biopsies were tested for IgA, IgG, IgM, and C3c at the basal membrane zone. Results from past studies have revealed little or no presence of immunoglobulin at the basal membrane zone in patients with PLE. In summary, these results did not allow any positive significant conclusions to be drawn about diagnostic significance or pathologic etiology of PLE related to LE. Microscopic analysis of skin tissue is mostly not necessary, but can be helpful where there is diagnostic difficulty. The diagnosis of PLE is made principally on clinical grounds based on the typical morphology of the eruption. Although the diagnosis is mainly clinical, provocative phototesting may be valuable in winter if no lesions are present, to confirm the diagnosis. The best way to do this is by using repetitive irradiations on the V area of the neck or forearms for 1-4 consecutive days. This can be done with high-intensity monochromatic UVA and UVB sources or with a solar simulator. The doses needed are not necessarily erythemal. Readings are made immediately and up to 72 h after the last irradiation. As mentioned above, abnormal reactions can be provoked in more than 60% of patients. In most studies more patients reacted to UVA than to UVB. In case of positive UVA or UVB test, the reaction does not necessarly correlate to PLE clinical features and not significant relationship with clinical disease severity has been showed (Janssens et al., 2007). There are no diagnostic laboratory tests available for PLE. Laboratory examinations are usually performed to exclude other dermatoses, such as photosensitive lupus erythematosus or erythropoietic protoporphyria. Subacute cutaneous lupus erythematosus, which is generally not itchy as PLE, must be excluded in some patients by determining antinuclear, Ro (SSA) and La (SSB) antibody titers. Persistent plaque-type PLE must also be differentiated from Jessner–Kanof's lymphocytic infiltration of the skin, while the photo-exacerbation of dermatoses such as atopic and seborrhoeic eczema may occur in susceptible subjects with the same time course as for PLE, but with differing and characteristic morphology. PLE treatment has to be subdivided into therapy for the acute exacerbation and prophylactic therapy before expected sun exposure. The mild disease of many patients is satisfactorily controlled by the moderation of sun exposure at times of high UV intensity, use of protective clothing, and the regular application of broad-spectrum sunscreens with high-protection factors including UVA filters. A combination of sunscreens with antioxidants was reported to be more effective than sunscreen alone, but this awaits further confirmation (Patel et al., 2000). Patients with fully developed disease require topical corticosteroids, in some cases in the form of wet dressings, for several days. More severe attacks may be treated effectively with a short course of systemic (oral or injection) corticosteroids (Patel et al., 2000). Because PLE will subside spontaneously and is not a life-threatening condition, all possible risks of therapy should be carefully considered. Many patients will agree to undergo some sort of preventive measures. Prophylactic treatment consists of several approaches. The mildly affected majority of patients will prevent their PLE, to significant degree, by control or avoidance of sunlight exposure and by using a topical high-factor broad-spectrum sunscreen. For others, gradual sun exposure in spring effects browning and thickening of the skin (so called hardening), which often helps to avoid PLE. Severely affected subjects, suffering frequent attacks throughout the summer may require courses of prophylactic phototherapy or photochemotherapy in the early spring before the expected sun exposure. At a first glance it appears somewhat bizarre to use light treatment to prevent a condition that is caused by light, and the mechanisms by which UVB and PUVA induce tolerance to sunlight are not completely understood. Pigmentation and thickening of the stratum corneum may be important factors for the protective effect, and UVB, high-dose UVA, and PUVA are efficient triggers of both. Although these local effects may provide some barrier against photosensitivity, they probably do not suffice to explain the degree of protection induced in many patients. Thus, other mechanisms may be involved, as photodermatoses do occur in dark-skinned subjects (Kontos et al., 2002). It is therefore now generally accepted that UVA, UVB, and PUVA therapy exert a variety of immunomodulatory effects on human skin and that this is of critical importance for the therapeutic efficacy of phototherapy. Janssens et al.. showed that UVB hardening significantly normalizes UV-induced cell migratory responses of Langerhans cells and neutrophils in patients with PLE. PUVA is a very effective preventive treatment. In approximately 70% of patients with this condition, a 3–4-week course of PUVA, 3 times a week, suffices to suppress the disease upon subsequent exposure to sunlight. The initial exposure and dose increments should be performed according to the guidelines outlined for psoriasis. PUVA induces pigmentation rapidly and intensively at relatively low suberythemogenic UVA doses that usually remain well below the threshold doses for eliciting PLE. About 10% of the patients develop typical lesions during the initial phase of PUVA. Interruption of treatment or reduction in the UVA dose is rarely required in such cases. Usually, brief symptomatic treatment with topical corticosteroids suffices. PUVA therapy protects only temporarily, and regularly repeated sun exposures are subsequently required to maintain protection. However, a considerable number of patients remain protected for 2–3 months, even after pigmentation has faded. The use of narrow-band 312 nm UVB phototherapy has become increasingly popular, being simpler to administer, perhaps safer than PUVA and of comparable efficacy. Also exposure of prophylactic UVB may sometimes trigger the eruption, particularly in severely affected subjects, necessitating occasionally concurrent systemic corticosteroid therapy. Commercial 'sun beds' are not recommended because they are most likely to provoke PLE rash. Patients who only develop their disorder during infrequent vacations, also generally have good result from preventive oral corticosteroids course. Other therapies, that are quite often listed in textbooks, are of uncertain efficacy. Such remedies include antimalarials, long been advocated, b-carotene, and nicotinamide, likewise probably only moderately effective are 0-3 polyunsaturated fatty acids (Murphy et al., 1987) (38). The efficacy of Escherichia coli filtration (Colibiogen) awaits further confirmation. Also systemic antioxidants were unable in reducing the severity of the disease (Eberlein-konig et al., 2000). The use of immunosuppressants should certainly be restricted to some rare severe disabling cases (Shipley, 2001). Recently, the photoprotective activity of oral polypodium leucotomos extract was shown to exert significant improvement in PLE patients (Caccialanza et al., 2007).

4. UV-induced skin cancers

Lifestyle changes during the past five decades, with increased sunlight exposure because of outdoor activities and worsening sunbathing habits, often result in skin cancers (SCs). Among Caucasians, intense early sunburns and blistering sunburns are closely associated with the development of melanoma. As a result of chronic UV exposure: skin aging, wrinkles, uneven skin pigmentation, loss of skin elasticity and a disturbance of skin barrier functions are nowadays well recognized. These changes in the skin that superimpose the alterations of chronological aging refer to photoaging. The development of squamous cell carcinomas, SCCs and BCCs, and malignant melanoma is often associated with painful sunburns. In fact, more than 1 severe sunburn in childhood is associated with a 2-fold increase in melanoma risk (Ma et al., 2007). Chronic exposure to UVR is known as the most important risk factor for the development of actinic keratoses (precursors of SCC). Exposure to UVR during childhood and adolescence plays a role in the future development of skin cancer. It was noted that in the US, most people receive 22.73% of their lifetime exposure to the sun by 18 years of age. This meant that during childhood (1–18 years of age), most people received approximately one-fifth of their total sun exposure. The total amount of sun received over the years, and overexposure resulting in sunburns are associated with skin cancers. The epidemiology implicating UV exposure as a cause of melanoma is further supported by biological evidence that damage caused by UVR, particularly damage to DNA, plays a central role in the development of melanoma. The relative risk of skin cancer is three times as high among people born in areas that receive high amounts of UVR than those who move to those areas in adulthood. Likewise, outdoor workers have a higher risk than indoor workers (Glanz et al., 2007). The aforementioned citations conclude that there is a dose-related relationship between sunlight exposure and the incidence of skin cancer. For the development of BCC and melanoma, intermittent intense exposures appear to carry a higher risk than lower level chronic exposures, even if the total UV dose is the same. By contrast, the risk for SCC is strongly associated with chronic UV exposure but not with intermittent exposure. Taken together, epidemiologic studies and experimental studies indicate that intermittent intense and chronic exposures to solar UVR are the primary cause of non melanoma skin cancer (NMSCs) and melanoma. Indeed photo-carcinogenesis plays a pivotal role in skin cancer occurrence in the general population and not only in high risk group such as patients affected by Gorlin's syndrome or Xeroderma pigmentosum. Other agents, relevant in the past such as arsenic are now extremely rare as population exposure manly ceased in the 1960s. Ionizing radiation is an ongoing cause of skin cancer, but overall ultraviolet radiation accounts for more than 90% of skin cancers. Ultraviolet radiation is a complete carcinogen which means that, on its own, it has the ability to cause skin cancer without the need for other factors, although other co-carcinogens may have an expediting effect on skin cancers leading to earlier onset or increasing SC number. Initiation of skin cancer comes about by DNA absorption of UVR, specific wavelengths which are similar to the ones able to induce erythema. Such absorbed photons lead to CPDs, which in case are not removed, they lead to errors in the transcribed DNA strand. The DNA repair mechanism is complex and comprises a series of enzymatically controlled steps whereby the DNA double helix is uncoiled, the cross-linked thymine dimer usually is repaired and DNA is reconstituted. DNA repair is an error-prone process and mutated genes may be retained. More than thirty different enzymatic steps contribute to the process of DNA repair involving nucleotide excision repair (NER), a specific response to the damage caused by absorption of UVR in human skin. Use of topically applied liposomal enzyme T4 endonuclease V which specifically removes CPDs in a clinical trial on xeroderma pigmentosum led to fewer basal cell carcinomas and actinic keratoses indicating the relevance of these lesions to carcinogenesis. Aging skin is less efficient at removing CPDs; this together with the accumulation of UV-induced DNA damage augments carcinogenesis. Though UVB is most efficient at inducing CPDs, UVA also induces these lesions participating in the carcinogenic UVR effect. As defence mechanism, apoptosis should help prevent SC. Cells carrying too much in the way of damaged DNA for easy repair, or accurate NER, are instructed, by complex cell signalling pathways caspase mediated, to self distruct: the so called programmed cell death. Damaged cells escaping repair or apoptosis proliferate and skin cancer arise. The genome guardian p53 has a key role in this process. Ultraviolet radiation induces p53 and it leads to p21 synthesis, able to stop the cell cycle in S1, enabling DNA repair to take place. MDM2 protein is also induced and serves as a mechanism for shutting off p53, and enabling its degradation via the ubiquitination pathway. The time course for these UVR-induced molecular events has been elucidated in vivo in human skin; further studies measured the time for apoptosis induction after 3 repeated MED exposures. Later, in the time course of the sunburn response the protein Bax is induced which leads to apoptosis and safe elimination of damaged cells. Skin cancer is the most common type of cancer in light skinned populations around the world. Skin cancers are mainly divided into melanoma, and non-melanoma skin cancers (NMSCs), the latter including basal and squamous cell carcinomas. Melanoma is responsible for most of the cancer related mortalities, and NMSCs are typically described as having a more benign course with locally aggressive features. Nevertheless, they represent ''the most common type'' of cancer in humans and they can result in significant disfigurement, leading to adverse physical and psychological consequences (Suarez, 2007). It is estimated that 2–3 million cases of NMSCs occur worldwide each year. The incidence varies with very high rates in the Caucasian populations. For incidence, the overall upward trend observed in most parts of Europe, Canada, USA and Australia shows an average increase between 3% and 8% a year (Rhee et al., 2007). The incidence of NMSCs is over 1.3 million cases each year in the U.S.; in fact, this incidence rate is expected to double in the next 30 years (Rhee et al., 2007). Approximately 30% of all newly diagnosed cancers in the U.S. are BCC, making it the most commonly diagnosed cancer in this country (Rittiè et al., 2007). BCC, which accounts for 80–85% of all NMSCs, rarely metastasizes to other organs. It is the most common malignancy in white people. Its worldwide incidence is increasing by up to 10% with highest rates in elderly men and increasing incidence in young women. Although mortality is low, this malignancy causes considerable morbidity and places a huge burden on worldwide healthcare systems. SCC, which accounts for 15–20% of all NMSCs, is more likely to invade other tissues and can cause death. As a result of the benign nature of NMSC characteristics, some patients may remain unregistered and undiagnosed, leading to an under-representation of the number of cases. Moreover, as NMSCs have localized symptoms and primarily manifest in older individuals, they may remain undiagnosed. BCC and SCC are usually found in sun exposed areas, especially the head and neck regions. They are both positively related to the amount of UVR received and inversely proportional to the degree of skin pigmentation in the population. Women have higher occurrences than men for both types of cancers on the legs, consistent with greater sun exposure at this site. In 2006, a study reported that the ratio of BCC to SCC is 4 : 1 for the head and neck (Gloster & Neal, 2006). The probability of getting SCC is less than getting BCC; however, SCC carries a > 10-fold higher risk of metastasis and mortality. It is estimated that 132,000 new cases of melanoma occur worldwide each year. Incidence rates are at least 16 times greater in Caucasians than African Americans and 10 times greater than Hispanics. The WHO also estimates that as many as 65,161 people a year worldwide die from malignant skin cancer, approximately 48,000 of whom are registered. Melanoma represents only about 3% of all skin cancers in the U.S., but it accounts for about 75% of all skin cancer deaths. The American Academy of Dermatology (AAD) in 2009, reported about 121,840 new melanoma cases in the U.S. with 8650 deaths (1 death every hour). This mortality value is remarkably high considering the fact that melanoma is nearly always curable in its early stages; however, this high number can be attributed to the late diagnosis of the disease in which the cancer spreads to other parts of the body. Over the last three decades, the incidence and mortality rates of melanoma have increased in the U.S. In particular, of all neoplasms, approximately 20–30% of skin cancers are diagnosed in Caucasians, 2–4% are in Asians and 1–2% are in blacks and Asian Indians. In 2006, of all skin cancers, melanoma represented 1–8% in blacks, 10–15% in Asian Indians and 19% in Japanese. Moreover, even though skin cancers are not as prevalent in individuals with darker skin, they can have more morbidity and fatalities as they may go undiagnosed for a while. Melanoma most often appears on the trunk of men and the lower legs of women, although it can be found on the head, neck, or elsewhere. As the incidence of skin cancer is increasing at an alarming rate, it is one of the greatest threats to public health.

5. PLE and skin cancer: Is one protective against the other?

For everything said so far, it would seem that the skin performs a 'balancing act' between adequate elimination of early cancerous cells and suppression of abnormal reactions against UV-exposed cells that may suffer transient aberrations. PLE appears to be associated with an 'imbalance' between UV-induced proinflammatory and UV-induced suppressive immunoreaction. Supporting the link between susceptibility to UV-induced immunosuppression and PLE incidence is the fact that PLE patients demonstrate a functional resistance to UV-induced immunosuppression, favouring a DTH response to potential UV-induced neo-antigens under certain circumstances (Palmer, 2004). High UV radiation dose (2 MED) resulted highly immunosuppressive in both, PLE patients and controls, leading to almost complete immune suppression by 93%. This might explain why PLE lesions are often provoked by exposure to low doses of UV radiation but rarely by severe sunburn PLE patients MED values do not differ significantly from those of normal subjects, although in some study it results lower. Further studies are required to fully elucidate these pathways. Another aspect of PLE that requires further investigation is the disproportionate incidence observed in females compared with males. Notably, it has been found that females are probably due to a more resistant to the immunosuppressive effects of UV radiation. Moreover, the results of a study by Widyarini et al. suggest that the sex difference in PLE may be due to protection from UV-induced immunosuppression afforded to females via signalling through the oestrogen receptor (Widyarini et al., 2006). Indeed, female hormone 17b-oestradiol may prevent UVR-induced suppression of the CHS response caused by the release of immunosuppressive cytokines (e.g. IL-10) from keratinocytes (Hiramoto et al., 2004). This might explain why PLE is more common in females than in males and why the risk decreases in women after the menopause. Because of these gender differences in UV-susceptibility together with the higher incidence of skin cancer in males, future studies must address the question of whether resistance to UV-induced immunosuppression lowers the skin cancer risk in PLE patients. Yoshikawa et al. compared normal healthy population versus NMSC patients. Using a protocol that achieved virtually complete depletion of epidermal LCs from UV irradiated skin, they found that approximately 60% of healthy volunteers developed a vigorous CHS to a given dose of DNCB painted on the UV-irradiated test site. These individuals were designated UVB-resistant, and were distinguished from other individuals who were designated UVB susceptible, by their failure to develop CHS. They then discovered that more than 90% of skin cancer patients exposed to UVB and DNCB failed to develop CHS, i.e. were UVB-susceptible. In subsequent experiments, epicutaneous application of the same dose of DNCB to unirradiated skin of UVB-susceptible individuals revealed a further distinction between normal persons and skin cancer patients. Approximately 45% of the latter (and none of the former) remained unresponsive, implying that they had been rendered immunologically tolerant. Because the incidence of UVB-susceptibility was significantly higher in skin cancer patients, and as specific unresponsiveness could be demonstrated only in these patients, it was proposed that UVB-susceptibility might be a risk factor for the development of skin cancer. Indeed, if patients with PLE have a general increased resistance to UV-induced immunosuppression, this may make them more resistant to UV carcinogenesis. In an earlier case–control study (Wolf et al., 1998), using a questionnaire for phenotypic markers and sunlight-related factors and habits, it was observed that UV-induced skin rashes indicative of PLE, were recalled by 12% (22/183) of melanoma patients compared with 18% (57/315) of healthy control subjects. Although not statistically significant, these results suggest that PLE-susceptible patients, possibly being more resistant to UV-induced immunosuppression, may have a lower melanoma risk. This hypothesis is supported by the results of a recent study by Lembo et al. who investigated the link between PLE and skin cancer prevalence. They performed two prospective case–control studies analysing a group comprising 214 patients with SC and 210 gender-and aged-matched controls (study A), and a group comprising 100 patients with PLE and 155 gender- and aged matched controls (study B). Skin type and cumulative exposure to UVR were documented. Three sun exposure levels, depending on lifestyle, were identified in different sections of the questionnaire designed for the survay, investigating work (in/outdoors) and free time (in/outdoors) activities. Their results showed that the prevalence of (histologically confirmed) SC in the PLE group was 4%; the prevalence of SC in the PLE matched control group was 7.1%, which is similar to the National Cancer Registry of Ireland figure of 6% prevalence of SC in the general population, with a cumulative risk of 12.5% by the 8th decade. These studies show that there is a reduced incidence of SC in patients with PLE compared with gender- and age-matched controls. There is less evidence of a reduced incidence of PLE in patients with SC compared with controls: the study size was too small to determine this and only a trend was observed.

One study of patients with melanoma showed sensitivity of LCs to the effects of solar-simulated radiation compared with controls. There has been much speculation as to the role of LCs in the induction of anti-tumour immunity. Whereas there is considerable circumstantial evidence that disruption in the density and function of these cells during the early stages of UVR-induced carcinogenesis may be important for enabling developing neoplasms to escape immune destruction, the role of the large number of LC infiltrating developed skin tumours is less clear. Interestingly, people "costumes and fashion" are not influenced by photoallergy or photoinduced SC. It might be expected that people change their behaviour in the sun after being affected by either SC or PLE. Surprisingly, as shown in multiple surveys, most subjects with a history of SC were not inclined to use regular sunscreen (Moloney et al., 2005). Awareness about sun exposure and SC risk does not necessarily influence patients' sun protection behaviour. Although people are aware of the risks of sunbathing, they continue to expose themselves to the sun without taking precautions, in accordance with the long-established habits of 'sun holidays' and sunbathing and the social belief that tanned skin is more aesthetically pleasing. Similarly, although patients with PLE might be expected to avoid the sun, many continued to go for sunny holidays despite their skin eruption. PLE patients recall more sun exposure than controls and in many cases have equivalent sun exposure to patients with SC.

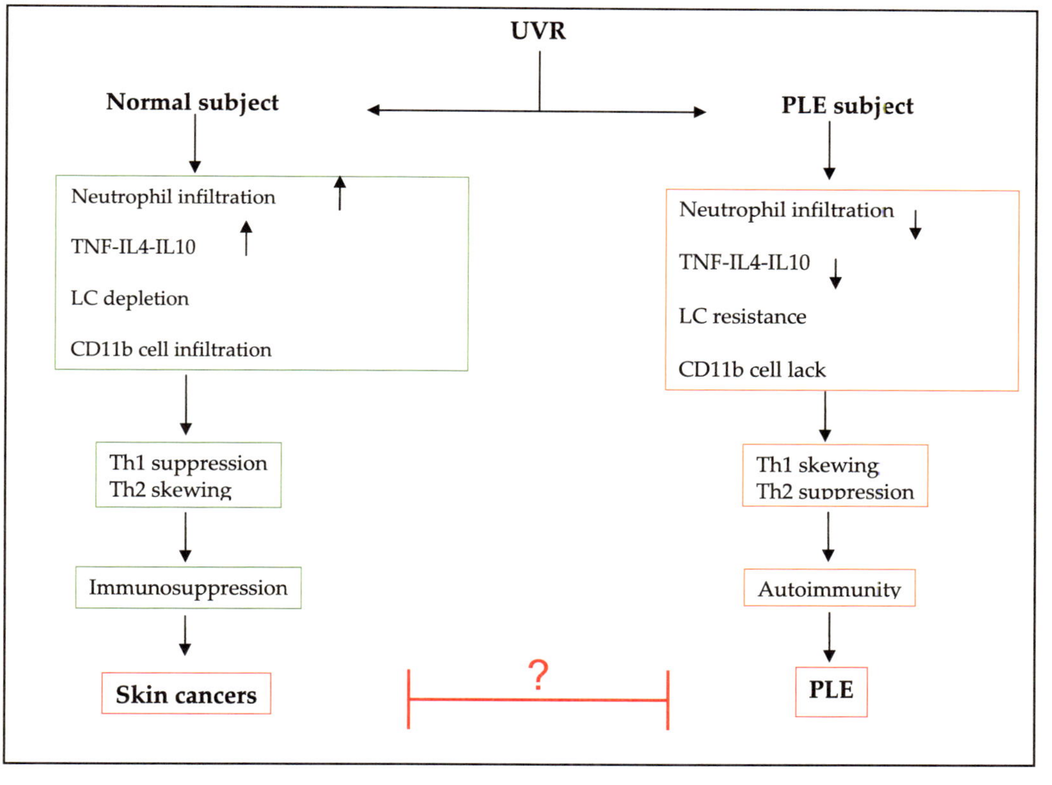

Fig. 2. Pathogenesis of skin cancers and PLE.

The schematic diagram highlights the potential pathway of inhibited ultraviolet radiation (UVR)-induced immune suppression in patients with polymorphic light eruption. In patients with PLE, a persistence of Langerhans cells and failure of UV-induced immune suppression may favour the occurrence of autoimmunogenic skin rashes. In normal subjects, concurrent UV-induced immunosuppression represent a risk factor for the skin cancers. The resistance to UVR-induce immunosuppression of PLE may prevent skin cancers risk as the immunosuppression that occurs in skin cancer may prevent PLE development.

6. Conclusion

A better understanding of UV-induce immunosuppression, leading to SC, and UV-induce immunoactivation, provoking PLE, may be helpful in preventing and treating these conditions. Therefore, it would be very useful to have a reliable cumulative sun exposure dose biomarker, which, related to every single case, could be a predictive factor for SC development. SC, up to date, remains the most common human malignancy and, its occurance is manly linked to UVR exposure. Immunosurveillance inefficiency or disruption of biological pathways of damage repair or programmed cells death, are additive mechanisms permitting progression of the neoplastic process initiated by UVR.
Despite these new insights, in fact, excessive and chronic natural, as well as artificial UVR exposure will, however, remain one of the major environmental threats for human health. Various skin cancer task forces have proposed several important guidelines to decrease the rising skin cancer incidence. These briefly include the following: (1) the establishment of policies that reduce exposure to UVR; (2) providing and maintaining physical and social environments, which support sun safety and are consistent with the development of other healthful habits; (3) professional pre-service and in-service skin cancer education for school administrators, teachers, physical education teachers and coaches, nurses, and others working in healthcare; (4) health services and organizations to increase skin cancer prevention education, sun-safety environments and making these policies readily available to the public; (5) lastly, the promotion of free skin cancer screening programs are also highly encouraged. Primary care physicians can have greater role in preventing skin cancer if they are trained to recognize it and able to educate patients to appropriate sun exposure and periodical dermatological consults. Therefore, there is a need for education related to UV exposure and skin cancer risk. To address this issue, it would be beneficial to implement educational programs tailored for schools/workplaces, homes and doctors' visits. Patient education can include advice pertaining to sunscreen usage, reapplication methods, risk factors and tanning bed dangers. In addition to this, visual aids can be valuable in physicians' offices, as they can display the results of people after receiving a great deal of UVR. Sun protection strategies utilized for promote safe sun behaviours are resumed in: (1) setting a date to end intentional tanning, (2) determining which past behaviors were helpful in protecting against sun exposure and trying to incorporate them (as well as other techniques) in the future, (3) making strategies to overcome obstacles and (4) involving family members so everyone would remind each other about using sun protection. Application and promotion of sun protective techniques in children will reduce their cumulative lifelong sun exposure and intense episodic sun exposure, hence reducing their risk for skin cancer.

7. References

Agar, N.S., Halliday, G.M., Barnetson, R.S., Ananthaswamy, H.N., Wheeler, M., Jones, A.M. (2004). The basal layer in human squamous tumors harbors more UVA than UVB fingerprint mutations: a role for UVA in human skin carcinogenesis. *Proc. Natl. Acad. Sci. U.S.A.*, Vol. , No. 14, (April 2004), pp. 4954–4959.

Andrews, F.J., Halliday, G.M., Muller, H.K. (1991). A role for prostaglandins in the suppression of cutaneous cellular immunity and tumour development in benzo(a)pyrene-treated mice but not dimethylbenz(a)anthracene-treated mice. *Clin. Exp. Immunol.*, Vol. 85, No. 1, (July 1991), pp. 9–13.

Arad, S., Konnikov, N., Goukassian, DA., Gilchrest, BA. (2006) T-oligos augment UV-induced protective responses in human skin. *FASEB J.*, Vol. 20, No. 11, (September 2006), pp. 1895–1897.

Balkwill, F., Mantovani, A. (2001). Inflammation and cancer: back to Virchow? *Lancet*, Vol. 357, No. 9255, (February 2001), pp. 539–545.

Beattie, PE., Dawe, RS., Ibbotson, SH., Ferguson, J. (2003). Characteristics and prognosis of idiopathic solar urticaria: a cohort of 87 cases. *Arch Dermatol.*, Vol. 139, No. 9, (September 2003), pp. 1149-1154.

Brenner M, Hearing VJ. (2008). The Protective Role of Melanin Against UV Damage in Human Skin. *Photochem Photobiol* Vol. 84, No. 3, (June 2008), pp. 539–549.

Caccialanza, M., Percivalle, S., Piccinno, R., Brambilla, R. (2007). Photoprotective activity of oral polypodium leucotomos extract in 25 patients with idiopathic photodermatoses. *Photodermatol Photoimmunol Photomed*, Vol. 23, No. 1, (February 2007), pp. 46–47.

Cooper, KD., Oberhelman, L., Hamilton, TA. (1992). UV exposure reduces immunization rates and promotes tolerance to epicutaneous antigens in humans: relationship to dose, CD1a-DR+ epidermal macrophage induction, and Langerhans cell depletion. *Proc Natl Acad Sci USA* Vol. 89, No. 18, (September 1992), pp. 8497- 8501.

Darvay, A., White, IR., Rycroft, RJ., Jones, AB., Hawk, JL., McFadden, JP. (2001). Photoallergic contact dermatitis is uncommon. *Photochem Photobiol*, Vol. 145, No. 4, (October 2001), pp. 532–536.

Diffey, BL. Sources and measurement of ultraviolet radiation. (2002). *Methods, Vol.* 28, No. 1, (September 2002), pp. 4-13.

Eberlein-Konig, B., Fesq, H., Abeck, D., Przybilla, B., Placzek, M., Ring, J. (2000). Systemic vitamin C and vitamin E do not prevent photoprovocation test reactions in polymorphous light eruption. *Photodermatol Photoimmunol Photomed,* Vol. 16, No. 2, (April 2000), pp. 50–52.

Epstein, JH. (1986). Polymorphous light eruption. *Dermatol Clin* Vol. 4, No. 2, (April 1986), pp. 243-251.

Fisher, MS., Kripke, ML. (1997). Systemic alteration induced in mice by ultraviolet light irradiation and its relationship to ultraviolet carcinogenesis. *Proc Natl Acad Sci U S A*, Vol. 74, No. 4, (April 1977), pp.1688-1692.

Ghoreishi, M., Dutz, JP. (2006). Tolerance induction by transcutaneous immunization through ultraviolet-irradiated skin is transferable through CD4+CD25+ T regulatory cells and is dependent on host derived IL-10. *J Immunol.,* Vol. 176, No.4, (February 2006) pp. 2635-2644.

Glanz, K., Buller, DB., Saraiya, M. (2007). Reducing ultraviolet radiation exposure among outdoor workers: state of the evidence and recommendations. *Environ Health, Vol. 8* (August 2007), pp. 22.

Gloster, HM., Neal, K. Skin cancer in skin of color. (2006). *J Am Acad Dermatol., Vol. 55,* No. 5, (November 2006), pp. 761-764.

Hampton, PJ., Farr, PM., Diffey, BL., Lloyd JJ. (2004). Implication for photosensitive patients of ultraviolet A exposure in vehicles. *Br J Dermatol,* Vol. 151, No. 4, (October 2004), pp. 873-876.

Hiramoto, K., Tanaka, H., Yanagihara, N., Sato, EF., Inoue, M. (2004). Effect of 17betaestradiol on immunosuppression induced by ultraviolet B irradiation. *Arch Dermatol Res* Vol. 95, No. 8, (February 2004), pp. 307–311.

Janssens, AS., Pavel, S., Ling, T., Winhoven, SM. (2007). *Arch Dermatol,* Vol. 143, No. 5, (May 2007), pp. 599–604.

Janssens, AS., Pavel, S., Out-Luiting, JJ., Willemze, R., de Gruijl, FR. (2005). Normalized ultraviolet (UV) induction of Langerhans cell depletion and neutrophil infiltrates after artificial UVB hardening of patients with polymorphic light eruption. *Br J Dermatol* Vol. 152, No. 6, (Jun 2005), pp. 1268–1274.

Jemal, A., Siegel, R., Ward, E., Murray, T., Xu, J., Thun, MJ. (2007). Cancer Statistics, 2007. *Cancer Journal for Clinicians,* Vol. 57, pp. 43–66.

Johnston, GA. (2002). Thiazide-induced lichenoid photosensitivity. *Clin Exp Dermatol* Vol. 27, No. 8, (November 2002), pp. 670 672.

K¨olgen, W., van Meurs, M., Jongsma, M, van Weelden, H., Bruijnzeel-Koomen, CA., Knol, EF., van Vloten, WA., Laman, J., de Gruijl, FR. (2004). Differential expression of cytokines in UV-B-exposed skin of patients with polymorphous light eruption: correlation with Langerhans cell migration and immunosuppression. *Arch Dermatol,* Vol. 140, No. 3, (March 2004), pp. 295–302.

Kontos, AP., Cusack, CA., Chaffins, M., Lim, HW. Polymorphous light eruption in African Americans: pinpoint papular variant. *Photodermatol Photoimmunol Photomed* Vol. 18, No. 6, (December 2002), pp. 303–306.

Lautenschlager, S., Wulf, HC., Pittelkow, MR. (2007). Photoprotection. *Lancet* Vol. 370, No. 9586, (August 2007), pp. 528–537.

Lembo, S., Fallon, J., O'Kelly, P., Murphy, GM. (2008). Polymorphic light eruption and skin cancer prevalence: is one protective against the other? *Br J Dermatol* Vol. 159, No. 6, (December 2008), pp.1342–1347.

Leverrier, S., Bergamaschi, D., Ghali, L. Ola, A., Warnes, G., Akgül, B., Blight, K., García-Escudero, R., Penna, A., Eddaoudi, A., Storey, A. (2007). Role of HPV E6 proteins inpreventing UVB-induced release of pro-apoptotic factors from the mitochondria. *Apoptosis* Vol. 12, No. 3, (March 2007), pp. 549–560.

Ma, F., Collado-Mesa, F., Hu, S., Kirsner RS. (2007). Skin cancer awareness and sun protection behaviors in white

Hispanic and white non-Hispanic high school students in Miami, Florida. *Arch Dermatol,* Vol. 143, No. 8, (August 2007), pp. 983–988.

McLoone, P., Simics, E., Barton, A. Norval, M., Gibbs, NK. (2005). An action spectrum for the production of cis-urocanic acid in human skin in vivo. *J Invest Dermatol,* Vol. 124, No. 5, (May 2005), pp. 1071–1074.

Moyal, D.D., Fourtanier, A.M. (2001). Broad-spectrum sunscreens provide better protection from the suppression of the elicitation phase of delayed-type hypersensitivity response in humans. J Invest. Dermatol., Vol. 117, No. 5, (November 2001), pp. 1186–1192.

Murphy GM. (2001). Diseases associated with photosensitivity. *J Photochem Photobiol* , Vol. 64, pp. 93–98.

Murphy, GM., Wright, J., Nicholls, DS., McKee, PH., Messenger, AG., Hawk, JL., Levene, GM. (1989). Sunbed-induced pseudoporphyria. *Br J Dermatol* Vol. 120, No. 4, (April 1989), pp. 555–562.

O'Connor, DP., Kay, EW., Leader M., Murphy, GM., Atkins, GJ., Mabruk, MJ. (2001). Altered p53e expression in benign and malignant skin lesions from renal transplant recipients and immunocompetent patients with skin cancer: correlation with human papillomaviruses? *Diagn Mol Pathol* Vol. 10, No. 32, (September 2001), pp. 190–199.

Ou-Yang, H., Stamatas, G., Saliou, C., Kollias, N. (2004). A chemiluminescence study of UVA-induced oxidative stress in human skin in vivo. *J Invest Dermatol.* Vol. 122, No. 4, (April 2004) , pp. 1020–1029.

Palmer, RA., Friedmann, PS. (2004). Ultraviolet radiation causes less immunosuppression in patients with polymorphic light eruption than in controls. *J Invest Dermatol* Vol. 122, No. 2, (February 2004), pp. 291–294.

Palmer, RA., Hawk, JL., Young, AR., Walker SL. (2005). The effect of solarsimulated radiation on the elicitation phase of contact hypersensitivity does not differ between controls and patients with polymorphic light eruption. *J Invest Dermatol* Vol. 124, No. 6, (June 2005), pp. 467–470.

Patel, DC., Bellaney, GJ., Seed, PT., McGregor, JM., Hawk, JL. (2000). Efficacy of short-course oral prednisolone in polymorphic light eruption: a randomized controlled trial. *Br J Dermatol* Vol. 143, No. 4, (October 2000), pp. 828–831.

Paulson, KG., Lemos, BD., Feng, B. Jaimes, N., Peñas, PF., Bi, X., Maher, E., Cohen, L., Leonard, JH., Granter, SR., Chin, L., Nghiem, P. (2009). Array-CGH reveals recurrent genomic changes in Merkel cell carcinoma including amplification of L-Myc. *J Invest Dermatol* Vol. 129, No. 6, (June 2009), pp. 1547–55.

Phillipson, R.P., Tobi, S.E.,. Morris, J.A, McMillan, T.J. (2002). UV-A induces persistent genomic instability in human keratinocytes through an oxidative stress mechanism, *Free Radic. Biol. Med.* Vol. 32, No. 5, (March 2002), pp. 474–480.

Rhee, JS., Matthews, BA., Neuburg, M., Logan BR., Burzynski, M., Nattinger, AB. (2007). The skin cancer index: clinical responsiveness and predictors of quality of life. *Laryngoscope* Vol. 117, No. 3, (March 2007), pp. 399–405.

Rittié, L., Kansra, S., Stoll, SW., Li, Y., Gudjonsson, JE., Shao, Y., Michael, LE., Fisher, GJ., Johnson, TM., Elder, JT. (2007). Differential ErbB1 signaling in squamous cell versus basal cell carcinoma of the skin. *Am J Pathol* Vol. 170, No. 6 (June 2007), pp. 2089–2099.

Ross JA, Howie SE, Norval M et al. Ultraviolet-irradiated urocanic acid suppresses delayed-type hypersensitivity to herpes simplex virus in mice. *J Invest Dermatol* 1986; 87:630–3.

Shipley, DR., Hewitt, JB. (2001). Polymorphic light eruption treated with cyclosporin. *Br J Dermatol* Vol. 144, No. 2, (February 2001), pp. 446–447.

Stratigos, AJ., Antoniou, C., Katsambas, AD. (2002). Polymorphous light eruption. *J Eur Acad Dermatol Venereol* Vol. 16, No. 3, (May 2002), pp. 193-206.

Suárez, B., López-Abente, G., Martínez, C., Navarro, C., Tormo, MJ., Rosso, S., Schraub, S., Gafà, L., Sancho-Garnier, H., Wechsler, J., Zanetti, R. (2007). Occupation and skin cancer: the results of the HELIOS-I multicenter case-control study. *BMC Public Health* Vol. 26, No. 7, (July 2007), pp. 180

Thompson, E.J., Gupta, A., Vielhauer, G.A., Regan, J.W., Bowden, G.T. (2008). The growth of malignant keratinocytes depends on signaling through the PGE2 receptor EP1, *Neoplasia* Vol. 3, No. 5, (September 2001), pp. 402-410.

Timares, L., Katiyar, SK., Elmets, CA. (2008). DNA damage, apoptosis and langerhans cells - Activators of UV-induced immune tolerance. *Photochem Photobiol* Vol. 84, No. 2, (April 2008), pp.422-436.

van de Pas, CB., Kelly, DA., Seed, PT., Young, AR., Hawk, JL., Walker, SL. (2004). Ultraviolet-radiationinduced erythema and suppression of contact hypersensitivity responses in patients with polymorphic light eruption. *J InvestDermatol* Vol. 122, No. 2, (February 2004), pp. 295-299.

Vural, P., Canbaz, M., Selcuki, D. (1999). Plasma antioxidant defense in actinic keratosis and basal cell carcinoma, *J. Eur. Acad. Dermatol. Venereol.* Vol. 13, No. 2 (September 1999), pp. 96-101.

Walterscheid, J.P., Ullrich, S.E.,. Nghiem, D.X. Plateletactivating factor, a molecular sensor for cellular damage, activates systemic immune suppression. (2002). *J. Exp. Med.* Vol. 195, No. 2, (January 2002), pp. 171-179.

Warren J.B. (1994). Nitric oxide and human skin blood flow responses to acetylcholine and ultraviolet light. *FASEBJ.*, Vol. 8, No. 2, (February 1994), pp. 247-251.

Whiteman, DC., Whiteman, CA., Green, AC. (2001). Childhood sun exposure as a risk factor for melanoma: a systematic review of epidemiologic studies. *Cancer Causes Control,* Vol. 12, No. 1, (January 2001), pp. 69-82.

Widyarini, S., Domanski, D., Painter, N., Reeve, V E. (2006). Estrogen receptor signalling protects against immune suppression by UV radiation exposure. *Proc Natl Acad Sci USA* Vol. 103, No. 34, (August 2006), pp. 12837-12842.

Wolf, P., Quehenberger, F., Mullegger, R., Stranz, B., Kerl, H. (1998). Phenotypic markers, sunlight-related factors and sunscreen use in patients with cutaneous melanoma: an Austrian case-control study. *Melanoma Res* Vol. 8, No. 4, (August 1998), pp. 370-378.

Wong, SN., Khoo, LS. (2003). Chronic actinic dermatitis as the presenting feature of HIV infection in three Chinese males. *Clin Exp Dermatol* Vol. 28, No. 3, (May 2003), pp. 265-268.

World Health Organization. Skin cancers [online]. Available from URL:
http://www.who.int/uv/faq/skin cancer/en/print.html.
[Accessed 2009 September 14].

Yoshikawa, T., Rae, V., Bruins-Slot, W., Van den Berg, J W., Taylor, J R., Streilein, J W. (1990). Susceptibility to effects of UVB radiation on induction of contact hypersensitivity as a risk factor for skin cancer in humans. *J Invest Dermatol* Vol. 95, No. 5, (November 1990), pp. 9530-9536.

2

Desmosomal Cadherins in Basal Cell Carcinomas

Justyna Gornowicz-Porowska,
Monika Bowszyc-Dmochowska and Marian Dmochowski
Cutaneous Histopathology and Immunopathology Section, Department of Dermatology, Poznan University of Medical Sciences, Poland

1. Introduction

During recent years desmosomal research has developed into a biomedical field focused on the role of desmosomal components in tissue development and homeostasis. Investigators' area of interest involves the influence of cell adhesion defects and abnormal cell signaling on cancer invasion and metastasis. Some data indicated that there is greater cell proliferation activity in basal cell carcinoma (BCC) than suggested by the clinically apparent slow growth of the tumor. Indeed, it may suggest that individual desmosomal cadherins play different roles in proliferation and differentiation in BCC. Thus, the functional importance of desmosomal cadherins in the adhesion of carcinoma cells and during destructive/invasive growth makes them a useful tool for the evaluation of the biological behaviour of BCC.

2. Basal cell carcinoma: Clinical and histological subtypes

BCC is the most common type of skin cancer with rising incidence trends. It originates from basal cell layers of epidermis and/or the pilosebaceous adnexa (Yu et al., 2008). It is usually slow growing and rarely metastasizes; however, it can cause clinically significant local destruction and disfigurement when neglected or inadequately treated (Wong et al., 2003, Telfer et al., 2008). Prognosis is excellent with proper therapy. Growth of BCC is usually localized to the area of its origin (Bath-Hextall et al., 2004). BCCs typically occur in adults, but the tumors can develop even in children (Kossard et al., 2006; Hakverdi et al., 2011). Furthermore, males show higher incidence of BCC than females (Bath-Hextall et al., 2004). The etiology of BCC is still unclear but appears to be of multifactorial origin, resulting from a complex interaction of both environmental and genetic factors (Hakverdi et al., 2011).
Still, little is known about the genetic mechanisms underlying BCC (Teh et al., 2005). The genetic predisposition can be associated with, for example, genomewide allelic changes such as losses of chromosomal fragments leading to losses of heterozygosity (LOH) from a single DNA sample (Greinert, 2009), which are the most frequent genetic alternation in BCC (Gailani et al., 1996). In BCCs LOH is usually restricted to chromosome arm 9q (Greinert, 2009) and *de novo* mutations in the Patched 1 (*PTCH*) were found in 69% BCCs with 9q LOH (Teh et al., 2005). It was suggested that mutations in gene on chromosome 9q22 may be a necessary event for basal cell carcinogenesis (Gailani et al., 1996). Genes of importance to BCC development

include *PTCH1, P53* and *MC1R,* and many other recently discovered genes, which probably also play a role in BCC pathogenesis (de Zwaan & Haass, 2010). Moreover, twin studies and other studies of familial aggregation suggest a genetic predisposition to this cancer (de Zwaan & Haass, 2010). BCC may be divided into various clinical and histological subtypes. Using cDNA microarrays it is suggested that phenotypic diversity of BCCs might be accompanied by a corresponding diversity in gene expression patterns (Yu et al., 2008).

Various types of cutaneous lesions may be a clinical manifestation of BCC. There have been also many histological subtypes of BCC described by various authors. The highest number, 26 subtypes was described by Wade et al. (Wade & Ackerman, 1978). Thus, the nosology system of BCC requires simplification and clustering which may lead to a more practical classification (Mosterd et al., 2009). Clinical and histological subtypes of BCC may exhibit different patterns of behaviour and may even have a different etiology (Yu et al., 2008). The distinction between different BCC variants is important for prognosis and treatment (Yu et al., 2008).

There are two basic criteria in histological classifications of BCC: the histological growth pattern and histological differentiation. The growth pattern of BCC is probably associated with its risk for recurrence (Vantuchová & Čuřík, 2006).

According to WHO classification 2006 (Kossard et al., 2006) BCC may be divided into eight subtypes (Table 1):

	Clinical subtypes	**Histological subtypes**
Superficial	Characterized by a flat, red, well-circumscribed plaque with slow centrifugal spread. It may present as multiple lesions. Different sizes: from a few millimeters to over 10 cm in diameter. A fine pearly border or central superficial erosions with a history of contact bleeding may be present. It develops most frequently in areas where skin is covered (especially on the trunk). 10-30% of BCC	Presence of superficial lobules of basaloid cells which project from the epidermis or from the sides of follicles or eccrine ducts into the dermis and are surrounded by loose myxoid stroma. Usually there appear to be multiple tumor foci, separated by areas of normal skin.
Nodular	Elevated pearly nodules associated with teleangiectasia. It may become ulcerated or cystic. It develops most frequently on the head. 60-80% of BCC.	Presence of large lobules of basaloid cells ("germinative cells") with peripheral palisading of the nuclei. The lobules may have associated mucinous degeneration with cysts or have an adenoid pattern.
Micronodular	Elevated or flat infiltrative tumor. It develops most frequently on the back.	Presence of small nodules that permeate the dermis. In contrast to nodular BCC the surgical margins of micronodular BCC may be underestimated.
Infiltrating	Pale, indurated, poorly-defined plaque. It is most often found on the upper trunk or face.	Presence of strands, cords and columns of basaloid cells with scant cytoplasm.
Fibroepithelial	Elevated flesh coloured or erythematous nodule that may resemble a seborrhoic keratosis or acrochordon. It develops most frequently on the back.	Presence of an arborising network of cords of basaloid cells that extend downwards from the epidermis and create a fenestrating pattern.
With adnexal differentiation	No distinguishing clinical features.	Presence of adnexal differentiation including basaloid buds, ductal, sebaceous, and trichilemmal elements.
Basosquamous	No distinguishing clinical features.	Presence of abundant cytoplasm with more marked keratinization than typical BCC. The nuclei have vesicular chromatin with pleomorphism.
Keratotic	It appears pearly and may be studded with small keratin cyst (milia).	It shares the overall features of a nodular BCC. Keratinization may be laminated.

Table 1. Subtypes of BCC

Still, it should be emphasized that individual BCCs, when their total mass is examined, may exhibit combined features of various histological subtypes.

3. Desmosomal cadherins: Molecular biology and distribution in physiological and pathological conditions

Desmosomal cadherins (DCs) are transmembrane glycoproteins, which belong to the group of calcium-dependent intercellular adhesion molecules. They may initiate and maintain cell-cell adhesion in the absence of any contribution from classical cadherins (Garrod et al., 2002). DCs involve two subfamilies: i) the desmogleins (DSGs), ii) the desmocollins (DSCs) (Bazzi et al., 2006; Ishii, 2007; Brennan et al., 2004, Koch et al., 1992). So far three isoforms, each in two splicing variants, of desmocollin (DSC1-3) and four isoforms of desmoglein (DSG1-4) are known in humans (Ishii, 2007; Brennan et al., 2004). An additional two DSGs, DSG5 and DSG6, are present in mice (Whittock, 2003). Alternative splicing of the cytoplasmic domain gives rise to a longer "a" and a shorter "b" form of each DSC isoforms (Garrod et al., 2002). It is known that DSG and DSC have approximately 30% amino acid identity with each other and with the classical cadherins. They all have homologic basic structure in their extracellular domains and possess in the amino-terminal EC1 ectodomain cell adhesion recognition (CAR) sites with a central alanine residue. In light of above, researchers, using transfected fibroblasts, shown that adhesion mediated by DSC2/DSG2 and DSC3/DSG3 could be specifically blocked by peptides (Garrod et al., 2002).

In humans the genes encoding DCs are clustered on the q arm of chromosome 18 (Fig.1), so the possibility exists that DC gene expression is controlled through a common locus control element (Smith et al., 2004). Each DCs arise from a distinct gene and they are generally expressed in a differentiation-specific manner. This may suggest that in addition to their adhesive function, they may have a direct or indirect role in regulating differentiation (Garrod et al., 2002). Thus, the correlation between DCs and the stage of differentiation/proliferation allows creating the hypothesis that changes in gene function resulting from mutations would lead to alternation in differentiation/proliferation of hair follicle and epidermal cells (Cserhalmi-Friedman et al., 2001; Smith et al., 2004). This idea is supported by the results of transgenic mice experiment in which mis-expression or target ablation of DCs has resulted in altered patterns of epidermal differentiation. The DSGs genes are arranged in the following order: DSG1, DSG4, DSG3, DSG2 from centromeric to telomeric direction in the cadherin gene locus (Mahoney et al., 2006). Interestingly, this organization of genes correlates with DSGs expression in the epidermis (Mahoney et al., 2006). Thus, DSG1 and DSG4 are expressed in the differentiated cells of epidermis while DSG3 and DSG2 are localized to the proliferative basal and suprabasal cells of epidermis (Mahoney et al., 2006).

Various studies on adult human and bovine tissues have established that the DSGs and DSCs are both expressed in tissue-specific and differentiation-dependent patterns (King et al., 1993, 1997). This type of DCs expression implies that desmosomes within different tissues are biochemically, and presumably functionally, distinct (Delava et al., 2011). Delava et al. demonstrated that the precise role for the tissue-specific expression patterns of desmosomal cadherins is not fully understood, but manipulation of their expression suggests that this regulation is critical to tissue homeostasis (Delava et al., 2011).

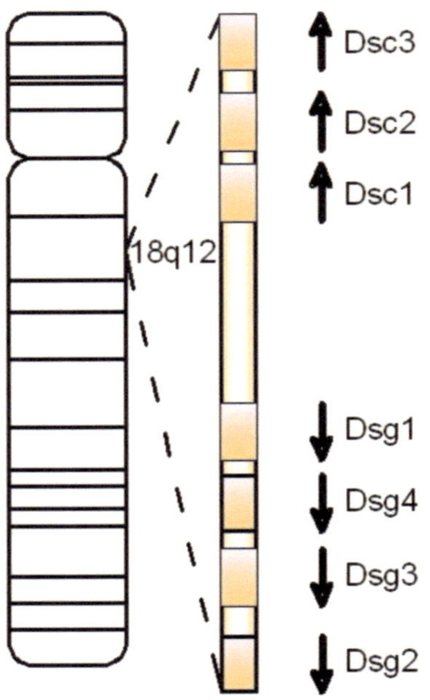

Fig. 1. Molecular biology of human desmosomal cadherins: genes reside in a genomic cluster on the q arm of human chromosome 18

3.1 Expression of desmosomal cadherins in normal tissue

The DCs show complex patterns of expression, particularly in intermediate layers where the majority of isoforms are expressed. However, the molecular mechanisms regulating DCs expressions are not well studied, particularly at the transcriptional level (Bazzi et al., 2006). Researchers, analyzing mRNA expression, suggested spatial patterns of DCs genes transcription and hierarchical expression of individual genes (King et al., 1997). However, most of the findings described the DC expression pattern at protein level. Nevertheless, Mahoney et al. (Mahoney et al., 2002) noticed that DSGs share high homology at both the gene and protein level and their expression is spatially and temporally regulated (existence of systems that provide both temporal and spatial control for transgene expression). This fact may potentially be contributing to significant role of DSGs in cell-cell adhesion during development (Mahoney et al., 2002). All desmosomes possess at least one DSC and one DSG but it appears to be no barrier to the presence of more than one of each (Chidgey, 2002; North et al., 1996; King et al., 1997). Data obtained with the use of mRNA and protein analyses shown that DCs are formed in the skin in relation to differentiation (Moll et al., 1997).

Expression pattern of DSGs in normal human epidermis was shown in Fig. 2. DSG1 and DSG3 are restricted to stratified epithelia (Brennan et al., 2010). DSG1 is more intensively expressed as the cells differentiate toward the stratum corneum, and very little detectable in the basal layer, whereas DSG3 is localized to the basal and immediate suprabasal layers (Wu et al., 2003). In normal human epidermis, DSG2 is expressed at low levels, and was reported to be restricted to the lowermost epidermis (Brennan et al., 2010). DSG2 expression fades with keratinocyte differentiation, whereas DSG3 expression decreases somewhat gradually from the basal into the spinous cell layers (Bowszyc-Dmochowska et al., 2010). DSG4 expression is restricted to the highly differentiated upper cell layers (Ishii, 2007), what is confirmed at both the mRNA and protein level (Bazzi et al., 2006). Expression of DSG4 may first be detected in the lower granular layers, increases in intensity upward into the horny layers, and terminates as the cells die to form the protective barrier (Mahoney et al., 2006). There is a hypothesis that DSG4 may coincide with the downregulation of DSG1 (Mahoney et al., 2006). Interestingly, the genes for DSCs are also differentially expressed. DSC1 is confined to the suprabasal cell layers, whereas DSC2 and 3 are found in desmosomes throughout the interfollicular epidermis (Moll et al., 1997).
Molecular cloning of DSGs and analysis of intron/exon organization of the DSG mice genes revealed significant conservation (Mahoney et al., 2002). Some studies indicated that expression of DSGs mRNA during mouse embryonic development and in various adult tissues are variable (Mahoney et al., 2002). This group of researchers shown that in adult mouse tissues, DSG2 is widely expressed while DSG1 and DSG3 expression is restricted to selected tissues (Mahoney et al., 2002).

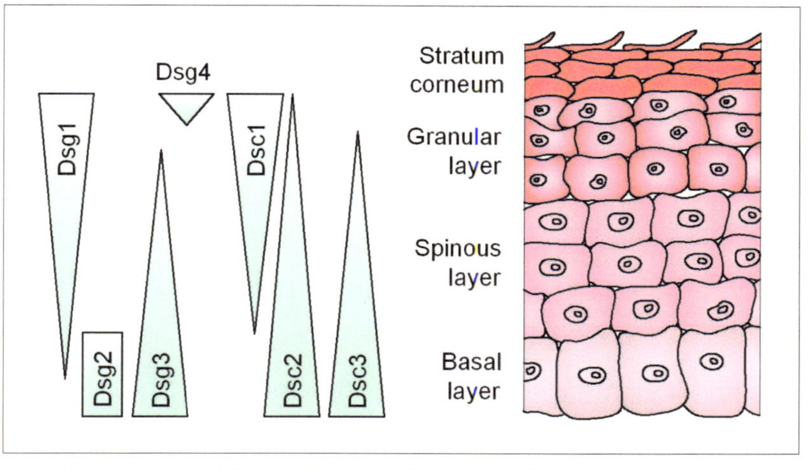

Fig. 2. Pattern of expression of desmogleins and desmocollins in normal human epidermis

Hair follicles exhibit morphological and ontogenic continuity with the epidermis. The distribution of DSGs in hair follicles (Fig. 3) has been described in some studies. Similar to epidermis, hair follicle is compartmentalized into a hierarchy of cells types based on the level of differentiation (Wu et al., 2003). DSG1 is expressed in the inner root sheath, and the innermost layers of the outer root sheath. There is a report that DSG2 is highly expressed by the least differentiated cells of the cutaneous epithelium, including the hair follicle bulge of fetus and adult, bulb matrix cells, and basal layer of the outer root sheath (Wu et al., 2003). Expression of DSG3 in hair follicle is correlated with different types of keratinization (all layers of outer root sheath in areas of trichilemmal keratinization and mainly the basal layer in areas of epidermal-like keratinization) (Wu et al., 2003). DSG4 is expressed specifically in hair shaft cortex, lower hair cuticle, and upper inner root sheath cuticle (Bazzi et al., 2009), what corroborated with findings based on *DSG4* mRNA obtained by Bazzi et al. (Bazzi et al., 2006). Probably this molecule is a key mediator of keratinocyte cell adhesion in hair follicle, where it coordinates the transition from proliferation to differentiation (Brennan et al., 2010). Analysis of expression of DSCs, with the use of monoclonal antibodies, in anagen hair follicles indicated that DSC1 is selectively localized in the inner root sheath. DSC2 is present in the area of cell borders of the central layer of the outer root sheath, while DSC3 shows increasing intensity with progressive differentiation (Kurzen et al., 1998).

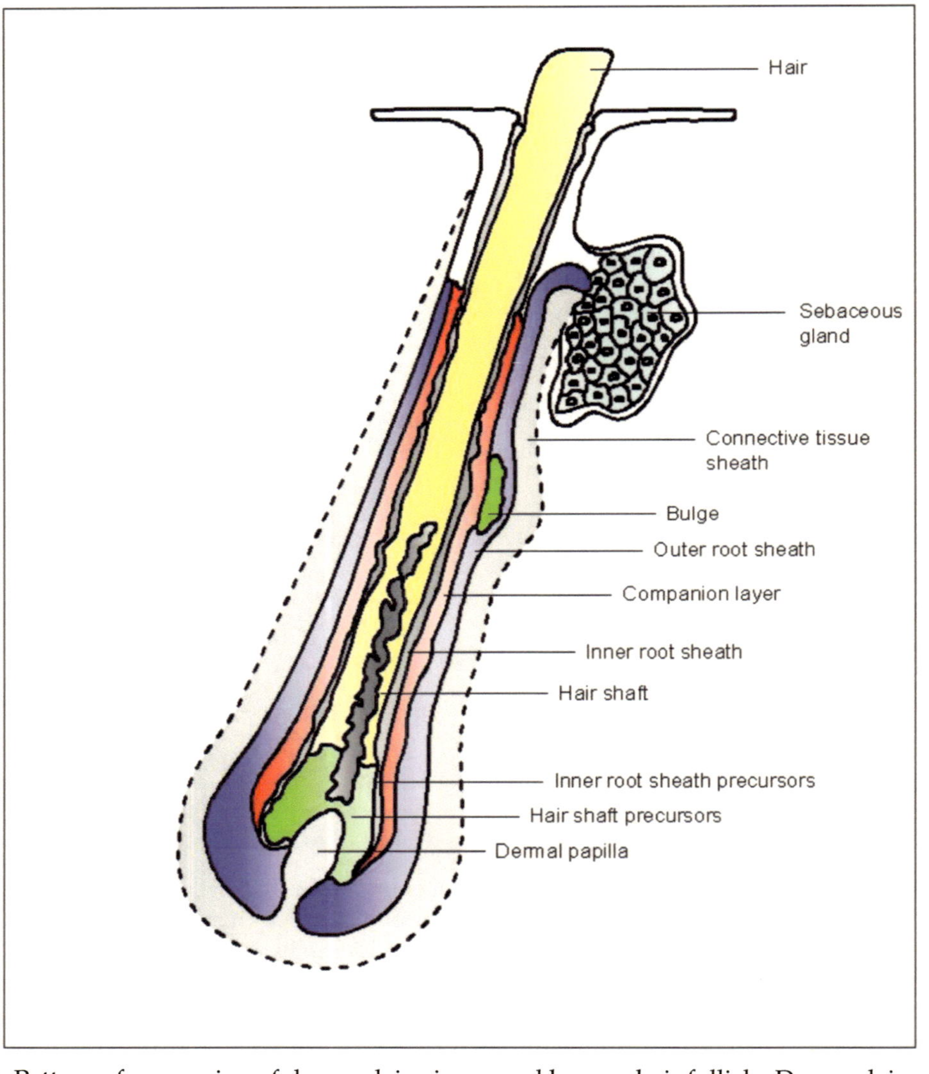

Fig. 3. Pattern of expression of desmogleins in normal human hair follicle. Desmogleins are marked as follows: red - DSG1, green - DSG2, blue - DSG3, yellow-DSG4

Recent studies have suggested that bulge region might be the reservoir of stem cells of hair follicles (Ma et al., 2004; Ohyama, 2007). Hair follicle stem cells are multipotent and having a superior clonogenicity and proliferative capacity. They are capable of giving rise to all cell types of hair, epidermis and sebaceous gland (Ma et al., 2004; Ohyama, 2007, Wu et al., 2003). Bulge cells might be susceptible to genetic alternation and be a source of carcinogenic mutations (Ohyama, 2007). Some data has suggested that several skin tumors, including BCC, might be derived from hair follicle cells, particularly from bulge cells (Ohyama, 2007). Most current data indicated (Grachtchouk et al., 2011) that probably there is a link between subtypes of BCC and its cell of origin, and constitutive hedgehog signaling activity.

3.2 Desmosomal cadherins and tumorigenesis

It is known that modulation or loss of intracellular junctions known as desmosomes has been implicated in tumorigenesis and contributes to the invasive and metastatic behavior of cancer cells (Teh et al., 2011). Beaudry et al. noted that probably desmosome loss does not promote tumorigenesis via a general trans-differentiation mechanism, but rather via more specific manner related to changes caused by complete desmosome-deficiency (Beaudry et al., 2010). However, studies about expression of desmosome components during human cancer progression have generated conflicting results (Beaudry et al., 2010). Thus, further genetic studies with animal models, such as knockout mice, to evaluate the functional consequence of desmosome alternation for tumorigenesis are necessary (Beaudry et al., 2010). Teh et al. found that downregulation of desmosomal components, particularly the DCs, precedes malignancy and is associated with desmosomal dysfunction (Teh et al., 2011). Beaudry et al. studying Perp-lacking mice demonstrated that Perp-deficiency indeed leads to accelerated skin tumorigenesis and PERP protein may be important as a tumor suppressor in humans (Beaudry et al., 2010).

Findings obtained by Teh et al. indicated that decreased assembly of desmosomes or down-regulation of desmosomal proteins, including DCs, is associated with several epithelial cancers (Teh et al., 2011). Studies on the role of DCs in BCC are relatively scanty in relation to squamous cell carcinoma (SCC), while it seems that BCC is the most common type of skin cancer. Better understanding of molecular basis of BCC may also lead to improvement therapeutic approaches. However, to the best of our knowledge, there have been no definitive data about the expression of all of DCs in BCC. Still, several reports (Mahoney et al., 2010; Bazzi & Christiano, 2007) indicated that the expression of DCs in tumor cells may be associated with the invasive or metastatic ability of various skin carcinomas, including BCC (Gornowicz et al., 2009). Although the mechanism by which DCs affect the tumorigenesis has not be fully elucidated and require further investigation (Tada et al., 2000). Consequently, the cell-cell adhesions of BCC represent an interesting field of examination (Moll et al., 1997).

Elegant study showed that, in SCC, during desmosome assembly, DSG3 first forms simple clusters at the cell surface (Garrod et al., 2002). Then the incorporation of desmosomal cadherin into the desmosomes was isoform-dependent (Ishii et al., 2001). Probably DSG2 and DSG3 were incorporated, but DSG1 and DSC1a were not. DSG1 normally expressed in the upper layers of epidermis, so the importance of a differentiation program for expression was stressed (Ishii et al., 2001).

Electron microscope studies of BCC revealed a significant reduction of desmosomes compared with normal basal cells and hair follicle keratinocytes (Krunic et al., 1997). Dysfunction or loss of desmosomal cadherins are also possible events in the BCC and these events may precede overt malignancy.

3.2.1 Expression of desmosomal cadherins in BCC

The desmosomal immunostainig (plakophilin 1) observed in BCC was very heterogeneous: in general, junctions in well-differentiated stratified tumor regions were more intensely stained than sections of poorly differentiated and invasively growing BCCs (Moll et al., 1997)

Tada et al. using immunofluorescence with monoclonal antibody revealed that expression of DSG1 in BCC was decreased or absent in tumor cells, whereas the expression of E-cadherin was strongly positive (Tada et al., 2000). Moreover, all of examined by Tada et al. (Tada et al. 2000) BCC cases showed no metastasis, then it is suggested that E-cadherin but not DCs may prevent the detachment of tumor cells from tumor nests. Bazzi et al. (Bazzi & Christiano, 2007) indicated that the links between classical cadherin (such as E-cadherin) downregulation and metastasis through epithelial-mesenchymal transition are well established. However, they noticed that still it remains to be determined whether a similar link between desmosomes and cancer exists and if so, which desmosomal components are involved (Bazzi & Christiano, 2007).

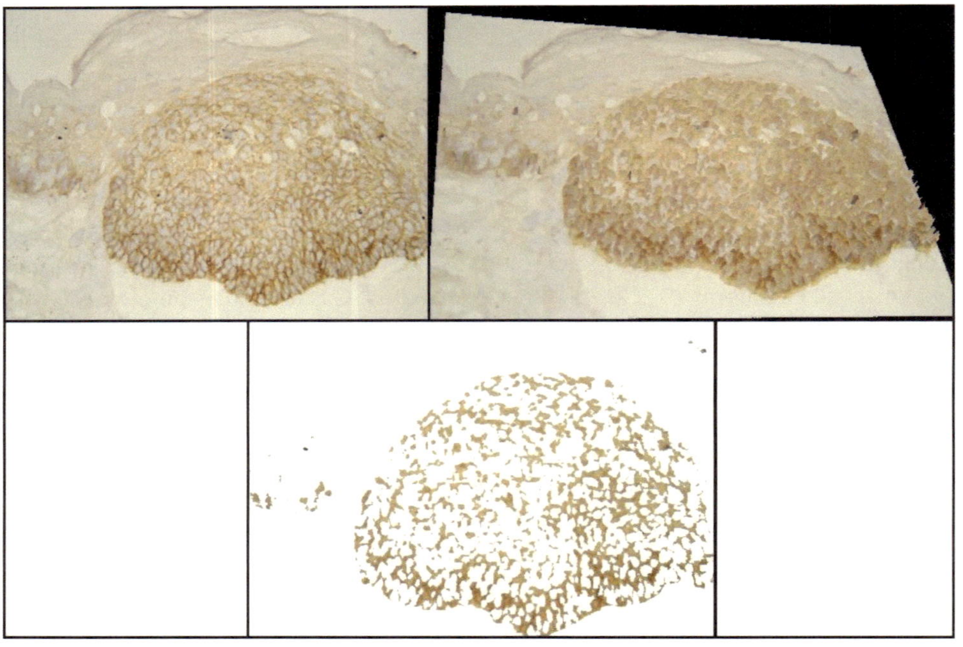

Fig. 4. Expression of DSG2 in BCC nests in patient with BCC. DSG2 expression in immunohistochemistry (top left) (immunoperoxidase staining on frozen sections), DSG2 expression processed with digital microscopic image analysis superimposed on DSG2 expression in immunohistochemistry (top right), intensity of DSG2 expression processed with digital microscopic image analysis (bottom) (original magnification x400).

It is suggested that only DSG2 may be found in tumors whereas the synthesis of other DSGs is much restricted. This hypothesis was corroborated by Schafer, who detected DSG2 in carcinoma cells with immunohistochemistry. Increased level of DSG2 in BCC was also observed in further investigation (Brennan & Mahoney 2009; Gornowicz et al., 2009). Brennan et al. identified DSG2 as a potential new marker for epithelial-derived malignancies and postulated that overexpression of DSG2 may deregulate multiple signaling pathways associated with increased growth rate, anchorage-independent cell survival, and the development of skin tumors (Brennan & Mahoney, 2009). In light of this, DSG2 overexpression may activate signal transduction pathways such as PI3K/Akt, MAPK, STAT3 and NFkappaB, which are often involved in cell proliferation and survival (Brennan & Mahoney, 2009). This group of researchers also noticed that the current dogma in cancer biology is that cell adhesion is reduced during malignant transformation, in turn allowing malignant cells to migrate, invade and metastasize. These data are compatible with our results (Bowszyc-Dmochowska et al., 2010, 2011), which demonstrated, with quantitative digital morphometry, an increased expression of DSG2 in BCC nest compared to normal epidermis (Fig. 4, Fig. 5). Furthermore, we found a significant correlation (r=+0.6092) between intensities of DSG2 and DSG3 expression in normal epidermis, but no significant correlation between those markers in BCC. However, still the potential value of DSG2-specific antibodies in tumor diagnosis as well as in studies of the mechanisms desmosomal cell coupling is discussed (Schäfer et al., 1996).

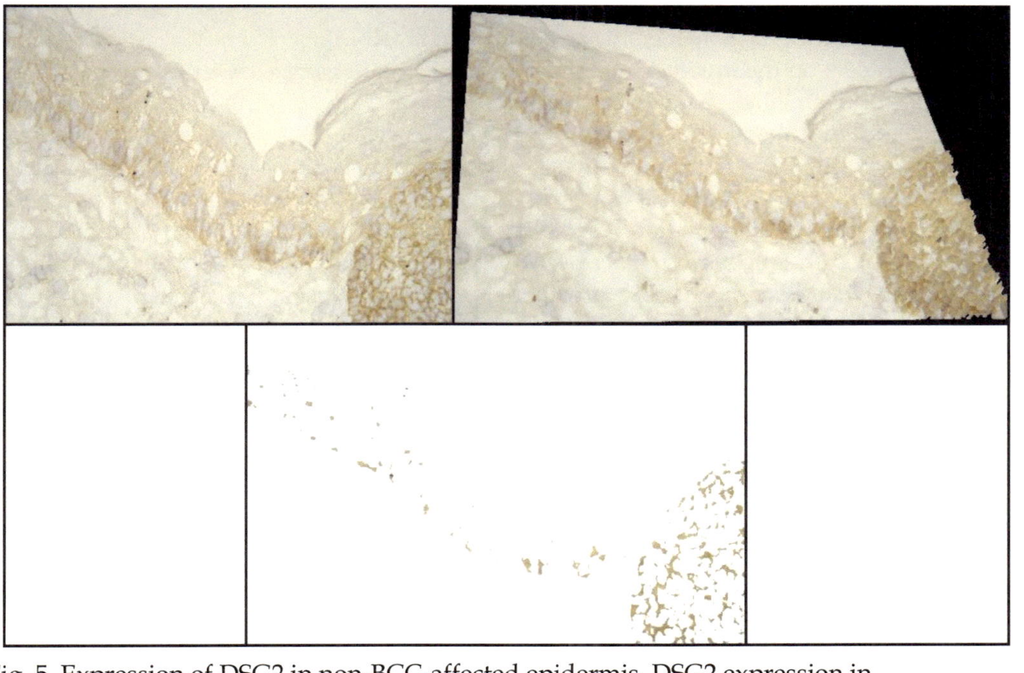

Fig. 5. Expression of DSG2 in non-BCC-affected epidermis. DSG2 expression in immunohistochemistry (top left) (immunoperoxidase staining on frozen sections), DSG2 expression processed with digital microscopic image analysis superimposed on DSG2 expression in immunohistochemistry (top right), intensity of DSG2 expression processed with digital microscopic image analysis (bottom) (original magnification x400).

The studies on the expression of DSG3 in human tumors are still scarce. Hence, the role and mechanism of DSG3 in cancer development remain to be elucidated. Study on expression of DSG3 in BCC (Gornowicz et al., 2009), using mathematical analysis of immunoperoxidase staining images, revealed that DSG3 expression is significantly decreased in BCC nest compared to both BCC-free epidermis in BCC patients (Fig. 6, Fig. 7) and patients with more benign tumors than BCC. Thus, these results seem to indicate that DSG3 might be involved in BCC pathogenesis as its decreased expression in BCC-affected epidermis might be responsible, in part, for locally invasive behavior of that tumor. The intriguing question arises what causes this decrease of expression of DSG3 in BCC, in other words whether it is a cause or result or somehow both of perturbed adhesion in BCC. It is noticed (Gornowicz et al., 2009) that the cooperation of p53/Perp (Kanellou et al., 2009; Bektas & Rubenstein 2009) pathways with DSG3 in regulating/disturbing keratinocyte adhesion in BCC is a sheer speculation at present, but this should be experimentally verified, especially as a role for Perp in DSG3-linked pemphigus vulgaris has recently been postulated (Nguyen et al., 2009). Alternatively, an exciting possibility is, giving the fact that tightly packed cancer cells showing a palisade arrangement on the periphery of the tumor are characteristic for BCC (Lever & Schaumburg-Lever, 1990), that the diminution/lack of DSG3-mediated adhesion is not enough for BCC cells to separate fully. In some cases of cancer the inhibition of tumor growth and invasion following the knockdown of DSG3 mediated by RNA interference (RNAi) was observed (Teh et al., 2011). RNAi is a powerful tool to dampen the level of proteins that are mutated or frequently overexpressed in skin diseases (Simpson et al., 2010). In BCC, perhaps, the DSG3 may be the target protein for RNAi.

There is no report on the involvement of DSG4 in BCC pathogenesis. Our own experiments using a commercially available anti-DSG4 antibody (unpublished data) with immunohistochemical staining, despite repetitive attempts under various conditions, gave no satisfying results. We found unequivocal DSG4 expression neither in BCC nests nor in normal epidermis, whereas DSG4 appeared to be expressed in sweat glands. It is known that BCC may show differentiation resembling the adnexal structures, such as hair follicles, sebaceous glands, or eccrine and apocrine sweat glands (Haushild et al., 2008). Interestingly, eccrine sweat glands are generally considered as a possible epidermal stem cell source (Biedermann et al., 2010). Birdermann described both *in vitro* and *in vivo* the capability of human eccrine sweat gland cells to form a stratified interfollicular epidermis. Little evidence for a sweat gland origin of the basal cell tumor has been presented by previous investigators (Zackheim, 1963). The origin of BCC from sweat gland ducts has been recorded, but probably its origin from sweat gland acini is extremely rare, if not actually unknown (Arnold, 1948). Still, a plausible link between DSG4 expression in sweat glands and BCC showing sweat gland-like structures should be explored.

Desmosomal and hemidesmosomal adhesion systems are downregulated in the hair matrix region of hair follicle and in BCC resulting from abnormal growth of developing hair follicles (Nanba et al., 2000). Some observation shown that the desmosomal adhesion system, in which the DCs of DSCs and DSGs function, is downregulated in hair placodes (Nanba et al., 2000). Furthermore, hair follicles, which physiologically express DSGs, apparently are involved in BCC pathogenesis (Gornowicz et al., 2009). Particularly, bulge cells are in the area of research interest, because of their possible role in tumorigenesis (Ohyama, 2007), including that of BCC. Several research groups have noted that some BCCs express K-15 that is usually expressed in human follicle bulge cells (Ohyama, 2007).

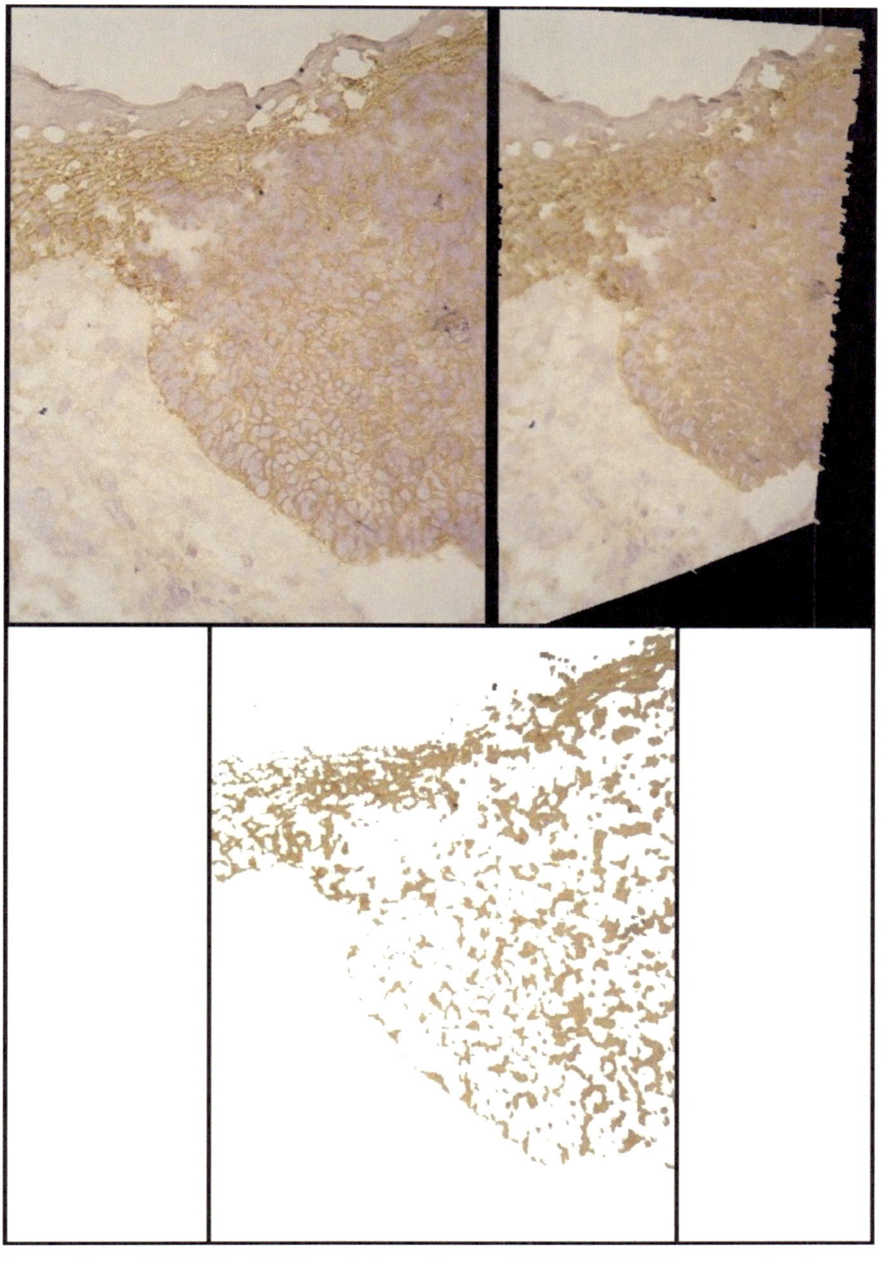

Fig. 6. Expression of DSG3 in BCC nests in patient with BCC. DSG3 expression in immunohistochemistry (top left) (immunoperoxidase staining on frozen sections), DSG3 expression processed with digital microscopic image analysis superimposed on DSG3 expression in immunohistochemistry (top right), intensity of DSG3 expression processed with digital microscopic image analysis (bottom) (original magnification x400).

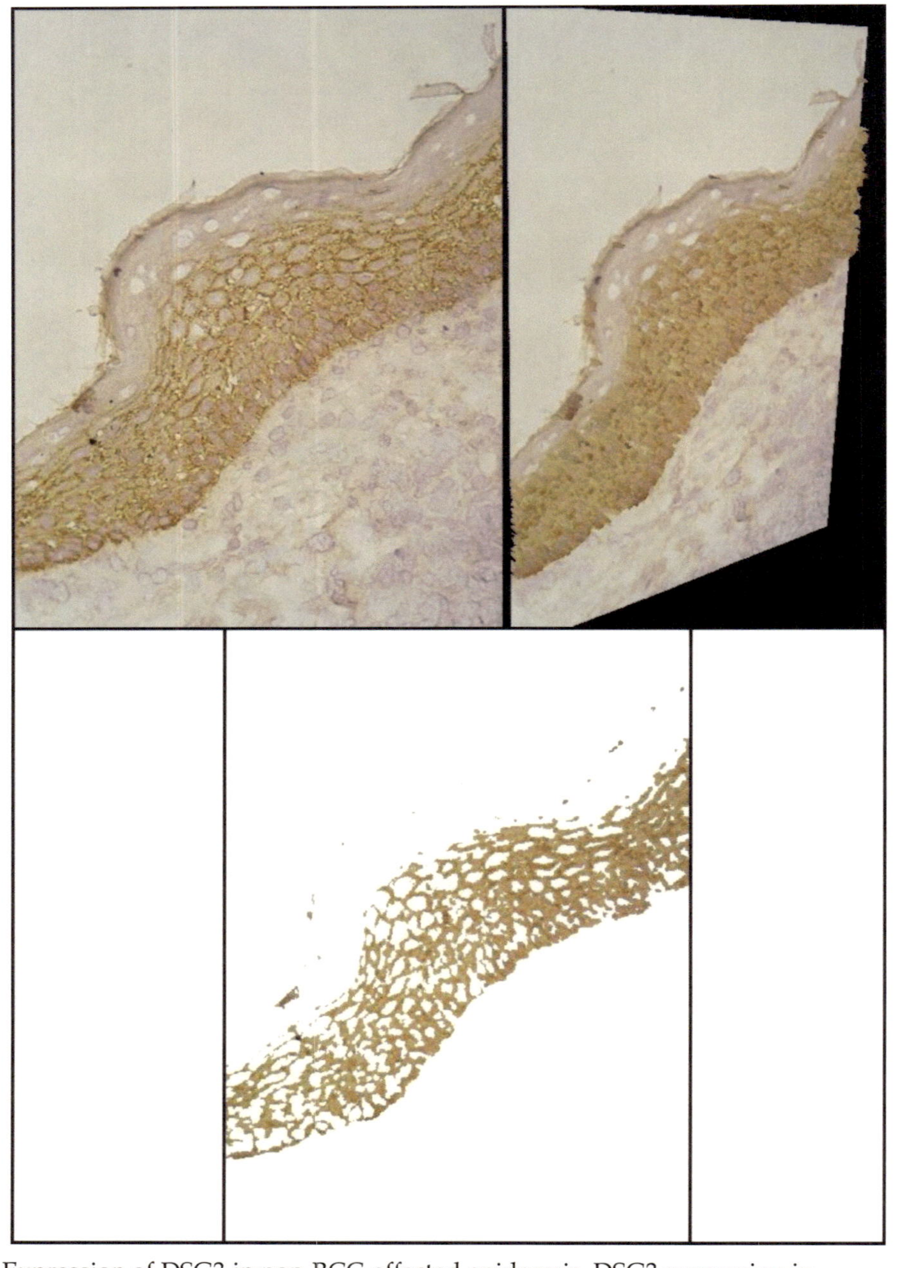

Fig. 7. Expression of DSG3 in non-BCC-affected epidermis. DSG3 expression in immunohistochemistry (top left) (immunoperoxidase staining on frozen sections), DSG3 expression processed with digital microscopic image analysis superimposed on DSG3 expression in immunohistochemistry (top right), intensity of DSG3 expression processed with digital microscopic image analysis (bottom) (original magnification x400).

Interestingly, it has been found that overexpression of *Shh* gene (sonic hedgehog), a gene essential for hair follicle morphogenesis, resulted in the formation of BCC like tumors (Ohyama, 2007). However, Youssef et al. using murine model (Youssef et al., 2010) have very recently revealed that BCC does not originate from bulge stem cells, as previously thought. With the use of clonal analysis they have found using mouse model of the disease that BCC arises from long-term resident progenitor cells of the interfollicular epidermis and the upper infundibulum (Youssef et al., 2010). Still, DSGs can be important in BCC pathogenesis regardless of the issue of BCC cellular origins as they are expressed in both bulge region and the upper infundibulum of hair follicle and interfollicular epidermis (Gornowicz et al., 2009).

Overall, what noticed Chidgey (Chidgey & Dawson, 2007), findings obtained by different authors demonstrate that alterations in DCs expression patterns, perhaps through modified intracellular signalling and/or changes in adhesive strength, have fundamental effects on cell behaviour, and can in some situations drive proliferation (Chidgey & Dawson, 2007). Thus, alterations in the expression of DCs in cancer could result in the release of plakoglobin from desmosomes, subsequent displacement of β-catenin from adherens junctions and increased Wnt/β-catenin signaling (Chidgey & Dawson, 2007).

3.3 Alternative splicing of DCs and tumorigenesis in BCC

Alternative splicing (AS) generates mRNA that encodes different polypeptides from a single gene. Different protein isoforms of a single gene may have distinct or even antagonistic functions, due to the insertion or deletion of key functional regions (Xing, 2007). AS is a common phenomenon and more than 90% human genes are alternatively spliced (Pan et al., 2008; Wang et al., 2008). It is known that AS is involved in numerous human diseases (Kim et al., 2007), thus accumulating evidence revealed that aberrant splicing contributes to human neoplasms (Miura et al, 2011; Xing, 2007; Kim et al., 2007; Venables, 2006; He et al., 2007; Srebrow & Kornblihtt, 2006). However, in only few cases it has been proved, e.g. breast and ovarian cancer, prostate cancer (Lixia et al., 2007; Rohlfs et al., 2000; Thorsen et al., 2008; Rajan et al., 2009). Kim et al. shown that cancerous tissues exhibit lower levels of AS than do normal tissues, what might be a result of disruption of splicing regulatory proteins (Kim et al., 2007).

AS is a fundamental molecular process which generates proteome functional diversity and may play a significant role in cell differentiation and proliferation, probably through the production of alternative transcripts of DCs. Srebrow et al. (Srebrow & Kornblihtt, 2006) indicated that the connection between the signaling pathways and splicing regulation can lead to the deregulation of proliferation and differentiation, which may contribute to cancer. The discovery of the events of AS in the DCs transciptome of BCC cells and understanding how AS contributes to tumorigenesis (Xing, 2007) may produce new medical implications, e.g. drug targets. However, the knowledge about AS in BCC is still limited. Some reports indicate that alternative splicing pattern of Mcl-1 (myeloid cell leukemia 1) may induce apoptosis in BCC (Shieh et al., 2009).

Both DSGs and DSCs exist in multiple isoforms (Hardman 2004). It is known that DSCs occur as "a" and "b" splice variants (Hardman et al., 2004; Cheng et al., 2003) and these alternative transcripts have different function. The "a" variant having slightly longer cytoplasmic domain can support desmosomal assembly (Hardman et al., 2004; Cheng et al., 2003). Some hypothesis indicate that "b" form mediates or regulates DSC signaling activity through its distinct cytoplasmic domain; however, Hardman et al. observed that DSC3b may be involved in epidermal differentiation regulation (Hardman et al., 2004).

Recent work revealed that the expression of DCs might be altered in cancers originating from keratinocytes (Lee et al., 2009). Lee et al. (Lee et al., 2009) examined expression of splicing variant of DSG3 in epidermal cancers, such as SCC and BCC. Their expression was highly increased in SCC, but not in BCC. These results suggest that splicing variant of DSG3 may disturb desmosome assembly components and weaken the cell-cel interaction (Lee et al., 2009). Thus, AS of DCs may affect signaling in the cell and regulate process of epidermal differentiation and proliferation.

Searching NCBI Gene Database by DSGs names revealed interesting issues. In humans, only *DSG4* gene is described as having alternative splicing form (DSG4 isoform 1 and DSG4 isoform 2). Interestingly, there is no NCBI data about AS in *DSG1, DSG2* and *DSG3* genes. However, some researchers (Lee et al., 2009) suggested that AS may generate a splicing variant of DSG3 (ΔNDg3). Thus, these results shown that molecular analyses of DCs should still be considered an important research area. It should be remembered that correct interpretation of genetic alternation and the investigation of aberrant transcripts is crucial for genetic diagnosis and molecular characteristics of neoplasms (Miura et al., 2011), including BCC. In light of this, oligonucleotide microarrays containing exon junction probes may be a powerful tool to investigate tissue-specific regulation of AS taking place in BCC (Nagao et al., 2005). Literature data may suggest that AS should be regarded as a potential source for new clinical diagnostic, prognostic and therapeutic strategies in cancer (He et al., 2007).

4. Conclusions

Thus, it seems that DCs might be involved in BCC pathogenesis. Seemingly, the expressions of DSG2 and DSG3, adhesion molecules that plausibly play different roles in proliferation and differentiation of epidermis, are coordinated in normal epidermis, but this apparent coordination is lost in BCC. That loss of coordination of DSG2 and DSG3 expressions, revealed with quantitative digital morphometry, in BCC might be a partial explanation of BCC behaviour as a locally invasive tumor.

There is still a very interesting issue, what role desmosomal adhesion and desmosomal components (particularly DSGs) play in carcinogenesis. The disturbance of desmosomal adhesion can result in tissue integrity damage and possibly induction of tumor cell migration and proliferation. Study on the role of DSG in BCC may suggest that in human skin DSG2-mediated adhesion appears to be more proliferation-associated, whereas DSG3-mediated adhesion seemingly is more differentiation-associated.

The impact of signaling pathway, involving DCs mediated adhesion, and cells of origin for BCC on different subtypes of BCC should be explained. Work with murine model, which was carried out by Grachtchouk et al. (Grachtchouk et al., 2011), shown that the level of expression of constitutive hedgehog pathway effector (GLI2*) is depended on histological BCC subtypes. Moreover, they indicated that phenotype of BCC may be determined by the cell of origin and tissue context. Thus, these connections may determine the different biological behavior of BCC.

Progress in these areas will lead to a better understanding of the role of desmosomes in normal tissue homeostasis and malignancy (Chidgey & Dawson, 2007).

5. Acknowledgment

Digital microscopic image analysis (Fig.4-7) courtesy of Prof. Elzbieta Kaczmarek and Agnieszka Seraszek-Jaros M.Sc.

6. References

Arnold H.R. (1948). Basal cell carcinoma of sweat gland origin. Archives of Dermatology and Syphilology, Vol.57, pp. 1042-1046

Bath-Hextall F., Bong J., Perkins W. & Williams H. (2004). Interventions for basal cell carcinoma of the skin: systematic review. British Medical Journal, Vol. 329, pp. 705

Bazzi H., Getz A., Mahoney M.G., Ishida-Yamamoto A., Langbein .L, Wahl J.K. & Christiano A.M. (2006). Desmoglein 4 is expressed in highly differentiated keratinocytes and trichocytes in human epidermis and hair follicle. Differentiation, Vol.74, No.2-3, pp. 129-140

Bazzi H. & Christiano A.M. (2007). Broken hearts, woolly hair, and tattered skin: when desmosomal adhesion goes awry. Current Opinion in Cell Biology, Vol.19, pp. 515–520

Bazzi H., Demehri S., Potter C.S., Barber A.G., Awgulewitsch A., Kopan R. & Christiano A.M. (2009). Desmoglein 4 is regulated by transcription factors implicated in hair shaft differentiation. Differentiation, Vol.78, No.5, pp. 292-300

Beaudry V., Jiang D., Dusek R.L., Park E.J., Knezevich S., Ridd K., Vogel H., Bastian B.C. & Attardi L.D. (2010). Loss of p53/p63 regulated desmosomal protein Perp promotes tumorigenesis. PloS Genetics, Vol. 6, No. 10, e1001168

Bektas M. & Rubenstein D.S. (2009). Perp and pemphigus: a disease of desmosome destabilization (commentary). Journal of Investigative Dermatology, Vol.129, pp. 1606-1608

Biedermann T., Pontiggia L., Böttcher-Haberzeth S., Tharakan S., Braziulis E., Schiestl C., Meuli M. & Reichmann E. (2010). Human eccrine sweat gland cells can reconstitute a stratified epidermis. Journal of Investigative Dermatology, Vol.130, pp. 1996-2009

Bowszyc-Dmochowska M., Gornowicz J., Seraszek A., Kaczmarek E. & Dmochowski M. (2010). Quantitative digital morphometry reveals decreased expression of desmoglein 3, but increased expression of desmoglein 2, in basal cell carcinomas. Journal of Investigative Dermatology, Vol.130, Suppl 2, S23

Bowszyc-Dmochowska M., Gornowicz J., Seraszek A., Kaczmarek Karczmarek. & Dmochowski M. (2011). Loss of correlation between desmoglein 3 and desmoglein 2 expressions, evaluated with quantitative digital morphometry, in basal cell carcinomas. 22nd World Congress of Dermatology, May 24-29, Seoul 2011

Brennan D., Hu Y., Kljuic A., Choi Y.W., Joubeh S., Bashkin M., Wahl J., Fertala A., Pulkkinen L., Uitto J., Christiano A.M., Panteleyev A. & Mahoney M.G. (2004). Differential structural properties and expression patterns suggest functional significance for multiple mouse desmoglein 1 isoforms. Differentiation, Vol.72, No., pp 434-449

Brennan D., Mahoney G. (2009). Increased expression of Dsg2 in malignant skin carcinomas: A tissue-microarray based study. Cell Adhesion & Migration, Vol.3, No.2, pp. 148-154

Brennan D., Hu Y., Medhat W., Dowling A. & Mahoney M.G. (2010). Superficial Dsg2 expression limits epidermal blister formation mediated by pemphigus foliaceus antibodies and exfoliative toxins. Dermatology Research and Practice, article ID 410278: 1-10. Available from: http://www.hindawi.com/journals/drp/2010/410278.html

Cheng X., Mihndukulasuriya K., Den Z., Kowalczyk A.P., Calkins C.C., Ishiko A., Shimizu A. & Koch P. (2004). Assessment of splice variant-specific functions of desmocollin 1 in the skin. Molecular and Cellular Biology, Vol.24, No.1, pp.154-163

Chidgey M. (2002). Desmosomes and disease: an update. Histology and Histopathology, Vol.17, pp.1179-1192

Chidgey M. & Dawson C. (2007). Desmosomes: a role in cancer? British Journal of Cancer, Vol.96, pp. 1783-1787

Cserhalmi-Friedman P.B., Frank J.A., Ahmad W., Panteleyev A.A., Aita V.M. & Christiano AM. (2001). Structural analysis reflects the evolutionary relationship between the human desmocollin gene family members. Experimental Dermatology, Vol.10, No.2, pp. 95–99

De Zwaan S.E. & Haass N.K. (2010). Genetics of basal cell carcinoma. Australasian Journal of Dermatology, Vol.51, pp. 81–94

Delva E.,Tucker D.K. & Kowalczyk A.P. (2009). The Desmosome. Cold Spring Harbor Perspectives in Biology, Aug;1(2):a002543Fjd_579

Gailani M.R., Leffell D.J., Ziegler A.M., Gross E.G., Brash D.E. & Bale A.E. (1996). Relationship between sunlight exposure and a key genetic alteration in basal cell carcinoma. Journal of the National Cancer Institute, Vol. 88. No. 6, pp. 349-354

Garrod D.R., Merritt A.J. & Nie Z. (2002). Desmosomal cadherins. Current Opinion in Cell Biology, Vol.14, No.5, pp. 537–545

Gornowicz J., Bowszyc-Dmochowska M., Seraszek A., Karczmarek E. & Dmochowski M. (2009). Quantitative digital morphometry reveals low expression of desmoglein 3 protein in basal cell carcinomas: relevance to pemphigus vulgaris pathogenesis? Clinical Dermatology, Vol.11, pp.191-194

Grachtchouk M., Pero J., Ermilov A.N., Michael L.E., Wilbert D., Lim S. & Dlugosz A.A. (2011). Basal cell carcinoma tumor subtype is defined by its cell of origin. Journal of Investigative Dermatology, Vol. 131, Suppl. 1, S29.

Greinert R. Skin cancer: new markers for better prevention. (2009). Pathobiology, Vol.76, No.2, pp. 64-81

Hakverdi S., Balci D.D., Dogramaci C.A., Toprak S. & Yaldiz M. (2011). Retrospective analysis of basal cell carcinoma. Indian Journal Dermatology Venerealogy and Leprology, Vol.77, No.2, pp. 251

Hardman M., Liu K., Avilion A.A., Merritt A., Brennan K., Garrod D.R. & Byrne C. (2005). Desmosomal cadherin misexpression alters beta-catenin stability and epidermal differentiation. Molecular and Cellular Biology, Vol.25, No.3, pp. 969-978

Hauschild A., Breuninger H., Kaufmann R., Kortmann R.D., Schwipper V., Werner J., Reifenberger J., Dirschka T. & Garbe C. (2008). Short German guidelines: Basal cell carcinoma. Journal der Deutschen Dermatologischen Gesellschaft, Vol.6, Suppl 1, S2-4

He C., Zuo Z., Chen H., Zhang L. Zhou F., Cheng H. & Zhou R. (2007). Genome-wide detection of testis- and testicular cancer-specific alternative splicing. Carcinogenesis, Vol.28, No.12, pp. 2484-2490

Ishii K., Norvell S.M., Bannon L.J., Amargo E.V., Pascoe L.T. & Greek K.J. (2001). Assembly of desmosomal cadherins into desmosomes is isoform dependent. Journal of Investigative Dermatology, Vol.117, pp. 26-35

Ishii K. (2007). Identification of desmoglein as a cadherin and analysis of desmoglein domain structure. Journal of Investigative Dermatology, Vol.127, E6-7

Kanellou P., Zaravinos A., Zioga M. & Spandidos D.A. (2009). Deregulation of the tumour suppressor genes p14ARF, p15INK4b, p16INK4a and p53 in basal cell carcinoma. British Journal of Dermatology, Vol.160, No.6, pp. 1215-1221

Kim E., Goren A. & Ast G. (2007). Insights into the connection between cancer and alternative splicing. Trends in Genetics, Vol.24, No.1, pp. 7-10

King I.A., Tabiowo A., Purkis P., Leigh I. & Magee A.I (1993). Expression of distinct desmocollin isoforms in human epidermis. Journal of Investigative Dermatology, Vol.100, pp. 373-379

King I.A., Angst B.D., Hunt D.M., Kruger M., Arnemann J. & Buxton R.S. (1997). Hierarchical expression of desmosomal cadherins during stratified epithelial morphogenesis in the mouse. Differentiation, Vol.62, No.2, pp. 83-96

Koch P.J., Goldschmidt M.D., Zimbelmann R., Troyanowsky R. & Franke W.W. (1992). Complexity and expression patterns of the desmosomal cadherins. Proceedings of the Natlional Academy of Sciens, Vol.89, pp. 353-357

Kossard S., Epstein E.H. Cerio, Yu L.L. & Weedon D. (2006). Basal cell carcinoma, In: World Health Organisation classification of tumors. Pathology and Genetics of Skin Tumors R.LeBoit P.E., Burg G., Weedon D. & Sarasin A. Lyon, France: IARC Press, pp. 10-33

Krunic A.L., Garrod D.R., Viehman G.E., Madani S., Buchanan M.D. & Clark R.E. (1997). The use of antidesmoglein stains in Mohs micrographic surgery. A potential aid for the differentiation of basal cell carcinoma from horizontal sections of the hair follicle and folliculocentric basaloid proliferation, Dermatologic Surgery, Vol.23, No.6, pp. 463-468

Kurzen H., Moll I., Schäfer S., Simics E., Amagai M., Wheelock M..J & Franke W.W. (1998). Compositionally different desmosomes in the various compartments of the human hair follicle. Differentiation, Vol.63, No.5, pp. 295-304

Lee J.S., Yoon H.K., Sohn K.C., Back S.J., Kee S.H., Seo Y.J., Park J.K., Kim C.D. & Lee J.H. (2009). Expression of N-terminal truncated desmoglein 3 (ΔNDg3) in epidermis and its role in keratinocyte differentiation. Experimental and Molecular Medicine, Vol.41, No.1, pp.42-50

Lever W.F. & Schaumburg-Lever G. (1990). Tumors of the epidermal appendages, In: Histopathology of the skin (Lever WF, Schaumburg-Lever G), 7th edition, Philadelphia: J.B. Lippincott Company, pp. 622-632

Lixia M., Zhijian C., Chao S., Chaojiang G. & Congyi Z. (2007). Alternative splicing of breast cancer associated gene BRCA1 from breast cancer cell line. Journal of Biochemistry and Molecular Biology, Vol.40, No.1, pp. 15-21

Ma D.R., Yang E.N. & Lee S.T. (2004). A review: The location, molecular characterization and multipotency of hair follicle epidermal stem cells. Annals Academy of Medicine, Vol.33, pp. 784-788

Mahoney M.G., Simpson A., Aho S., Uitto J. & Pulkkinen L. (2002). Interspecies conservation and differential expression of mouse desmoglein gene family. Experimental Dermatology, Vol.11, No.2, pp. 115-125

Mahoney M.G., Hu Y., Brennan D., Bazzi H., Christiano A.M. & Wahl J.K. (2006). Delineation of diversified desmoglein distribution in stratified squamous epithelia: implications in diseases. Experimental Dermatology, Vol.15, No.2, pp. 101–109

Mahoney M.G., Müller E. & Koch P. (2010). Desmosomes and desmosomal cadherin function in skin and heart diseases—advancements in basic and clinical research. Deramtology Research and Practice, 2010. pii: 725647.

Miura K., Fujibuchi W. & Sasaki I. (2011). Alternative pre-mRNA splicing In digestive tract malignach. Cancer Science, Vol.102, No.2, pp. 309-316.

Moll I., Kurzen H., Langbein L. & Franke W.W. (1997). The distribution of the desmosomal protein, plakophilin 1, in human skin and skin tumors. Journal of Investigative Dermatology, Vol.108, pp. 139-146

Mosterd K., Arits A., Thissen M. & Kelleners-Smeets N. (2009). Histology-based treatment of basal cell carcinoma. Acta Dermato-Venereologica , Vol.89, No.5, pp. 454-458

Nagao K., Togawa N., Fujii K., Uchikawa H., Kohno Y., Hamada M. & Miyashita T. Detecting tissue-specific alternative splicing and disease-associated aberrant splicing of the *PTCH* gene with exon junction microarrays. Human Molecular Genetics, Vol.14, pp. 3379-3388

Nanba D., Hieda Y. & Nakanishi Y. (2000). Remodeling of desmosomal and hemidesmosomal adhesion systems during early morphogenesis of mouse pelage hair follicles. Journal of Investigative Dermatology, Vol.114, pp. 171-177

Nguyen B., Dusek R.L., Beaudry V.G., Marinkovich M.P. & Attardi L.D. (2009). Loss of the desmosomal protein perp enhances the phenotypic effects of pemphigus vulgaris autoantibodies. Journal of Investigative Dermatology, Vol.129, pp. 1710-1718

North A., Chidgey M., Clarke J.P., Bardsley W.G. & Garrod D.R. (1996). Distinct desmocollin isoforms occur in the same desmosomes and show reciprocally graded distributions in bovine nasal epidermis. Proceedings of the Natlional Academy of Sciens, Vol.93, pp. 7701-7705

Ohyama M. (2007). Hair follicle bulge: A fascinating reservoir of epithelial stem cells. Journal of Dermatological Sciences, Vol.46, No.2, pp. 81-89

Pan Q., Shai O., Lee L.J., Frey B.J. & Blencowe B.J. (2008). Deep surveying of alternative splicing complexity in the human transcriptome by high-throughput sequencing. Nature Genetics, Vol. 40, No.12, pp. 1413-1415.

Rajan P., Elliott D.J., Robson C.N. & Leung H.Y. (2009). Alternative splicing and biological heterogeneity in prostate cancer. Nature Reviews Urology, Vol.6, No.8, pp. 454-460

Rohlfs E.M., Puget N., Graham M.L., Weber B.L., Garber J.E., Skrzynia C., Halperin J.L., Lenoir G.M., Silverman L.M. & Mazoyer S. (2000). An Alu-mediated 7.1 kb deletion of BRCA1 exons 8 and 9 in breast and ovarian cancer families that results in alternative splicing of exon 10. Genes, Chromosomes and Cancer, Vol.28, No.3, pp. 300-307

Schäfer S., Stumpp S. & Franke W.W. (1996). Immunological identification and characterization of the desmosomal cadherin Dsg2 in coupled and uncoupled epithelial Wells and In human tissues. Differentiation, Vol.60, No.2, pp. 99-108

Shieh J.J, Liu K.T., Huang S.W., Chen Y.J. & Hsieh T.Y. (2009). Modification of alternative splicing of Mcl-1 pre-mRNA using antisense morpholino oligonucleotides induces apoptosis in basal cell carcinoma cells. Journal of Investigative Dermatology, Vol.129, No.10, pp. 2479-2506

Simpson C.L., Kojima S. & Getsios S. (2010). RNA interference in keratinocytes and an organotypic model of human epidermis. Methods in Molecular Biology, Vol.585, pp. 127-146

Smith C., Zhu K., Merritt A., Picton R., Youngs D., Garrod D. & Chidgey M. (2004). Regulation of desmocollin gene expression in epidermis: CCAAT/enhancer binding proteins modulate early and late events in keratinocyte differentiation. Biochemical Journal, Vol.15, pp. 757-765

Srebrow A. & Kornblihtt A.R. (2006). The connection between splicing and cancer. Journal of Cell Science, Vol.119, pp. 2635-2641

Tada H., Zatoko M., Tanaka A., Kuwahara M. & Muramatsu T. (2000). Expression of desmoglein I and plakoglobin in skin carcinomas. Journal of Cutaneous Pathology, Vol.27, No.1, pp. 24–29

Teh M.T., Blaydon D., Chaplin T., Foot N.J., Skoulakis S., Raghavan M., Harwood C.A., Proby C.M., Philpott M.P., Young B.D. & Kelsell D.P. (2005). Genomewide single nucleotide polymorphism microarray mapping in basal cell carcinomas unveils uniparental disomy as a key somatic event. Cancer Research, Vol. 65, No. 19, pp. 8597-8603

Teh M.T., Parkinson E.K., Thurlow J.K., Liu F., Fortune F. & Wan H. (2011). A molecular study of desmosomes identifies a desmoglein isoform switch in head and neck squamous cell carcinoma. Journal of Oral Pathology and Medicine, Vol.40, No.1, pp. 67–76

Telfer N.R., Colver G.B. & Morton C.A. (2008). Guidelines for the management of basal cell carcinoma. British Journal of Dermatology, Vol.158, No.7, pp. 35-48

Thorsen K., Sorensen K.D., Brems-Eskildsen A.S., Modin C., Gaustadnes M., Hein A.M., Kruhoffer M., Lauberg S., Borre M., Wang K., Brunak S., Krainer A.R., Torring N., Dyrskjot L., Andersen C.L. & Orntoft T.F. (2008). Alternative splicing in colon, bladder, and prostate cancer identified by exon array analysis. Molecular & Cellular Proteomics, Vol. 7, No. 7, pp. 1214-1224

Vantuchová Y. & Čuřík R. (2006). Histological types of basal cell carcinoma. Scripta Medica (BRNO), Vol. 79,pp. 261-270

Venables J.P. (2006). Unbalanced alternative splicing and significance in cancer. BioEssays, Vol.28, pp. 378-386

Wade T,R. & Ackerman A.B. (1978). The many faces of basal cell carcinoma. The Journal of Dermatologic Surgery and Oncology, Vol. 4, pp. 23-28

Wang E.T., Sandeberg R., Luo S., Khrebtukova I., Zhang L., Mayr C., Kingsmore S.F., Schroth G.P. & Burge C.B. (2008). Alternative isoform regulation in human tissue transcriptomes. Nature, Vol.456, No.7221, pp. 470-476

Whittcok N.V. (2003). Genomic sequence analysis of the mouse desmoglein cluster reveals evidence for six distinct genes: characterization of mouse DSG4, DSG5, and DSG6. Journal of Investigative Dermatology, Vol. 120, pp. 970-980

Wong C.S.M, Strange R.C. & Lear J.T. (2003). Basal cell carcinoma. British Medical Journal, Vol.327, No.7418, pp. 794-798

Wu H., Stanley J.R. & Cotsarelis G. (2003). Desmoglein isotype expression in the hair follicle and its cysts correlates with type of keratinization and degree of differentiation. Journal of Investigative Dermatology, Vol.120, pp. 1052-1057

Xing Y. (2007). Genomic analysis of RNA alternative splicing in cancers. Front Biosci, Vol.12, pp. 4034-4041

Youssef K.K., Van Keymeulen A., Lapouge G., Beck B., Michaux C., Achouri Y., Sotiropoulou P.A. & Blanpain C. (2010). Identification of the cell lineage at the origin of basal cell carcinoma. Nature Cell Biology, Vol.12, pp. 299-305

Yu M., Zloty D., Cowan B., Shapiro J., Haegert A., Bell R.H., Warshawski L., Carr N. & McElwee K.J. (2008). Superficial, nodular, and morpheiform basal-cell carcinomas exhibit distinct gene expression profiles. Journal of Investigative Dermatology, Vol.128, No.7, pp. 1797-1805

Zackheim H.S. (1963). Origin of the human basal cell epithelioma. Journal of Investigative Dermatology, Vol.40, pp. 283-297

3

Basal Cell Carcinoma

Yalçın Tüzün, Zekayi Kutlubay, Burhan Engin and Server Serdaroğlu
Istanbul University, Cerrahpaşa Medical Faculty, Department of Dermatology
Turkey

1. Introduction

Basal Cell Carcinoma (BCC) is the most common malignant tumour of the skin. It is also the most common cancer in humans in some countries. BCC is malignant neoplasm derived from nonkeratinizing cells originating in the basal layer of the epidermis. The histology of the tumour and the surrounding stroma is characteristic.

Basal cell carcinoma was first described in 1824 by *Jacob* who called it "*ulcus rodens*"; its current nomenclature was proposed by *Krompecher* in 1903. It is the most common type of nonmelanoma skin cancer (80% of all skin cancers) and most common malignancy in humans. It is delivered from the basal layer of the epidermis or pluripotent bazaloid cells of adnex and almost seen in the areas of sun exposure and hairy parts of the skin. There are many factors in its etiology including genetic predisposition, immune deficiency and chronic sun exposure (Adisen & Gurer, 2007). Recently published studies major on genetic and molecular aspects of the pathogenesis of basal cell carcinoma. Metastasis is rare in BCC and local destruction and disfigurement are much more common (Sikar et al., 2011). BCC usually appears as a flat, firm, pale area that is small, raised, pink or red, translucent, shiny, and waxy, and the area may bleed following minor injury. Tumor size can vary in diameter. Treatment options include electrodesiccation and curettage, surgical excision, cryosurgery, 5-fluorouracil, 5% imiquimod cream, and superficial radiographic therapy. Electrodesiccation and curettage are the most common treatments. Cure rate in these options is approximately 95%.

Nevoid basal cell carcinoma syndrome or *Gorlin-Goltz* syndrome is an autosomal dominant disorder characterized by multiple basal cell carcinoma, multiple keratocystic tumors, and skeletal anomalies (Bader, 2011).

2. Epidemiology

Frequency of BCC has been increasing in many countries around the world. *The American Cancer Society* reports that it is the most common cancer in the *United States*. Approximately 1 million new cases diagnosed in a year and more than 10,000 deaths occur (2% of all cancer deaths). The observed increase in incidence rates may be because of increased detection and skin cancer awareness in health policy. Increased longevity may also affect the increased incidence of BCC; recent data also suggest that incidence is also increasing in the young population.

Because of its high frequency, the disease has been accepted to be a public health issue. Despite low mortality rates and the rare occurrence of metastases, the tumor may be locally invasive and relapse after treatment, causing significant morbidity. In BCC knowledge of risk factors, early diagnosis and treatment is the major point.

BCC incidence varies all around the world. In states near the equator, such as *Hawaii*, BCC incidence is approaching 3-fold more often than that of states in the Midwest, such as *Minnesota* (Bader, 2011). The highest rates of skin cancer occur in *South Africa* and *Australia.* In these areas exposure to UV radiation is in high dose.

Ramani and *Bennett* reported a significantly higher incidence of BCC in *World War 2* servicemen stationed in the *Pacific* theater than in those stationed in *Europe* (Carucci & Leffell, 2008).

BCC is seen in all skin types, but dark-skinned individuals are rarely affected, and more common in fair-skinned individuals (type 1 or type 2 skin types). People who have *Fitzpatrick* type 1 skin are very fair and have red or blond hair and freckles; these individuals always burn and never tan. People who have type 2 skin are fair and burn easily and tan minimally.

Incidence is low in blacks, *Asians*, and *Hispanics* (Machado et al., 1996). Also it was found that approximately 13 million white non-*Hispanics* living in the USA in early 2007 had at least one non-melanoma skin cancer.

Among to gender men are affected twice as women. The higher incidence in men might be because of occupational exposure to the sun.

BCC frequency increases with age. Except of basal cell nevus syndrome, BCC is rarely found in patients younger than 40 years. Approximately 5-15% of cases of BCC occur in patients aged between 20 and 40 years. Aggressive-growth of basal cell carcinoma (AG-BCC) is more frequently noted in patients younger than 35 years than in older individuals. Aggressive-growth of basal cell carcinoma includes morpheaform, infiltrating, and recurrent BCCs (Bader, 2011).

3. Etiology and pathogenesis

Its etiology is still unclear, but both constitutional and environmental factors and genetic predispotion are accused in BCC etiopathogenesis. The most important risk factor for basal cell carcinoma is exposure to UV-radiation (Bauer et al., 2011). Almost all basal cell carcinomas occur on parts of the body excessively exposed to the sun especially the face, ears, neck, scalp, shoulders, and back. Outdoor workers with a long history of work-related UV-exposure are at increased risk of developing BCC. Other risk factors include light skin phototypes, advanced age, family history of skin carcinoma, light-coloured eyes and blond hair, freckles in childhood and immunosuppression. Behavioral aspects such as occupational sun exposure, rural labor and sunburns at a young age also play a role (Bader, 2011). CYLD is a deubiquitination enzyme that regulates different cellular processes, such as cell proliferation and cell survival. Mutation and loss of heterozygosity of the CYLD gene causes development of cylindromatosis, a benign tumour originating from the skin. *Kuphal* et al. suggested that suppression of CYLD has a significant role in basal cell carcinoma progression (Kuphal et al., 2011).

Between 30% and 75% of the sporadic cases are associated with patched hedgehog gene (PTCH) which is a tumor suppressor gene located in the 9q22 (PTCH1) and 1p32 (PTCH2) location. This gene is almost with all cases associated with basal cell nevus syndrome. Other genetic changes are also described like experiments with activation of the hedgehog signaling pathway in different compartments of the epidermis and on the expression of cytokeratins 5, 14, 15, 17 and 19 with a follicular pattern, which has defined it as a malignant neoplasm of follicular germinative cells (trichoblasts) (Chinem, 2011; Youssef, et al., 2010).

Furthermore, there is an association of BCC with abnormalities of the sonic hedgehog gene (Donovan, 2009). This hypothesis is further strengthened by the rarity of palmoplantar and mucosal lesions, where no hair follicles are found (Betti, 2005; Orsini 2001). *Baskurt* et al. have reported two brothers who have albinism and synchronous developed BCC on their trunk region. That means development of the same malignancy in the same life period at the similar localizations reminds the importance of genetic predisposition (Baskurt, 2011).
BCC can rarely develop on unexposed areas. In some case reports, BCC of the prostate has been reported. Contact with arsenic, tar, coal, paraffin, certain types of industrial oil, and radiation are some factors playing role in BCC etiology (Kwasniak & Zuazaga 2011).
BCC can also be associated with scars (eg, burn complications), xeroderma pigmentosum, previous trauma, vaccinations, or even tattoos (Bader, 2011).
Lee et al. published a case report about expression of RUNX3 (Runt-related transcription factor 3) in skin cancers. They found that higher expression of RUNX3 is seen in several cancers, including basal cell carcinoma. Expression of RUNX3 is reduced in a large number of cancers. As a result they suggest that RUNX3 has an oncogenic potential and does not act as a tumour suppressor in skin cancers (Lee et al., 2011).
Activation of Gli-1 factor, induces the transcription of several oncogenes involved in the development of BCC and other malignancies. An other gene in BCC etiology is SMO gene which is a protein located in the membrane - smoothened -expressed by the SMO gene. *Chinem* et al. reported that mutations in the SMO gene are present in 10-21% of sporadic BCCs and mutations in the p53 gene are present in more than 50% of cases, although the p53 gene is more related to the progression than the origin of BCC (Chinem & Miot, 2011).
Fernandez –Flores reported a case about D2-40 immunoexpression in BCC etiology. They suggested that this immunoexpression was a prognostic connotation in carcinomas of organs other than the skin. In their case rapid grown had been seen over the last few months (Fernandez –Flores, 2011).
Involvement of the trunk and development of multiple BCCs were related to genetic polymorphisms in glutathione S-transferase, NADPH and cytochrome P-450. Also trisomy of chromosome 6 was linked to increased aggressiveness of BCC (Chinem & Miot, 2011).
Kwasniak et al. reported that BCC is one of the cancers most strongly associated with the atomic bombing in Japan. It is reported that residents of *Nagasaki* who were not exposed to atomic bomb radiation, the incidence of BCC was 3.1 per 100,000 while the survivors incidence was 9.4 per 100,000 people per year (Kwasniak & Zuazaga 2011).
Tang et al. reported in their study that topical vitamin D3 treatment of existing murine BCC tumors significantly decreases Gli-1 and Ki-67 staining. Thus, vitamin D3 acting via its *Hedgehog* inhibiting effect may hold promise as an effective anti-BCC agent (Tang et al., 2011).

4. Clinical manifestations

Basal cell carcinoma patients often present with a slowly growing, nonhealing sore of varying duration. The lesions are typically seen on the face (Figure 1), ears (Figure 2), scalp, neck, or upper trunk. Mild trauma initially may cause bleeding. A history of chronic sun exposure is commonly elicited. The early tumours are commonly small, translucent or pearly, raised and rounded areas located on a few dilated, superficial vessels. There are six subtypes of BCC that include nodular, superficial, pigmented, morpheaform, cystic and fibroepithelioma of *Pinkus*.

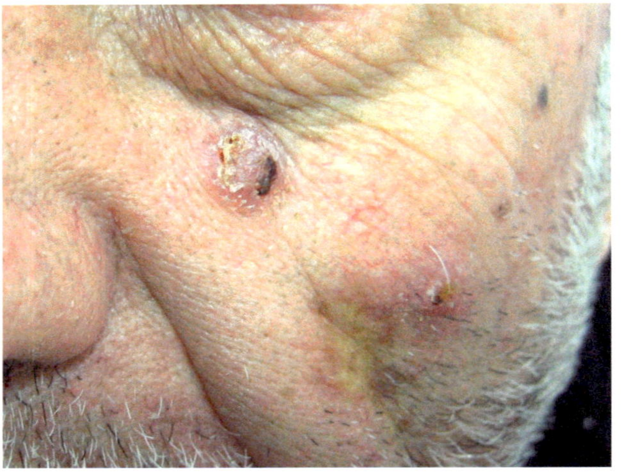

Fig. 1. Basal cell carcinoma as nonhealing sore on face.

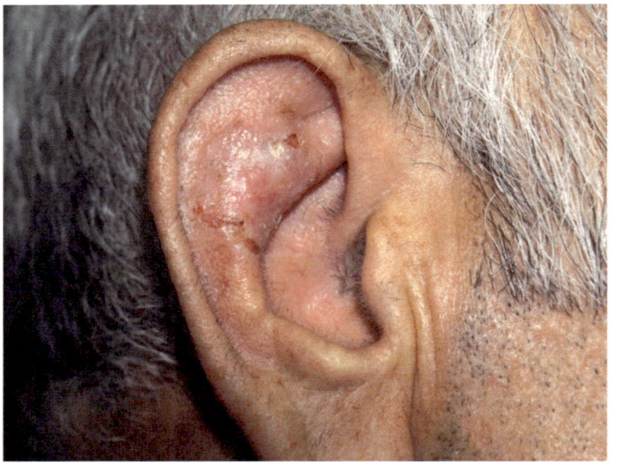

Fig. 2. Superficial spreading basal cell carcinoma located on ears.

4.1 Nodular Basal Cell Carcinoma

Nodular BCC is the most common subtype, accounting for more than 60% of all tumors. Lesions are clinically found on the head and neck regions. BCC can also be seen in sun-protected areas. The nodular form of BCC appears as red or pink papules with raised, rolled borders that slowly enlarge (Figure 3 & 4). Red papules have a pearly or waxy appearance and telengiectasias are seen. On the microscopic examination; BCC is composed of well-defined, smooth-bordered basophilic staining islands of neoplastic cells. Melanin pigmentation of tumor cells and adjacent stromal histiocytes may be seen. Mitoses and individual cell necrosis are uncommon. The surrounding stroma showing myxoid change, is rarely fibrotic and may show calcification in discrete islands of tumour or in adjacent stroma. This subtype of BCC grows slowly; however if left untreated for enough time, it can invade structures and increase morbidity (Miller, 2008; Nouri, 2007 & Schwartz, 2008).

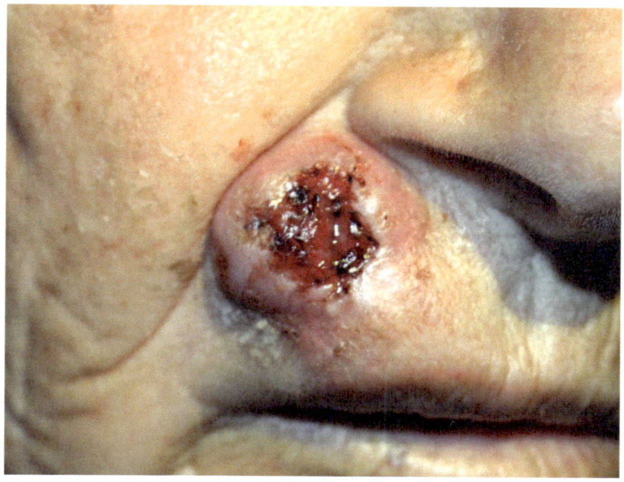

Fig. 3. Rodent ulcer type of basal cell carcinoma

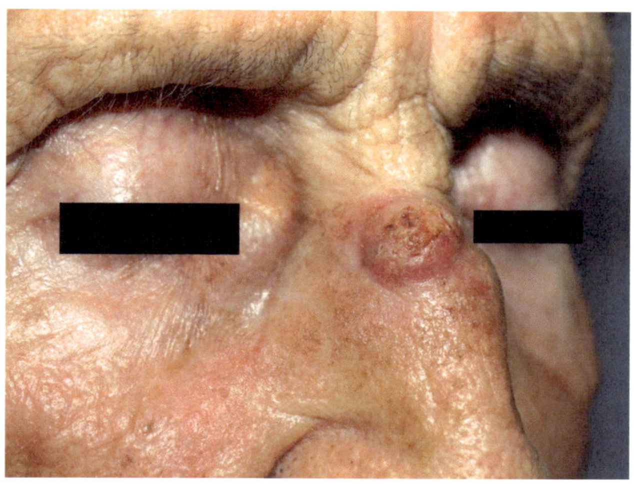

Fig. 4. Nodular type of basal cell carcinoma.

According to some authors multinodular BCC is accepted as an another subtype of BCC. It manifests a plaque-like indurated lesion with poorly demarcated contour. Lesions may be difficult to remove and so have an increased incidence of recurrence. In the pool data, subjects with a micronodular BCC had a mean age comparable with subjects with a superficial BCC but were younger than subjects with nodular or an infiltrative BCC (Betti et al., 2010).

In one study, it was found that nodular BCC is associated with increased hyluronan homeostasis, when compared with normal skin. Also chondroitin sulphate were significantly higher, whereas dermatan sulphate was significantly lower in BCC when compared with normal skin. There may be a relationship between the proliferative activity of tumour cells and the stromal occurrence of hyaluronan and that this proliferative activity differed in the various types of BCC (Tzellos et al., 2010).

4.2 Pigmented Basal Cell Carcinoma

This form of BCC consists of a brown, black, or gray blue color that can present on the head, neck, trunk or extremities. It appears as a hyperpigmented, translucent papule, which may also be eroded (Figure 5). These are usually extremely slow in evolving. This type is seen more frequently in dark-complexioned people such as *Latin Americans* or *Japanese*. Pigmented type constitutes approximately 6% of all BCC. Pigmented nevi, melanoma, pigmented *Bowen*'s disease are the most frequent clinical differential diagnosis for such lesions. Pigmented BCC shows similar histologic features with nodular type but there are large amounts of melanin. In dermoscopy; maple leaf like areas, spoke-wheel areas, large, blue-gray ovoid nests, multipl blue-gray globules, arborizing (tree-like) telangiectasia and ulceration may be seen (Carucci, 2008; Odom, 2000 & Menzies 2002).

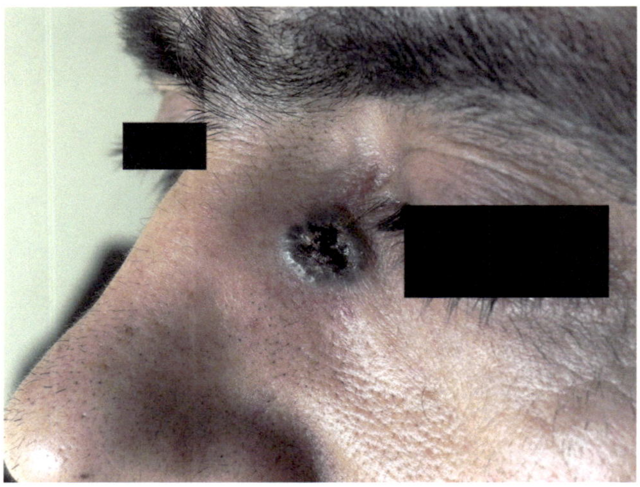

Fig. 5. Hyperpigmented nodular basal cell carcinoma

4.3 Superficial Basal Cell Carcinoma

This subtype is the second common one and seen mostly on the trunk and extremities. Lesions are clinically flat, red to pink, scaly patches with ulcerations and crusting. The borders can be elevated or rolled. This thin threadlike border facilitates distinction from a plaque of *Bowen*'s disease or of psoriasis. It also presents at younger age than nodular type (average age is 57.5 vs 65.5 years). Superficial BCC usually do not extend into the deep dermis, and a nonspecific inflammatory infiltrate may be seen in the papillary dermis. They usually grow laterally, and can reach unstantial sizes. Horizontal growth allows these tumours to extend significantly beyond the clinical borders (Figure 6)..

Superficial BCC is characterized microscopically by buds of malignant cells extending into the dermis from the basal layer of the epidermis. The peripheral cell layer shows palisading. Tumour cells may colonize the hair follicle and rarely the ecrine adnexal structures. Mitoses are infrequent, and apoptotic cells are rare in the atypical basaloid buds. When seen in the setting of a biopsy for suspect superficial BCC, a band-like lymphoid infiltrate should prompt a careful search through multipl levels looking for foci of superficial BCC (Nouri, 2007; Schwartz, 2008 & Tzellos 2010).

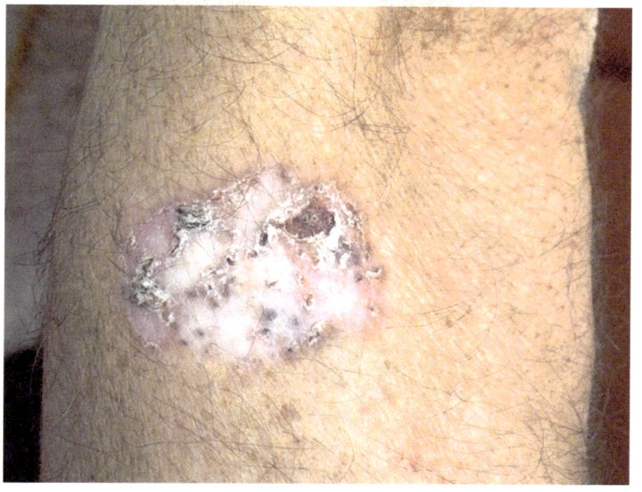

Fig. 6. Slightly elevated borders of superficial type of basal cell carcinoma.

In dermoscopy; according to a study, shiny white to red areas were seen in 100% of the lesions, while approximately 86% revealed short fine telangiectasias; they also described small surface ulcerations or erosions in about 78% of the lesions. Other dermoscopic criteria, such as leaf-like areas, arborizing telangiectasias, blue-gray globules, and large blue-gray ovoid nests, are not strongly associated with the diagnosis of superficial BCC (Scalvenzi et al., 2008).

4.4 Morpheaform Basal Cell Carcinoma

This type of BCC demonstrates waxy white sclerotic plaques occuring in the head and neck region, with a conspicious absence of a rolled edge. The exact margin of the lesion is impossible to define, but palpation reveals a firm skin texture that extends irregularly beyond the visible changes. Ulceration and crusting are also absent, whereas telangiectasia is prominent. The surface is smooth and may be slightly depressed below the normal level. The colour is yellowish, pink or white and may appear as a smooth shiny scar. These lesions are reported to be more frequent on the face in women and may be associated with smoking. The morpheaform BCC tends to develop at a younger age compared with other types, sometimes during adolescence. These lesions are usually misdiagnosed, leading to greater tumour growth and delayed treatment. This is an aggressive growth variant of BCC (Mackie, 2004; Nouri, 2007; Schwartz, 2008 & Tzellos 2010).

In histopathology; there is a fibrotic dermis that contains small, linear, and branching collections of basal cells. Morpheaform BCC islands typically are not well circumscribed and do not demonstrate prominent peripheral palisading of nuclei. Individual cell necrosis and mitotic activity are brisk considering the relative tumor volume and the neoplasms themselves are poorly demarcated, showing widespread invasion of the reticular dermis and penetration into the subcutaneus tissue (Nouri, 2007 & Tzellos 2010).

4.5 Cystic Basal Cell Carcinoma

This type of BCC is uncommon. It is usually seen around the eyes. This tumour shows differentiation towards the hair follicle infundibulum. A sebaceous component is usually absent. It may appear as a blue-gray cystic nodule suggestive of an apocrine hidrocystoma. It has two subtypes. One is small cyst of light blue-gray coloration; other one is variable in size and may be quite large. Both subtypes are interfere with benign cutaneous cysts. It can not be clinically separated from hidrocystoma, as it too has a broad base, fine telangiectasias and a blue tint. Any cyst or inflammatory lesion of the eyelid which does not resolve within a reasonable period should be examined histologically (Braun-Falco, 2000; Nouri, 2007 & Tzellos 2010).

4.6 Fibroepithelioma of Pinkus

This type of BCC was first described by *Pinkus* in 1953. This is an uncommon variant of BCC. Fibroepitheliomas are usually soft pink or flesh-colored nodules or plaques on the trunk, especially the lumbosacral region. They are extremely rare on sunlight-exposed sites and do not ulcerate but erosions may be seen. They may be broad-based flat plaques or pedunculated, tending to be smooth surfaced with a pink or reddish colorationn, and characteristically appear on the lower back. They may be pigmented. They may follow many years after local X-ray therapy.

Histopathologic findings include lacy strands of basaloid cells extending into a fibrous stroma. Some authors regard the fibroepithelioma as a form of fenestrated trichoblastoma, a lesion held to be a benign analogue of BCC that shares many morphological features of BCC but has not to date been shown to manifest PTCH mutations and dominantly affects sun-protected skin (Braun-Falco, 2000; Nouri, 2007 & Repertinger, 2008).

There are other rare clinical types of BCC. These are wild-fire BCC, giant-pore BCC, angiomatous BCC, lipoma-like BCC, and metatypical BCC. In wild-fire type; plaques expands rapidly with crusting, ulceration, and scarring. The giant pore BCC appears on the face as a 2-10 mm orifice, usually skin colored. It could represent a localized follicular abnormality. The angiomatous BCC is bluish or violaceous nodule with a somewhat cystic quality and is exceedingly rare. The lipoma-like BCC displays a remarkable clinical resemblance to the lipoma. Metatypical BCC is very rare and may simply be a subset of BCC that is radiation-resistant. They tend to be large aggressive tumors that usually have been unsuccessfully irradiated. They are seen on the back and nose (Braun-Falco, 2000; Hakverdi, 2011 & Ting, 2005).

5. Biological behavior

5.1 Local Invasion

Local invasion is the most important problem of BCC (Carucci, 2008 & Schwartz, 2008). It grows in a "silent" way into immediately adjacent tissue (Figure 7). It rarely metastasizes. The doubling time is between 6 months and 1 year. There may be irregular intrusions into certain tissues: dermis, fascial planes, periosteum, perichondrium, embryonic fusion planes and nerve sheath (Carucci, 2008). Tumor progression is slow in anatomic fusion planes. BCC located in embryonic fusion planes, periauricular region, tends to be at high risk of deep extension. It has been shown that the highest risk tumors which exhibit extensive subclinical spread are basosquamous and morpheaform BCC found on nose and morpheaform BCC on cheek and those with a preoperative size greater than 25 mm (Batra, 2002 & Schwartz, 2008). The tendency of BCC to spread into the dermis is understandable, because it develops immediately beneath the epidermis. Intradermal invasion may be clinically inapparent and moreover may prove quite asymmetrical, being several times larger on side of BCC than on the other. Inapparent extensions often result in tumor recurrence after removal (Schwartz, 2008).

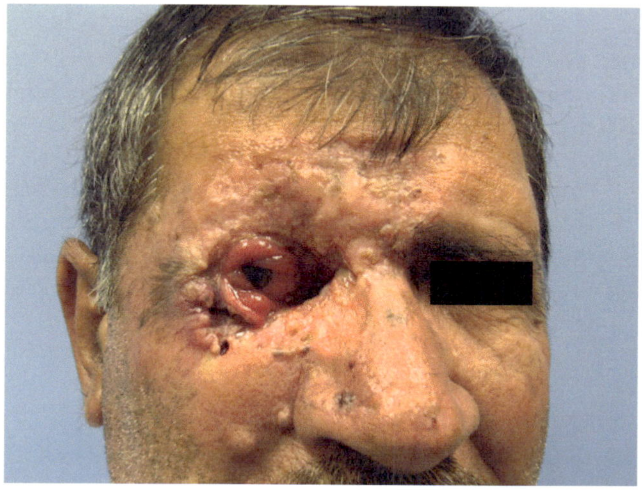

Fig. 7. Advanced and invazive basal cell carcinoma of the right periorbital region.

When BCC penetrates the dermis, additional expansion patterns may ocur (Schwartz, 2008). The biological behavior of the micronodular, infiltrating and sclerosing (morpheaform) variants of BCC are known to be more aggressive than that of the nodular and superficial forms. These three "agressive growth" subtypes are characterized by an infiltrative growth pattern that has poor circumscription (Miller, 2008).

BCC may spread along perichondrium of the nose or ear as the cutaneous and subcutaneous tissues are so thin there. The cartilage of the nose is quite irregular, small pockets of tumor spread in auricular and periauricular region appear to correspond to embryonic fusion planes (Schwartz, 2008).

Stromal reaction tends to be sclerotic rather than fibroblastic or myxoid. The attraction of BCC for connective tissue is well recognized but not well understood. This stromal dependency is one of the basic characteristics of BCC (Miller, 2008).

5.2 Perineural invasion

The reported rate of perineural spread in all BCC is between 0.18% and 3%, and is present more often in deep specimens (Walling et al., 2004). Perineural invasion is more common in the aggressive subtypes of BCC (micronodular, infiltrating and sclerosing variants) (Brown & Perry, 2000).

What is the true incidence of perineural invasion among skin carcinomas? Considering large published series that encompass all 'ordinary' BCCs, it seems rather uncommon, oscillating from 0.19% to 0.49% . Some authors reported an increased frequency of 3.8% in cancers treated by *Mohs'* micrographic surgery (Cernea et al., 2009).

The cancer may extend cylindrically, several cells thick, around the nevre beneath the perineurum (Schwartz, 2008). The low resistance cleavage plane of the perineural sheath may allow rapid and broad tumor extension. 'Skip' areas along nerves are also common, and spread may be proximal or distal along fibers (Walling et al., 2004).

Diagnosis of perineural involvement in many cases requires micrographic analysis, as patients frequently exhibit no neurological symptoms. Those who do demonstrate sensory or motor findings, however, are at particularly high risk of a poor outcome (Walling et al., 2004).

Neurotrophic factors that influence the interaction between cancer cells and nerves are suspected. p75NGFR immunostaining increased detection of perineural invasion compared with H&E. p75NGFR could serve as an alternative to S-100 in the detection of perineural invasion, or as part of an immunostaining panel for perineural invasion detection (Lewis et al., 2006). Usually, however, perineural spread is less extreme but may produce a neuropathy. Rarely, the neuropathy may be the presenting sign of a recurrent skin cancer, with no cutaneous tumor evident (Morris & Joffe, 1983). Involvement of the trigeminal nerve may produce pain; involvement of the facial nerve may cause facial muscle weakness (Schwartz, 2008).

5.3 Metastasis

Despite the large number of primary BCCs diagnosed each year, the rate of metastatic BCC (MBCC) ranges from 0.0028% to 0.5% (Malone et al., 2000 & Soleymani et al., 2008). Since MBCC was first reported in 1894 by *Beadles*, there have been more than 240 cases reported in the literature. Of these cases, 66–85% of MBCCs arise from primary lesions in the head and neck region (Soleymani et al., 2008 & Ting et al., 2005).

The primary tumor must originate from the skin and not the mucosa, metastasis must occur at a site distant from the primary tumor without evidence of direct extension, and the primary and metastatic tumors must have similar histopathology. These are the criteria needed for the true diagnosis of MBCC (Soleymani et al., 2008). Metastases occur in males and females in a 2:1 ratio, most often involving dissemination to regional lymph nodes and hematogenous spread to lungs, bone, and skin (Ting et al., 2005).

Risk factors associated with the rare occurrence of metastasis include tumor size of less than 2cm, multiple primary tumors in the region of the head and neck, significant tumor depth, fair skin, middle age, and male gender (Ozgediz et al., 2008). Mean survival for patients with metastatic disease is 8 months (Snow et al., 1994), although those with spread limited to the lymph nodes alone have an average survival of up to 3.6 years (Soleymani et al., 2008).

There is no consensus as to whether any one histologic subtype of the primary tumor predisposes to MBCC. Nodular, micronodular, morpheaform, metatypical or basosquamous, and infiltrative histologies have all been reported (Soleymani et al., 2008).

In a retrospective review of 5270 morpheaform or invasive BCCs over a 50-year period did not reveal an increased rate of metastasis compared to other histologic subtypes (Soleymani et al., 2008). It is very difficult to predict the metastatic potentiality of BCCs by histopathology (Kinoshita et al., 2005). In a case report it was shown that the tumor cells were bcl-2 negative and positive for Ber-EP4. The negative expression of bcl-2 correlates with the aggressive nature of this tumor and Ber-EP4 confirms the diagnosis of BCC (Richard et al., 2010).

In a literature search of cases of black patients with metastatic BCC revealed eight cases. In these cases, the most obvious common predisposing factor seems to be large lesion size, with all of the cases having at least one dimension greater than 5 cm (Saladi et al., 2004).

6. Diagnosis

Diagnosis of BCC is accomplished by accurate interpretation of the skin biopsy results (Carucci, 2008). It should be remembered that the diagnosis of any cancer is always a histologic one; clinical acumen cannot replace histologic documentation (Schwartz, 2008).
The tumor growth pattern is importatnt information that is impossible to determine if only a superficial fragment is submitted to the laboratory. Deep shave, punch, incisional or excisional biopsy can all give sufficient dermis for the evaluation.
A number of non-invasive imaging technologies are being investigated to delineate tumor depth and extent preoperatively and thus guide treatment. Confocal microscopy, infrared spectroscopy and ultrasound are some of them but for the moment they remain experimental.
If a BCC may have been neglected and reached a size such that direct bony invasion occurred a preoperative CT scan should be considered.
Dermoscopy is a noninvasively method that has been reported to be a useful tool for the early and accurate recognition of pigmented lesions of the skin . However, nodular lesions can lack specific dermoscopic criteria being completely or partially featureless in their appearance. Reflectance confocal microscopy (RCM) is an emerging noninvasive diagnostic tool that provides *in vivo* tissue images at nearly cellular histological resolution. In a study four patients with nodular lesions have been examined clinically and dermoscopically equivocal a RCM examination allowed for a rapid and accurate prebiopsy diagnosis (Carucci, 2008 & Schwartz, 2008).

7. Differential diagnosis

A lot of benign appendageal tumors may cause confusion, as may rare malignant appendageal cancers, SCCs, atypical fibroxanthomas, melanocytic nevi, Merkel cell carcinoma and rarely melanoma. A hemispheric nodule clinically indistinguishable from a BCC may be a trichoepithelioma, a benign appendageal tumor. A small yellowish papule with a central dell may be confused with an early BCC; sebaceous hyperplasia is quite common and often displays telangiectasia, additionally reminiscent of the BCC.
Granulomatous lesions may need a distinction from BCC, examples of which include tuberculosis; syphilis; deep fungal infections. Other types of BCC besides the noduloulcerative type expand the list of differential diagnoses. Sclerosing-type BCCs may be mistaken for scars or small plaques of localized scleroderma (morphea) (Table 1) (Schwartz, 2008).

8. Histopathology

BCC have in common proliferations of basaloid keratinocytes in various configurations with a variable fibromyxoid stroma. Epidermal origin is usually evident and an inflammatory infiltrate is variably present (Miller, 2008).
Under the microscope, BCC appears as irregular dermal masses of variable sizes and shapes, surrounded by a layer of peripheral tumor cells with palisading nuclei. The individual tumor cells are usually rather uniform in appearance and lack atypia .When nuclear atypia and multiple mitotic figures are rarely present, this does not alter the clinical course of these BCCs (Schwartz, 2008).

- Nodular basal cell carcinoma:
    - Squamous cell carcinoma
    - Seborrheic keratosis
    - Intradermal nevus
    - Sebaceous hyperplasia
    - Fibrous papule
    - Molluscum contagiosum
    - Keratoacanthoma
    - Scar tissue
- Superficial basal cell carcinoma:
    - Discoid eczema
    - Psoriasis
    - Actinic keratosis (solar keratosis)
    - *Bowen*'s disease
    - Squamous cell carcinoma
    - Seborrhoeic keratosis
- Pigmented basal cell carcinoma:
    - Melanoma
    - Lentigo maligna melanoma
    - Appendegeal tumor
    - Compound nevus
    - Blue nevus
- Morphoeic basal cell carcinoma:
    - Scar tissue
    - Localised scleroderma
    - Trichoepithelioma
- Fibroepihtelioma of *Pinkus*:
    - Skin tag
    - Papillomatous dermal nevus
    - Fibroma

Table 1. Differential diagnosis according to the types of basal cell carcinoma (Carucci, 2008).

Traditionally, BCCs have been classified as solid (or undifferentiated) vs those tumors that manifest specific differentiation features (ie to eccrine, sebaceous or other cell lines). However, the only proven histologic prognosticator of biologic behavior, and therefore a major determinant of what constitutes an appropriate therapeutic approach, is the architectural growth pattern (Crowson, 2006).

The nuclei in basal cell carcinoma as a rule have a rather uniform, nonanaplastic appearance. They usually show no variation in size or intensity of staining and no abnormal mitoses, even in the rare instances of BCC with metastases (Kirkham & Elder 2005). Cellular borders are indistinct and desmosomes are inapparent. Apoptotic cells are common. The fibromyxoid stroma is intimately associated with the tumor islands, often showing increased cellularity (Miller, 2008).

8.1 Special types of histological patterns include

1. Keratotic BCC with parakeratotic stratum corneum
2. Sebaceous differentiation of the sebaceous epithelioma (also called BCC with sebaceous differentiation, a possible marker for *Muir-Torre* Syndrome of multiple sebaceous neoplasms, keratoacanthomas, and multiple low-grade visceral malignancies)
3. Adenoid histologic-type BCC, with its lace-like pattern of interconnected tumor strands, producing a glandlike structure
4. Sclerosing BCC with abundant dense stroma with multiple islands of compressed tumor cells
5. Pigmented BCC with histologic evidence of melanocytes with large amounts of melanin
6. Superficial-type BCC with superficial tumor buds that appear to originate at multiple foci from the overlying attached epidermis
7. Fibroepithelioma, with its long, thin anastomosing tumor cell strands
8. Granular cell–type BCC
9. Signet-ring–type BCC
10. Clear cell–type BCC
11. Cystic BCC, which may mimic other cysts, including inclusion cysts due to penetrating injury, mucoceles, apocrine hidrocystoma, and necrotic metastatic tumors
12. BCC with eccrine differentiation
13. MTC with tumor lobules more irregular and peripheral palisading less pronounced but focally present. Stromal proliferation is more prominent.

Areas of typical BCC may be seen to merge into a metatypical region. The most important histologic finding that confirms the metatypical carcinoma (MTC) diagnosis is the absence of a transition zone between the basal cell and squamous cell types. This is the reason why MTC is not a collision between a BCC and a SCC (Kirkham & Elder 2005; Schwartz, 2008).

8.2 Nodular Basal Cell Carcinoma

The nodular form of BCC is characterized by discrete large or small nests of basaloid cells in either the papillary or reticular dermis accompanied by slit-like retraction from a stroma in which the fibroblasts do not appear to be plump or proplastic . Any of the differentiated elements (eccrine, sebaceous, etc) may be seen in nodular tumors and roughly one-third of cases will show a coexistent superficial component.

The surrounding stroma shows myxoid change, is rarely fibrotic and may show calcification in discrete islands of tumor or in adjacent stroma. Mitoses and individual cell necrosis are uncommon. The presence of abundant slit-like retraction may cause tumor nests to drop out from the stroma during processing yielding empty spaces with a rounded contour in the mid or deep dermis. This is an important clue to the diagnosis in the setting of the nodular and/or infiltrative growth patterns. A significant proportion of BCCs with a nodular component manifests a variable admixture of superficial and/or micronodular morphologies. Melanin pigmentation of tumor cells and adjacent stromal histiocytes may be seen (Crowson, 2006).

In larger tumor islands, central areas of necrosis may develop, leading to the formation of cystic spaces. True cystic or nodulocystic BCCs form on the basis of mucin pools within tumors (Miller, 2008).

8.3 Micronodular Basal Cell Carcinoma

Micronodular BCC manifests a plaque-like indurated lesion with a poorly demarcated contour. They are composed of smaller tumor islands than those of nodular BCC. The cellular features are similar (Miller, 2008). The micronodular BCC has been reported to have a higher incidence of local recurrence and may penetrate more deeply into the reticular dermis and/or subcutis (Crowson, 2006).

8.4 Infiltrative growth Basal Cell Carcinoma

Infiltrating BCC is poorly circumscribed with jagged, irregular contours and tumor strands which may invade beyond the dermis. Peripheral palisading is absent, inflammation is minimal, and the surrounding stroma is often fibrous. There is evidence that many of these multifocal buds connect in a net-like pattern, so most are not truly multifocal (Miller, 2008). Infiltrative tumors, in particular, have been found to have a relatively higher growth fraction as ascertained by Ki-67 immunohistochemistry (Walling et al., 2004).

8.5 Keratotic Basal Cell Carcinoma

Also known as pilar BCC as it appears to differentiate along pilosebaceous lines, the keratotic BCC manifests large basaloid tumor nests that are rounded and show central keratinization and degeneration. The central cysts typically lack a granular cell layer and are filled with keratin and parakeratotic debris; a granular cell layer is present in some cases and the cysts may show central calcification surrounded by the basaloid tumor cells.True hair production is absent (Crowson, 2006). Infundibulocystic BCC may appear similar but usually has a more anastomosing pattern of tumor nets (Miller, 2008). Keratotic BCC shares with trichoepithelioma the presence of horn cysts, and it is sometimes difficult to decide whether a lesion represents a keratotic BCC or a trichoepithelioma (Kirkham & Elder 2005).

8.6 Morpheaform Basal Cell Carcinoma

Morpheaform or sclerosing BCC is characterized by columns of basaloid cells one to two cells thick enmeshed in a densely collagenized stroma containing proplastic fibroblasts (Crowson, 2006). A peripheral palisaded pattern of tumor cells is absent and stromal retraction is also frequently not evident (Miller, 2008 ; Walling et al., 2004). Individual cell necrosis and mitotic activity considering the relative tumor volume and the neoplasms themselves are poorly demarcated, showing widespread invasion of the reticular dermis and penetration into the subcutaneous tissue (Crowson, 2006). Morpheaform BCC has been associated with greater subclinical depth of extension , and morpheaform and infiltrating BCC are associated with a greater rate of recurrence (Walling et al., 2004).

8.7 Fibroepithelioma of Pinkus

Described by Pinkus in 1953 the fibroepithelioma typically arises above the natal cleft or on the lower trunk as a pink or flesh colored nodule with a constricted inferior margin suggesting a seborrheic keratosis. In this tumor, elongated basaloid epithelial strands manifesting slit-like retraction from stroma are enmeshed in a myxoid matrix or a background of proliferating spindle cells with abundant collagen (Crowson, 2006 & Miller, 2008). Peripheral palisading is less prominent, as is peritumoral retraction.

Only rarely will one find areas of the tumor with more classic findings for BCC. Some consider fibroepithelioma as a benign tumor while others view it as very low-grade of BCC (Braun-Falco et al., 2000). In differential diagnosis ecrine syringofibroadenoma and reticulated seborrheic keratosis should be considered (Miller, 2008).

8.8 Subtypes according to histopathological growth pattern and potential for aggression

Less aggressive

- Superficial
- Nodular

More aggressive

- Infiltrative
- Micronodular
- Morphoeic

Other types (uncommon)

- Basosquamous (metatypical) - BCC with squamous differentiation. Probably more aggressive with a greater chance of metastasis than other forms of BCC.
- Adenoid
- Cystic
- Pigmented
- Cornifying/keratotic
- Fibroepithelioma
- Follicular/infundibulocystic

9. Treatment

For basal cell carcinoma, the goal of treatment is elimination of the tumor with maximal preservation of function and physical appearance according to the 2011 National Comprehensive Cancer Network (NCCN) clinical practice guidelines in oncology. As such, treatment decisions should be individualized according to the patient's particular risk factors and preferences. Evaluating all of the cases, the recommended treatment modality for basal cell carcinoma is surgery. Treatments vary according to cancer size, depth, and location on the body. Dermatologists may perform nearly all of the therapeutic options in an outpatient setting. Most therapies are well established and widely applied; nevertheless, researchers are studying some additional options (photodynamic therapy with photosensitizers etc and awaiting further reports.

Local therapy with chemotherapeutic and immune-modulating agents is useful in some cases of BCC. In particular, small and superficial BCC may respond to these compounds. Topical 5% imiquimod is approved by the US Food and Drug Administration (FDA) for the treatment of nonfacial superficial BCCs that are less than 2 cm in diameter. Likewise, topical fluorouracil is approved by the FDA for the treatment of superficial BCC. Both imiquimod and fluorouracil may be used topically for prophylaxis or maintenance in patients who are prone to having many BCCs.

For tumors that are more difficult to treat (infiltrative, morpheaform, micronodular, and recurrent BCCs) or those in which sparing normal (noncancerous) tissue is paramount, *Mohs* micrographic surgery should be preferred.

For metastatic BCC, the 2011 NCCN guideline recommends clinical trials of systemic chemotherapy, particularly platinum-based combination therapy. Clinical trials of investigational biologic modifiers such as hedgehog pathway inhibitors are also recommended (Bader, 2011).

9.1 Mohs Micrographic Surgery

Mohs micrographic surgery (MMS) is a procedure based on the principles of microscopic margin control and tissue sparing (Alam et al., 2010). *Mohs* micrographic surgery was first reported in 1941 by *Mohs* (Samarasinghe et al., 2011). At first the tumor tissue is removed at an angle of about 45°, and then tumor tissue is instantly frozen and cut horizontally from the base to the surface, and all margins, especially lateral and basal margins, examined histologically whether tumor cells are still present or not. If the tumor cells detected, additional excisions are performed until all the tumor tissue has been disappeared (Wetzig et al., 2009). This method almost requires local anesthesia (Telfer et al., 2008).
This specialized surgical procedure is commonly used in a patient with large (> 2 cm) tumors, high-risk morphea-type BCC tumors, recurrent tumors, or tumors located in cosmetically sensitive locations (Ceilley Del & Rosso, 2006). There are three important matter for compliance with the method of *Mohs* micrographic surgery for BCCs: i) location and size, ii) histology, iii) pre-treatment preferences. If BCC lesion is located on the head and neck, if some of the histological types are present (shown in Table 2) and if the lesion is previously untreated, MMS is preferable. The most common indication for MMS is BCC located on the head and neck. Because these sites of the body are the most cosmetically sensitive regions and also recurrence risk is considerably high. BCC lesions in some parts of the body such as eyelids, lips, ears, nose, H-zone, genitalia, fingers and toes are generally treated by *Mohs* micrographic surgery (Wood & Ammirati, 2011). Aggressive histological subtypes of BCC include metatypical, morpheaform, micronodular, and infiltrative have a higher risk for recurrence, for this reason MMS is recommended in the treatment of these lesions with this certain histology (Cumberland, 2009). The indications for Mohs micrographic surgery are shown in Table 3 (Telfer et al., 2008).
Most of the methods of treatment except MMS do not include microscopic evaluation of tumor margins, such as curettage and desiccation, cryosurgery, radiation therapy and topical chemotherapy (Cumberland, 2009). The advantages over other surgical procedures this surgical procedure enables for greater tissue conservation and margin control (Ceilley Del & Rosso, 2006). *Muller* and his colleagues have shown that MMS is more tissue sparing compared to surgical excision (Muller et al., 2009). Also the 5- year recurrence rate is approximately 1% and 6-10% for primary BCC and recurrent BCC, respectively (Ho & Byrne, 2009). In another study conducted in recent years, very low recurrence rates and excellent cure rates have been reported in both primary and recurrent BCC by *Wetzig* et al (Wetzig et al., 2010).

- BCC with poorly defined clinical margins
- Syndromic multiple BCCs
- Large and deeply penetrating BCC
- Basosquamous (metatypical) BCC
- Morphea-form, sclerotic, micronodular, infiltrative, recurrent BCC
- BCCs with local invasion (perichondral, perivascular, periosteal, and perineural invasions)
- Superficial multicentric BCC
- BCC arising within a scar
- BCC within an existing lesion

Table 2. MMS is preferred in the treatment of some specialized subtypes (Wood & Ammirati, 2011).

In recent years, high-resolution ultrasound has been used for some tumoral lesions before Mohs micrographic surgery and is indicated for small lesions of BCC (Marmur et al., 2010). It is a non-invasive technique and it can detect how deep tumors spread into the skin (Wood & Ammirati, 2011).

Also in recent years immunostaining techniques have been used to detect tumor cells when histological features are nonspecific or is masked histologically by dense inflammation. Sometimes immunostaining can increase the efficacy of the margins evaluation but it is very expensive (Cumberland, 2009).

Complications of Mohs micrographic surgery include postoperative bleeding, scarring, wound infection, flap or graft necrosis (Samarasinghe et al., 2011).

- Tumor site cosmetically sensitive locations (especially central face, around the eyes, nose, lips and ears)
- Undefined tumor margins
- Tumor size (any size, but mainly > 2 cm)
- Histological subtype (especially morpheaform, infiltrative, micronodular and basosquamous subtypes)
- Recurrent lesions
- Local invasions (perineural or perivascular involvement)

Table 3. Indications for Mohs micrographic surgery (Telfer et al., 2008).

9.2 Standard surgical excision

Surgical excision is the main treatment modality for basal cell carcinoma and is usually applied as a standart method (Rogers & Bentz, 2011). This method is one of the most commonly used techniques in the treatment of nodular BCC and superficial BCC. Tumor tissue plus surrounding normal tissue area should be excised in this method (Ceilley Del & Rosso, 2006). A four millimeter excision margin is currently recommended for small, well demarcated BCC's (Sherry et al., 2010). The deep margins should contain the fascia (forehead), the perichondrium (ear, nose), or the periosteum (scalp) (Dandurand et al., 2006). Then, whether the presence of tumor cells in extracted material margins, should be verified by histopathological examination. Nevertheless, the incidence of incomplete excision can be increased up to 10% approximately. Some factors such as experience of surgeon, histologic subtypes and excision margins play an important role in the success of the operation (Ceilley Del & Rosso, 2006).

Its effectiveness is quite higher for primary BCC and also cosmetic results are usually well. Peripheral excision margins for primary BCC of 3–5 mm and 5-10 mm for recurrent BCC have been suggested. Due to high recurrence risk excision should be wider in recurrent BCC (Telfer et al., 2008). In contrast to small primary BCCs, morphoeic and large BCCs require wider surgical margins, between 5-15 mm, for complete histological resection (Pua et al., 2009). *Gulleth* et al. reported that 3-mm surgical margin can be safely used for nonmorpheaform basal cell carcinoma lesions 2 cm or smaller (Gulleth et al., 2010).

The cure and recurrence rates are variable. *Wetzig* et al. reported high cure rates for primary and recurrent BCCs, 99,5% and 97,1% respectively, at the end of 5-year follow-up (Wetzig et al., 2010). *Szeimies* et al. reported that clinical lesion response 99,2% and cosmetic outcome 59,8% 3 months and 12 months after surgical excision for superficial basal cell carcinoma, respectively. 12 months after surgical excision, reccurence has not been reported (Szeimies et

al., 2008). *Rhodes* et al. found that surgical excision is more effective than photodynamic therapy for the treatment of nodular basal cell carcinoma as a result of 5-year follow-up and recurrence rate was reported as 4%. (Rhodes et al., 2007). In 2008 a randomised controlled study of surgical excision versus fractionated 5-aminolevulinic acid-photodynamic therapy by *Mosterd* et al. found that 88 primary nodular BCC excised with 3 mm margins, the cumulative incidence of failure was 2,3% after 3-years of treatment (Mosterd et al., 2008).
There are some disadvantages of this method such as scars, bleeding and risk of infections (Szeimies et al., 2008). Also incomplete excision is another complication of the surgical excision which is correlate with the cure and recurrence rate, the patients morbidity and/or mortality, and the overall cost of treatment. *Pua* et al. reported that the overall incomplete excision rate was 1,54% (Pua et al., 2009). For this reason, surgical excision should be done by experienced surgeons (Szeimies et al., 2008).

9.3 Chemotherapy

Chemotherapy is generally used in two conditions: i) for the management of uncontrolled local disease, ii) for patients with metastatic BCC. Both conditions are extremely rare and are rapidly fatal position.
Various drugs can be used in metastatic BCC, including cyclophosphamide, etoposide, 5-fluorouracil, methotrexate, bleomycin, doxorubicin, and cisplatin but their effectiveness is variable. Cisplatin is the most effective chemotherapeutic agent in the treatment for patient with metastatic or locally advanced BCC, alone and/or combined. *Carneiro* et al. reported that a case of BCC metastatic to the lungs treated with the combination of carboplatin and paclitaxel (Carneiro et al., 2006). Also *Jefford* et al. observed that this treatment regimen was less neurotoxic effect and could provide rapid symptomatic relief (Jefford et al., 2004).
Paclitaxel, which is a chemotherapeutic agent, shown to be effective in a patient with nevoid BCC syndrome. Most of the aggressive BCC lesions of the patient which had not responded to treatment with intravenous cisplatin healed after 19 cycles intravenous paclitaxel treatment (Russo, 2005).
Snipes et al. reported that there was improvement with systemic 5-fluorouracil(5-FU) in a 52-year-old male patient with nodular BCC (Snipes et al., 2006).

9.4 Curettage and desiccation

Electrodesiccation and curettage (ED&C) is the most common method used by dermatologists to treat primary nodular and superficial BCC tumors < 1,5 cm in diameter (Ceilley Del & Rosso, 2006; Jefford et al., 2004). Initially tumor tissue is curetted and then the area is treated with electrosurgery (electrodesiccation or coagulation) to control bleeding until clinically normal tissue is appeared and all of tumor cells are eliminated. This method is repeated two or three times for achieving the success (Ceilley Del & Rosso, 2006). The wound heals within 4-6 weeks by secondary intention (Ho & Byrne, 2009).
While electrodesiccation and curettage are generally used for the treatment of low-risk lesions, they are generally contraindicated for the treatment of high-risk lesions because of their high recurrence risk (Telfer et al., 2008). This method can be applied in selected cases whom patients with multiple, superficial tumors on the trunk. Nevertheless, this method is contraindicated for facial tumors and in high-risk lesions (Wetzig et al., 2009). Disadvantages of this treatment option include to leave residual tumor tissue which may be demonstrated with histopathological examination and to develop hypertrophic scarring at

lesion site (Wu et al., 2006). There is a risk of development of hypertrophic scarring or white scar tissue formation after the procedure and this probability increases with the number of treatment cycles (Ceilley Del & Rosso, 2006). Some complications such as ulceration, hypopigmentation, blistering, edema, pain, secondary infection and recurrence can be seen immediately after the treatment or a later period (Dixon, 2005). Despite all of these possibilities cosmetic outcomes are usually pleasurable (Murchison et al., 2011).
The cure rates for primary basal cell carcinoma were reported between 88%-99% (Murchison et al., 2011). Also *Barlow* et al. reported that results of curettage alone were successful for nonaggressive basal cell carcinomas (Barlow et al., 2006).

9.5 Cryosurgery

The aim of this method is destruction of tumor cells using liquid nitrogen spray or probe. Cryosurgery is usually suitable for BCC lesions with well-defined borders (Ceilley Del & Rosso, 2006). Liquid nitrogen has a boiling point of -195°C, making it a very effective cryotherapy agent (Moesen et al., 2010). Two freeze-thaw cycles (30 seconds each cycle duration) with a tissue temperature of -50 °C are recommended (Ceilley Del & Rosso, 2006). While double freeze-thaw cycles are generally suggested for the treatment of facial BCC, superficial truncal lesions may need only one treatment cycle (Telfer et al., 2008). At first the diagnosis should be confirmed by biopsy. Preliminary curettage may be done before cryosurgery except superficial basal cell carcinoma. Thermocouple needles are useful to measure the temparature inside the tumor. When the desired temperature was achieved within the tumor, freezing process is interrupted until the frozen ring is resolved, and then freezing-thawing cycle was repeated (Kuflik, 2004). The success rate increases when the procedure used the treatment of correct lesions by the experienced people (Telfer et al., 2008). One of the advantage is that this method does not require local anesthesia. Other advantages are outpatient, inexpensive and no requirement of patient sedation (Murchison et al., 2011).
Some factors include rate of temperature fall, speed of tissue thaw, solution concentration, time of subzero temperature exposure, lowest temperature achieved in the target tissue and the number of freeze–thaw cycles can change the degree of tissue destruction. If the freezing occurs quickly, further tissue damage happens according to slow freezing (Murchison et al., 2011).
Two distinct technique, open also known as spray and closed also known as probe or contact, are preferred for malignant lesions. Some sensitive areas, e.g. eyelids, the use of probes is quite favorable, because periocular structures can be damaged with spray technique. Therefore, when using the spray technique, it should be noted to avoid damage to unaffected areas by the dermatologists (Murchison et al., 2011). In the treatment of primary periocular BCCs, cryosurgery with nitrous oxide probe may be an alternative treatment modality in the absence of appropriate surgical procedures. The disadvantage of this procedure is higher recurrence rate, approximately 8%, compared with other treatment modalities (Moesen et al., 2010). But *Emanuel* and her colleagues reported that 5-years cure rate and 30-years cure rate for basal cell carcinoma after cryosurgery were 99% and 98,6% respectively (Kuflik, 2004). This noninvasive method was compared with topical methyl aminolaevulinate photodynamic therapy, recurrence rates were similar but cosmetic results were worse than photodynamic therapy (Basset-Seguin et al., 2008).
Adverse events such as peri/postoperative pain, tenderness, vesicle and/or bullae, erythema, sloughing of necrotic tissue or eschar formation, localized edema, scarring,

hypo/hyperpigmentation may occur during or after the procedure (Ceilley Del & Rosso, 2006). Posttreatment pain may require the use of narcotic drugs especially within the first few days (Murchison et al., 2011). Severe edema may occur in some locations such as periorbital region, around the temples and on the forehead and therefore the patients should be warned (Wetzig et al., 2009).

Cryosurgery should be avoided in areas of hair growth and in patients with conditions sensitive to temperature, including *Raynaud*'s syndrome, cold panniculitis, and cryoglobulinemia (Ceilley Del & Rosso, 2006). Some body sites such as hair-bearing scalp, nasolabial fold, tragus, retroauricular groove, upper lip and distal portion of the lower leg are relatively contraindicated locations. Cryotherapy is not recommended for sclerodermiform BCC (Wetzig et al., 2009).

9.6 Topical treatment of Basal Cell Carcinoma

9.6.1 Imiquimod cream

Topical imiquimod 5% cream (Aldara 3M Pharmaceuticals, St Paul, MN) is a Toll-like receptor agonist that acts as an immune-response modifier (Raasch, 2009 & Robinson et al., 2003). Imiquimod 5% cream is approved by the United States Food and Drug Administration (FDA) for the treatment of external genital and perianal warts; nonhyperkeratotic actinic keratosis and superficial BCCs mostly in patients in whom surgery is not an option. Imiquimod promotes the innate immune response and the cell-mediated immune pathway, potentiating its antiviral, antitumoral, and immunoregulatory properties (Amini et al., 2010). The mechanism of action of imiquimod is thought to occur through the binding to cell surface receptors, such as Toll-like receptor 7 which leads to activation of macrophages and other cells (Ceilley Del & Rosso, 2006). Toll like receptor 7 (TLR-7) is found on dendritic cells and monocytes (McGillis & Fein, 2004). Binding to TLR-7 receptor induces proinflammatory cytokine secretion (e.g.interferon-alpha and tumor necrosis factor-alpha, IL-1, IL-12, IL-6, IL-8, and IL-10) that favors type 1 helper T-cell-mediated immune response (Robinson et al., 2003). These cytokines play role in the activation of the adaptive immune response toward the TH-1 or cell-mediated pathway and inhibit the TH-2 pathway. By this immunmodulation, imiquimod is believed to be important for control of tumors (Navi & Huntley, 2004). Data have shown that imiquimod 5% cream may induce Fas (CD95) receptor (FasR) mediated apoptosis in BCC cells (Berman et al., 2003). Normally in BCC cells FasR expression is not seen so cell apoptosis via a FasR–Fas ligand interaction is prevented (Ceilley Del & Rosso, 2006). *Berman* et al. demonstrated that BCC cells in 3 of 4 patients treated with imiquimod 5% cream applied five times per week for up to 2 weeks were positive for FasR, leading to an infiltration of T lymphocytes (i.e. suggesting cell apoptosis), while all 5 vehicle-treated patients had FasR negative BCC cells at the end of the treatment period (Berman et al., 2003). Therefore, imiquimod 5% cream acts by inducing FasR in the treatment of BCC.

Imiquimod has been approved in the United States by the FDA for the treatment of superficial BCC (sBCC) in immunocompetent adults with tumors >0.5 cm^2 in area and <2 cm in diameter located on the trunk and extremities (Krown, 1991). Initial trials of imiquimod 5% cream for the treatment of skin cancer focused on sBCC. In a multicenter 6-week dose-response trial, complete histological clearance was seen in 87.9 % (29/33) of patients in the once-daily three-times-per-week regimen, 73.3 % (22/30) of patients in twice-daily three-times-per-week regimen, and 69.7 % (23/33) of patients in the once-daily, three-

times-per-week regimen. The median duration of treatment for complete clearance was 10-16 weeks (Marks et al., 2001).
Patients with sBCC were enrolled in a randomized, double-blind,vehicle-controlled study to determine the efficacy of longer treatment regimens and treated with imiquimod for 12 weeks once daily seven times per week (n =31), once daily five times per week (n =26), or once daily three times per week (n =29) (Geisse et al., 2002). In this study, histologic clearance rates in the three groups were 87%, 81%, 52%, respectively. These histologic clearance rates for imiquimod were similar to those reported in the 6-week study (Marks et al., 2001), suggesting that an additional 6 weeks of treatment may not be necessary for efficacy.
In addition to sBCC, imiquimod also has been demonstrated efficient in the treatment of nBCC (Shumack et al., 2002). One such study was a Phase II clinical trial comparing efficacy of various dosing regimens in a 6-week study in *Australia* and *New Zealand* and a 12-week study in *United States*. In both studies histological examination of lesion site on 6-weeks post-treatment showed the highest clearance rate in the once daily for 7 days per week groups, with 71% of patients in the 6-week study and 76% of patients in the 12-week study having complete response following treatment. The authors pointed out that these response rates were lower than the nearly 88% response rates seen in studies of superficial BCC lesions (Shumack et al., 2002).This type of treatment modality applies better for those patients in which surgery, radiotherapy, or cryotherapy are not an option.
The side effects from use of imiquimod are mainly local site reactions. In a phase II study, the most common local skin reactions were erythema, crusting, flaking, and erosion (Marks et al., 2001). However, these dose-related side-effects were generally well tolerated, and none of the patients discontinued because of local skin reactions.
In addition to monotherapy, imiquimod 5% cream may also be useful as adjunctive therapy in the treatment of BCC. *Torres et al.* have reported on a randomized, double-blind, vehicle-controlled phase II study (n = 72) of imiquimod 5 days per week for 2–6 weeks before excision with MMS in the treatment of sBCC and nBCC. Treatment with imiquimod significantly reduced the size of the target tumor and thereby resulted in a smaller cosmetic defect from the MMS excision compared with vehicle (Torres et al., 2003).

9.6.2 Topical 5- Fluorouracil

Fluorouracil (5-FU) is an antineoplastic pyrimidine analog which decreases cell proliferation and induces cellular death, particularly in cells with high mitotic rates, through inhibition of thymidylate synthetase, which interferes with DNA synthesis. Evidence suggests that 5-FU used as a topical chemotherapeutic agent in NMSC has been effective for the treatment of superficial BCC, insitu SCC, and AKs. Due to lack of penetration through the dermis, 5-FU is generally not recommended for invasive BCCs and SCCs (Chakrabarty & Geisse, 2004). Published studies have indicated that 5-FU monotherapy has low clearance rates compared with other modalities. In a small study, 44 sBCC tumors were treated with a high concentration of medication, administered as a 25% fluorouracil paste, with occlusion that was changed once weekly for 3 weeks (Ebstein, 1985). This treatment regimen resulted in a 5-year recurrence rate of 21%. Although rigorous data are lacking, reports of 5-FU in combination with curettage or cryotherapy have suggested that combination therapy may be more effective than monotherapy (Ebstein, 1985; Tsuji et al., 1993). In the same study, 51 light curettage of 244 sBCC tumors before the 25% fluorouracil regimen resulted in a 5-year

cumulative recurrence rate of 6%, compared with the above-noted 21% for the fluorouracil regimen alone. Because limited data are available, the actual clearance rate for the topical treatment of sBCC with 5-FU is currently unknown.
In another study,superficial BCC treated with fluorouracil, thirty-one tumors were treated twice daily for an average of 11 weeks. A 90% clearance rate was observed on the basis of histologic evaluation results 3 weeks after treatment. No clinical follow-up was provided (Gross et al., 2007).
Application of 5-FU causes severe local skin reactions, including pain and burning, pruritus, irritation, inflammation, swelling, tenderness, hyperpigmentation, and scarring (Ebstein, 1985).

9.7 Radiation Therapy

Radiation therapy (RT) has been a useful alternative to surgical treatments. Radiotherapy (RT) can be effective for primary BCC, recurrent BCC or as adjuvant for incompletely excised BCC in patients where further surgery is neither possible nor appropriate (Samarasinghe et al., 2011). It has been particularly useful in the treatment of elderly patients and for larger tumors or tumors in difficult-to treat locations, such as the eyelids or pinna of the ear. Lower risk areas, such as the trunk and extremities, as well as the genitalia, hands, and feet are usually not treated with this modality (Ceilley Del & Rosso, 2006). RT is a complex mixture of different techniques including superficial RT (generated at up to 170 kV) which is suitable for lesions up to ~6 mm in depth, electron beam therapy (generated at higher energies) which penetrates deeper tissues, and brachytherapy which is useful for lesions arising on curved surfaces (Telfer et al., 2008). The total dose and treatment regimen (e.g. number of fractionated doses) depend on many factors including tumor location, size, type, and depth (Ceilley Del & Rosso, 2006). Radiotherapy is contraindicated in radiotherapy recurrent BCC, genetic syndromes predisposing to skin cancer and connective tissue disease. Significant side effects are radionecrosis, atrophy, and telangiectasia. Skin cancers can arise from radiotherapy field scars and should be avoided in younger age groups (Samarasinghe et al., 2011).
A study of BCC irradiated by a 'standardized' X-ray therapy schedule indicated an overall 5-year recurrence rate of 7.4% for primary (n =862) and 9.5% for recurrent (n =211) BCC (Silverman et al., 1992).
Surgical excision (91% with frozen section margin control) of 174 primary facial BCCs < 4 cm in diameter has been compared with RT (mix of interstitial brachytherapy, contact therapy and conventional RT) for 173 lesions (Avril et al., 1997). The 4-year recurrence rates were 0-7% (surgery) and 2-5% (RT).
Radiation therapy is contraindicated in certain genetic disorders, which predispose patients to skin cancers (e.g. patients with *Gorlin*'s syndrome, xeroderma pigmentosum, or connective tissue diseases, such as lupus and scleroderma) (Ceilley Del & Rosso, 2006).

9.8 Photodynamic Therapy

Photodynamic therapy (PDT) is performed by topical application of the prodrug 5-aminolaevulinic acid (ALA) or methyl aminolaevulinic (MAL) to the BCC lesion. The prodrug is converted intracellularly into a potent photosensitizer, protoporphyrin IX (PpIX), and, when exposed to oxygen and an appropriate light source, a cytotoxic reaction via oxygen radicals occurs within cells containing these precursors.(Ceilley Del & Rosso, 2006;

Samarasinghe et al., 2011). The light source is usually either 410nm blue light or 630nm red light to match the absorption peak for PpIX. Red light may be preferred with the lipophilic MAL for deeper tissue penetration (Samarasinghe et al., 2011). PDT induces intense inflammation through the release of cytokines, chemokines and other immunological proteins by the injured and apoptotic cells. PDT has also been demonstrated to act as a biologic response modifier (Oseroff, 2006). In addition to damaging target cells directly, PDT, through upregulated cytokine production, enhances the innate and adaptive immune responses in immunocompetent individuals (Oseroff, 2006).

In a study of 95 patients with sBCC, the primary response rate with ALA PDT was 86%, with a 44% recurrence rate after a median follow up of 19 months and a projected disease-free rate of only 50% (Fink-Puches et al., 1998). In a long-term study of 350 sBCC and nBCC lesions treated with methyl 5-ALA PDT, 89% of lesions cleared with an overall cure rate of 79% after a mean follow-up of 35 months (Soler et al., 2001).

For nodular BCC a study comparing MAL PDT with surgical excision in 101 patients showed a MAL PDT cure rate of 76% compared to 96% for surgical excision. Cosmetis result was better for PDT with 87% of patients rated as good cosmetic outcome in comparison to 54% for surgery (Rhodes et al., 2004).

When undergoing PDT, patients often complain of stinging, burning, and itching at the site of treatment. Erythema, scaling, and crusting may be evident after treatment, but usually the area heals with no evidence of scarring (Neville et al., 2007).

Although one advantage of PDT is that multiple BCC tumors can be treated simultaneously, PDT is a relatively inconvenient treatment option. Treatment involves a two stage process requiring several office visits. Because single PDT treatment demonstrates poor efficacy in BCC, multiple visits to a healthcare provider's office are required. Photosensitivity is also associated with this treatment regimen. After application of topical agents, patients should avoid exposure to sunlight or bright indoor light until after controlled exposure to the light source that completes treatment. Treatment with PDT is contraindicated in patients with porphyria, known allergies to porphyrins, and patients with photosensitivity to wave lengths of applied light sources (Ceilley Del & Rosso, 2006).

9.9 Immunotherpy

9.9.1 Intralesional Interferon

Interferon (IFN) works by binding to receptors located on target cells. The exact mechanism of action of these cytokines remains unclear, but interferons are known to have many important effects for the treatment of skin cancer, including antiproliferative effects (i.e., inhibition of mitosis and growth factors, activation of pro-apoptotic genes, and promotion of antiangiogenic activity) and upregulation of the immune system in the skin (Amini et al., 2010).

The mechanism by which IFN causes regression of BCCs has also been investigated. In IFN-treated BCCs, a considerable increase in the number of CD41 T cells infiltrating the dermis and surrounding the BCC nests was observed. As CD41 T cells have been shown to be capable of inducing apoptosis in their target cells via the CD95 receptor–CD95 ligand interaction, the expression of this ligand and receptor was subsequently analyzed in IFN-treated BCCs. In untreated patients, BCCs were found to express the CD95 ligand but not the receptor. In IFN-treated patients, BCCs expressed both the CD95 ligand and CD95 receptor, indicating that this signaling pathway may be capable of inducing apoptosis within these tumors by CD95 interactions with CD95 ligand (Buechener et al., 1997).

Intra- and perilesional IFN represent effective nonsurgical alternatives to treat BCCs, obtaining clearance rates between 70 to 100% (Telfer et al., 1999; Tucker et al., 2006). Its use is limited by its cost, safety profile, and the inconvenience of returning to a physician's office for multiple injections. A multicenter randomized controlled trial where IFN-α2b was used to treat 172 patients with biopsy proven BCC found the optimal dose to be 1.5 million IU intralesionally administered 3x/wk for three weeks. Significant clinical and histological clearance was obtained when compared with placebo (Greenway et al., 1986).

Twenty BCCs received treatment with intralesional IFN-α2b 3x/wk for three weeks at a dose of 1.5 million IU for lesions less than 2cm in diameter and three million IU for lesions 2cm or greater in diameter. More than half of lesions completely responded clinically and histologically at eight weeks of follow up. In those lesions that completely responded, only one recurrence was reported at five years of follow up (Bostanci et al., 2005).

Treatment with IFN can cause flulike symptoms including headache, myalgia, and fever, which can be alleviated by taking acetaminophen (Neville et al., 2007).

Even though several studies have demonstrated IFN's biologic potential for the treatment of BCC, it is not an established treatment option for BCC. This is because the clearance rates (approximately 70%) do not approach those achieved with surgical interventions, and it is also time consuming and costly to perform, as injections have to be administered by a healthcare professional up to five times per week. In addition, there have been no definitive large-scale studies that have determined the initial and long-term efficacy of this treatment option (Gaspari & Sauder, 2003).

9.10 Special management issues

9.10.1 Incompletely Excised Basal Cell Carcinoma

Various prospective and retrospective reviews of incompletely excised BCC suggest that not all tumours will recur. Studies using approximately 2–5 years of follow up have reported recurrence rates following histologically incomplete excision of 38%, (Richmond & Davie, 1987) and 41% (De Silva & Dellon, 1985). Patients should undergo re-treatment of incompletely excised lesions especially when they involve critical midfacial sites, where the deep surgical margin is involved, the surgical defect has been repaired using skin flaps or skin grafts and where histology shows an aggressive histological subtype (Mackie & Quinn, 2004). If the decision is made to re-treat rather than observe, re-excision (with or without frozen section control) or MMS are the treatments of choice. Patients should be treated at the time of diagnosis, because delay will likely result in increased local tissue damage. Patients should be evaluated for XRT if they are unable to undergo re-excision (Carucci & Leffell, 2008).

9.10.2 Neurotropic Basal Cell Carcinoma

Perineural invasion is not a common finding in basal cell carcinomas, with an estimated incidence that, depending on the series, varies between 0.17% and 3.8% (Ratner et al., 2000). The frequency is higher in more aggressive histological subtypes and in recurrent tumors. Due to the high risk of local recurrence, basal cell carcinomas with perineural invasion require specific management. The majority of authors agree on the use of *Mohs* surgery as the treatment of choice for this type of tumor; however, the use of other therapeutic options, such as adjuvant radiotherapy, or performing an additional Mohs stage after obtaining negative margins (Leibovitch et al., 2005), continues to be a subject of debate. Patients with gross perineural invasion manifesting neurologic symptoms would benefit from preoperative magnetic resonance imaging to assess extent of tumor spread (Carucci & Leffell, 2008).

9.10.3 Metastatic Basal Cell Carcinoma

While the lifetime risk of basal cell carcinoma is high, it is well known to physicians that metastasis is relatively rare. Studies have indexed a metastasis rate of 0.0028% to 0.5% (Von Domarus & Stevens, 1984). In a review by *Randle*, tumors with any of the following characteristics should be considered high-risk for metastatic potential: long duration, location in the mid face or ear, diameter larger than 2 cm, aggressive histological subtype, previous treatment, neglected, or history of radiation (Randle, 1996). There is a 2% incidence of metastasis for tumors larger than 3 cm in diameter.

Increased tissue invasion and extension of the tumor into adjacent anatomical structures also enhance metastatic potential (Snow et al., 1994). Immunosuppression and evidence of perineural spread or invasion of blood vessels have also been implicated as risk factors for metastasis (Robinson & Dahiya, 2003).

For patients with metastatic disease, morbidity and mortality remain exceedingly high. The biggest risk factors for metastasis are tumor size, depth, and recurrence, despite optimal treatment. Primary basal cell carcinoma metastasizes usually via lymphatics, although it also spreads hematogenously. Metastasis most commonly occurs in regional lymph nodes, lung, and bone.

If nodal disease is suspected on surgical examination, lymph node biopsy and imaging studies, as well as evaluation by medical and surgical oncologists, are indicated. Platinium-based chemotherapy has been used with modest results in treatment of metastatic BCC; however rapid clinical response was reported using a combination and paclitaxel (Carucci & Leffell, 2008).

10. Course and prognosis

The prognosis of basal cell cancer is very good. Patient's survival rate is 100% without metastasis. However, rare in advanced cases can lead to serious morbidity and cosmetic problems.

The incidence of basal cell carcinoma is increasing with each passing day, consequently increases in the rate of metastatic BCC (MBCC). Therefore, the prognosis is important for early detection and treatment of cases of BCC.

Metastatic BCC is extremely rare. Rates reported in the literature of metastatic BCC are between 0.0028% and 0.5% (Berlin et al., 2002; Cotran, 1961; Malone et al., 2000). Criteria for the diagnosis of metastatic BCC were first described in 1951 by Lattes and Kessler. These are as follows:

1. Primary tumor is originated from the skin and not from mucous membranes or other glands
2. Metastasis occurred to a distant site from the primary tumor and could not result from direct extension
3. Both metastatic and primary tumors have identical histopathology
4. No squamous cell features may be present (Ozgediz et al., 2008).

BCC metastases could be occured by lymphatic, hematogenic, or direct infiltration of subcutaneous tissue (Von Domarus & Stevens, 1984).

The most common areas of metastasis are lymph nodes, lungs, bone, skin (Berlin et al., 2002), and parathyroid glands (Wadhera et al., 2006). 85-90% of metastatic BCC is due to head and neck region (Wadhera et al., 2006). More than 300 cases of metastatic BCC have been reported in the literature (Spates et al., 2003).
The median age of the first sign of metastasis has been reported as 59, with the interval from onset of primary tumor to the time of metastasis ranging from <1 to 45 years.
A limited number of reviews have elucidated several possible risk factors for developing MBCC (Table 4).
The prognosis of metastatic BCC is usually very poor. The median survival time was 8 months after the first metastasis, although it has been reported in patients with longer survival time (Boswell et al., 2006). Only those with lymph node metastasis have limited survival time as 3.6 years (Pfeiffer et al., 1990).
The risk of metastasis increases with the size of primary tumor. Those with primary tumor size greater than 3 cm, 2% increases the risk of developing metastasis, 25% for those greater than 5 cm in, 50% for those greater than 10 cm in diameter (Snow et al., 1994).

- Size of tumor > 2 cm
- Head and neck locations
- Tumor recurrence refractory to treatment
- Previous radiation therapy
- Multiple primary tumors
- Increased depth of tumor
- Invasion of perineural space and blood vessels
- Fair skin
- Male

Table 4. Generally Accepted Risk Factors of Metastatic Basal Cell Carcinoma.

Some BCC species and locations are more likely to metastasize. Today, very large size attained is reported cases of BCC. Giant BCC is rarely seen and constitute 1% of all cases of BCC. Rates of local invasion and metastasis of making Giant BCC is higher (Varga et al., 2011). Early diagnosis and treatment can not be done in cases of localized BCC. Periorbital BCC may lead to blindness as a result of orbit propagation. Cases of BCC in the medial region of cantus deep seated and tend to be invasive. BCC cases of this type of may lead to perineural invasion and neural dysfunction (Bader, 2011).
Poor prognosis could be avoided by early diagnosis and treatment, various patient's self sufficient treatments and sun protection (Wong et al., 2003). Oral retinoid therapy may prevent or delay the development of new BCC lesions in patients with a high degree of actinic damaged skin, Gorlin syndrome patients and renal transplant patients (Hodak et al., 1987).

11. Recurrence

5-year recurrence rate of BCC is approximately 4-5% (Kyrgidis et al., 2010). Tumour localization, T-stage, histologic subtype (Pieh et al., 1999) and the choice of treatment are significant predictors of the risk of recurrence. The relapse rate for primary basal cell carcinomas on the T-region of the face and nose is highest. T2 and T3 tumours show a 2- and

3-fold increased relapse rate, respectively, compared with T1 basal cell carcinomas. Patients with chronic skin diseases have a 50% lower risk of relapse than healthy patients. Recurrent basal cell carcinomas have a higher relapse rate than primary lesions. Patients treated in a specialized skin cancer unit have a 6,4-fold higher cure rate compared with those treated by less experienced physicians (Bogelund et al., 2007). Recurrence 5-year rate due to various treatments is summarized in the following table 5.

- Surgical excision - 10.1%
- Radiation therapy - 8.7%
- Curettage and electrodesiccation - 7.7%
- Cryotherapy - 7.5%
- All non-Mohs modalities - 8.7%
- Mohs micrographic surgery - 1%

Table 5. Recurrence rate according to the treatment choices

Reported rates of incomplete excision of basal cell carcinoma (BCC) range from 5% to 25% (Farhi et al., 2007; Su et al., 2007). Incomplete excision and repeated surgical excisions are increased recurrence rate. A positive pathologic margin has an average recurrence rate of 21-32,2 percent (Santiago et al., 2010).

Following BCC patients after their treatment procedure, the probability of occuring the new tumor in their first 3 years is 35%, and in 5 years that ratio is 50% (Mc Loone et al., 2006). The median time free of second primary tumour was 7 years, while the median time free of recurrence was 12 years (Kyrgidis et al., 2010). For that reason, following up BCC patients after their treatment procedure is very important (Mc Loone et al., 2006). Recurrence of incompletely excised BCC was significantly higher in younger patients, in aggressive histological types and in localizations like postauricular and nasogenian folds (Santiago et al., 2010).

A 3-mm surgical margin can be safely used for BCC to attain 95% cure rates for lesions 2 cm or smaller (Gulleth et al., 2010). Issued as a clean surgical magrin, recurrence develops in approximately 1% in cases of BCC. Average 36.6 months of development time to recurrence is needed after surgery (Wetzig et al., 2010).

Located on the face of recurrent BCC and aggressive subtypes of the best treatment is Mohs surgery (Mosterd et al., 2009). 5-year recurrence rate after Mohs surgery for recurrent BCC is approximately 5.6%. This rate is 4 times more than the other treatment modalities (surgical excision, radiotherapy, cryotherapy, curettage and electrodesiccation) (Rowe et al., 1989).

A recurrence of BCC should be suspected when one of the following conditions occurs:

- Nonhealing ulceration
- Tissue destruction
- Scar tissue that becomes red, scaled, or crusted or enlarges with large adjacent telangiectasia
- Scar tissue that slowly enlarges over time (months)
- Development of papule/nodule within a scar

Histologic types of BCC at higher risk for recurrence include morpheaform (sclerotic), micronodular, infiltrative, and superficial (multicentric). Other conditions that contribute to a higher recurrence rate include recurrent tumors that have been treated previously, large tumors (>2 cm), and deeply infiltrating tumors (Bader, 2011).

In immunocompromised patients, the risk of developing BCC is 10-16 times higher than the normal population. The risk of BCC in patients with renal transplant recipients is approximately 15% and female patients are at greater risk of BCC development. Recurrence rate after surgery is 10% (Mertz et al., 2010). However, placement and choice of treatment in these patients revealed no difference in terms of the normal population and does not seem to act more aggressively (Lott et al., 2010).

12. References

Adisen, E. & Gurer, MA. (2007). Basal Cell Carcinoma. *Turkiye Klinikleri J Int Med Sci*, 3, 22, pp.10-19, ISSN 1300-0292

Alam, M.; Berg, D.; Bhatia, A.; Cohen, JL.; Hale, EK.; Herman, AR.; Huang, CC.; Jiang, SI.; Kimyai-Asadi, A.; Lee, KK.; Levy, R.; Rademaker, AW.; White, LE. & Yoo, SS. (2010). Association between number of stages in Mohs micrographic surgery and surgeon-, patient-, and tumor-specific features: a cross-sectional study of practice patterns of 20 early- and mid-career Mohs surgeons. *Dermatol Surg*, 36, 12, pp. 1915-1920 ISSN 1524-4725

Amini, S.; Viera, MH.; Valins, W. & Berman, B. (2010). Nonsurgical Innovations in the Treatment of Nonmelanoma Skin Cancer. *J Clin Aesthetic Dermatol*, 3, 6, pp. 20–34

Avril, MF.; Auperin, A. & Margulis, A. (1997). Basal cell carcinoma of the face: surgery or radiotherapy? Results of a randomized study. *Br J Cancer*, 76, 100–106, *ISSN* 0007-0920.

Bader, RS. (n.d.). Basal Cell Carcinoma, In: *Emedicine*, 20.06.2011, http://emedicine.medscape.com/article/276624-overview.

Barlow, JO.; Zalla, MJ. & Kyle, A. (2006). Treatment of basal cell carcinoma with curettage alone. *J Am Acad Dermatol*, 54, pp. 1039-1045, *ISSN*:0190-9622

Baskurt, H.; Celik, E.; Yeşiladali, G. & Tercan, M. (2011). Importance of Hereditary Factors in Synchronous Development of Basal Cell Carcinoma in Two Albino Brothers: Case Report. *Ann Plast Surg*, Mar 14, [Epub ahead of print], *ISSN*:0148-7043

Basset-Seguin, N.; Ibbotson, SH. & Emtestam, L. (2008). Topical methyl aminolaevulinate photodynamic therapy versus cryotherapy for superficial basal cell carcinoma: a 5 year randomized trial. *Eur J Dermatol*, 18, pp. 547-553, *ISSN*: 1167-1122.

Batra, RS. & Kelley, LC. (2002). Predictors of extensive subclinical spread in nonmelanoma skin cancer treated with Mohs micrographic surgery. *Arch Dermatol*, 138, pp. 1043–1051, *ISSN* (printed): 0003-987X. *ISSN* (electronic): 0096-5359

Bauer, A.; Diepgen, TL. & Schmitt J. (2011). Is occupational solar UV-irradiation a relevant risk factor for basal cell carcinoma? A systematic review and meta-analysis of the epidemiologic literature. *Br J Dermatol*. May 23, [Epub ahead of print], ISSN 1365-2133, *ISSN*: 1365-2133.

Berlin, JM.; Warner, MR. & Bailin, PL. (2002). Metastatic basal cell carcinoma presenting as unilateral axillary lymphadenopathy: report of a case and review of the literature. *Dermatol Surg*, 28, pp. 1082-1084, *ISSN*: 1524-4725

Berman, B.; Sullivan, T. & De Araujo, T. (2003). Expression of Fasreceptor on basal cell carcinomas after treatment with imiquimod 5% cream or vehicle. *Br J Dermatol*, 149, (Suppl. 66), pp. 59–61, *ISSN*: 1365-2133.

Betti, R.; Facchetti, M.; Menni, S. & Crosti, C. (2005). Basal cell carcinoma of the sole. *J Dermatol*,32, pp. 450-453, *ISSN*: 1167-1122

Betti, R.; Menni, S.; Radaelli, G.; Bombonato, C. & Crosti, C. (2010). Micronodular basal cell carcinoma: A distinct subtype? Relationship with nodular and infiltrative basal cell carcinomas. *J Dermatol*, 37, 7, pp. 611-616, *ISSN*: 1167-1122

Bøgelund, FS.; Philipsen, PA. & Gniadecki, R. (2007). Factors affecting the recurrence rate of basal cell carcinoma. *Acta Derm Venereol*, 87, pp. 330-334, *ISSN*:0001-5555 (Print); 0001-5555

Bostanci, S.; Kocyigit, P. & Alp, A. (2005). Treatment of basal cell carcinoma located in the head and neck region with intralesional interferon alpha-2a: evaluation of long-term follow-up results. *Clin Drug Investig*, 25, 10, pp. 661–667, *ISSN* 1173-2563.

Boswell, JS.; Flam, MS.; Tashjian, DN. & Tschang, TP. (2006). Basal cell carcinoma metastatic to cervical lymph nodes and lungs. *Dermatol Online J*, 31, 12: 9, *ISSN*:1087-2108 (Electronic) ; 1087-2108 (Linking).

Braun-Falco, O.; Plewig, G.; Wolff, HH. & Burgdorf, WHC. (2000). In: *Braun-Falco's Dermatology*, 2nd Ed. pp. 1463-1489, Springer-Verlag, ISBN 978-3-540-59452-3 Berlin

Brown, CI. & Perry, AE. (2000). Incidence of perineural invasion in histologically aggressive types of basal cell carcinoma. *Am J Dermatopathol*, 22, pp. 123–125, *ISSN*: 1533-0311

Buechner, SA.; Wernli, M.; Harr, T.; Hahn, S.; Itin, P. & Erb, P. (1997). Regression of basal cell carcinoma by intralesional interferon-alpha treatment is mediated by CD95 (Apo-1/Fas)-CD95 ligand-induced suicide. *J Clin Invest*, 100, 2691–2696, *ISSN*:0021-9738 (Print) ; 1558-8238 (Electronic)

Carneiro, BA.; Watkin, WG.; Mehta, UK. & Brockstein, BE. (2006). Metastatic basal cell carcinoma: complete response to chemotherapy and associated pure red cell aplasia. *Cancer Invest*, 24, pp. 396-400, *ISSN* (printed): 0735-7907. *ISSN* (electronic): 1532-4192

Carucci, J. & Leffell, D. (2008). Basal cell carcinoma. In: *Fitzpatrick's Dermatology in General Medicine.* Wolf, K.; Goldsmith, L.; Gilchrest, B.; Paller, A. & Leffell, D. pp. 1036-1042, Mc Graw Hill, ISBN 0-07-146690-8, New York

Ceilley, RI. & Del Rosso, JQ. (2006). Current modalities and new advances in the treatment of basal cell carcinoma. *Int J Dermatol*, 45, pp. 489-498, Print *ISSN*: 0011-9059. Online *ISSN*: 1365-4632

Cernea, CR.; Ferraz, AR.; de Castro, IV.; Sotto, MN.; Logullo, AF.; Bacchi, CE.; Plopper, C.; Wanderlei, F.; de Carlucci, D Jr. & Hojaij, FC. (2009). Perineural Invasion in Aggressive Skin Carcinomas of the Head and Neck. Potentially Dangerous but Frequently Overlooked. *ORL J Otorhinolaryngol Relat Spec*, 71, 1, pp. 21-26, *issn*/03011569

Chakrabarty, A. & Geisse, JK. (2004). Medical therapies for nonmelanoma skin cancer. *Clin Dermatol*, 22, 3, pp. 183–188, *ISSN*: 0738-081X (Print) 1879-1131

Chinem, VP. & Miot, HA. (2011). Epidemiology of basal cell carcinoma. *An Bras Dermatol* 86, 2, pp.292-305 ISSN 0365-0596

Cotran, RS. (1961). Metastasizing basal cell carcinomas. *Cancer*, 14, pp. 1036-1040

Crowson, AN. (2006). Basal cell carcinoma: biology, morphology and clinical implications. *Mod Pathol*, 19, Suppl 2, pp. 127-147, *ISSN*: 0893-3952

Cumberland,L.; Dana, A. & Liegeois, N. (2009). Mohs micrographic surgery for the management of nonmelanoma skin cancers. *Facial Plast Surg Clin North Am*, 17, pp. 325-335, *ISSN*:1064-7406

Dandurand, M.; Petit, T.; Martel, P. & Guillot, B. (2006). Management of basal cell carcinoma in adults Clinical practice guidelines. *Eur J Dermatol*, 16, PP. 394-401, *ISSN*: 1167-1122

De Silva, SP. & Dellon, AL. (1985). Recurrence rate of positive margin basal cell carcinoma: results of a five-year prospective study. *J Surg Oncol*, 28, pp. 72–74, *ISSN*:0975-7651

Dixon, AJ. (2005). Multiple superficial basal cell carcinomata--topical imiquimod versus curette and cryotherapy. *Aust Fam Physician*, 34, pp. 49-52, *ISSN*: *0300-8495*

Donovan, J. (2009). Review of the hair follicle origin hypothesis for basal cell carcinoma. *Dermatol Surg*, 35, pp.1311-1323, *ISSN*: 1524-4725

Epstein, E. (1985). Fluorouracil paste treatment of thin basal cell carcinomas. *Arch Dermatol*, 121, pp. 207–213, *ISSN* (printed): 0003-987X. *ISSN* (electronic): 0096-5359

Farhi, D.; Dupin, N.; Palangié, A.; Carlotti, A. & Avril, MF. (2007). Incomplete excision of basal cell carcinoma: rate and associated factors among 362 consecutive cases. *Dermatol Surg*, 33, pp. 1207-1, *ISSN*: 1524-4725

Fernandez -Flores, A. (2011). Study of D2-40 Immunoexpression of the Spindle Cell Areas of a Metaplastic Basal Cell Carcinoma (Sarcomatoid Basal Cell Carcinoma). *Appl Immunohistochem Mol Morphol*, May 19, [Epub ahead of print], *ISSN*:1541-2016

Fink-Puches, R.; Soyer, HP. & Hofer, A. (1998). Long-term followup and histological changes of superficial nonmelanoma skin cancers treated with topical delta-aminolevulinic acid photodynamic therapy. *Arch Dermatol*, 134, pp. 821– 826, *ISSN* (printed): 0003-987X. *ISSN* (electronic): 0096-5359

Gaspari, AA. & Sauder, DN. (2003). Immunotherapy of Basal Cell Carcinoma: Evolving Approaches. *Dermatol Surg*, 29, pp. 1027–1034, *ISSN*: 1524-4725

Geisse, JK.; Rich, P. & Pandya, A. (2002). Imiquimod 5% cream for the treatment of superficial basal cell carcinoma: a doubleblind, randomized, vehicle-controlled study. *J Am Acad Dermatol*, 47, pp. 390–398, *ISSN*:0190-9622

Greenway, HT.; Cornell, RC. & Tanner, DJ. (1986). Treatment of basal cell carcinoma with intralesional interferon. *J Am Acad Derm*, 15, pp. 437–443, *ISSN*:0190-9622

Gross, K.; Kircik, L. & Kricorian, G. (2007). 5% 5-Fluorouracil cream for the treatment of small superficial basal cell carcinoma: efficacy, tolerability, cosmetic outcome, and patient satisfaction. *Dermatol Surg*, 33, 4, pp. 433-440, *ISSN*: 1524-4725

Gulleth, Y.; Goldberg, N.; Silverman, RP. & Gastman, BR. (2010). What is the best surgical margin for a Basal cell carcinoma: a meta-analysis of the literature. *Plast Reconstr Surg*, 126, pp. 1222-1231, *ISSN*: 1529-4242

Hakverdi, S.; Balci, DD.; Dogramaci, CA.; Toprak, S. & Yaldız, M. (2011). Retrospective analysis of basal cell carcinoma. *Indian J Dermatol Venereol Leprol*, 77, 2, 251, *ISSN*:0378-6323

Ho, T. & Byrne, PJ. (2009). Evaluation and initial management of the patient with facial skin cancer. *Facial Plast Surg Clin North Am*, 17, pp. 301-307, *ISSN*:1064-7406

Hodak, E.; Ginzburg, A.; David, M. & Sandbank, M. (1987). Etretinate treatment of the nevoid basal cell carcinoma syndrome. Therapeutic and chemopreventive effect. *Int J Dermatol*, 26, pp. 606-609, Print *ISSN*: 0011-9059. Online *ISSN*: 1365-4632

Jefford, M.; Kiffer, JD.; Somers, G.; Daniel, FJ. & Davis, ID. (2004). Metastatic basal cell carcinoma: rapid symptomatic response to cisplatin and paclitaxel. *ANZ J Surg*, 74, pp. 704-705, *ISSN*: 1365-2168

Kinoshita, R.; Yamamoto, O.; Yasuda, H. & Tokura, Y. (2005). BBasal cell carcinoma of the scrotum with lymph node metastasis: report of a case and review of the literature. *Int J Dermatol*, 44, pp. 54-56, Print *ISSN*: 0011-9059. Online *ISSN*: 1365-4632.

Kirkham, N. (2005). Tumors and Cysts of the epidermis. In: *Lever's Histopathology of the Skin*, Elder, DE, pp. 805-866, 9th Ed., Lippincott Williams & Wilkins, ISBN 0-7817-3742-7 Philadelphia

Krown, SE. (1991). "Interferon and other biologic agents for the treatment of Kaposi's sarcoma," *Hematology/Oncology Clinics of North America*, vol. 5, no. 2, pp. 311–322, *ISSN*: 0889-8588.

Kuflik, EG. (2004). Cryosurgery for skin cancer: 30-year experience and cure rates. *Dermatol Surg*, 30, pp. 297-300, *ISSN*: 1524-4725

Kuphal, S.; Shaw-Hallgren, G.; Eberl, M.; Karrer, S.; Aberger, F.; Bosserhoff, AK. & Massoumi R. (2011). GLI1-dependent transcriptional repression of CYLD in basal cell carcinoma. *Oncogene*. May 16, [Epub ahead of print], *ISSN: 0950-9232*

Kwasniak, LA. & Zuazaga, JG. (2011). Basal cell carcinoma: evidence-based medicine and review of treatment modalities. *International Journal of Dermatology*, 50, pp. 645–658, *ISSN 0011-9059*,

Kyrgidis, A.; Vahtsevanos, K.; Tzellos, TG.; Xirou, P.; Kitikidou, K.; Antoniades, K.; Zouboulis, CC. & Triaridis, S. (2010). Clinical, histological and demographic predictors for recurrence and second primary tumours of head and neck basal cell carcinoma. A 1062 patient-cohort study from a tertiary cancer referral hospital. *Eur J Dermatol*, 20, pp. 276-282, *ISSN*: 1167-1122

Lee, JH.; Pyon, JK.; Kim, DW.; Lee, SH.; Nam, HS.; Kang, SG.; Kim, CH.; Lee, YJ.; Chun, JS. & Cho, MK. (2011). Expression of RUNX3 in skin cancers. *Clin Exp Dermatol*, May 30, ISSN 0307-6938 [Epub ahead of print], *ISSN*: 1365-2230

Leibovitch, I.; Huilgol, SC.; Selva, D.; Richards, S. & Paver, R. (2005). Basal cell carcinoma treated with Mohs surgery in Australia III. Perineural invasion. *J Am Acad Dermatol*, 53, pp. 458-463, *ISSN*:0190-9622

Lewis, KR.; Colome-Grimmer, MI.; Uchida, T.; Wang, HQ. & Wagner, RF Jr. (2006). p75NGFR Immunostaining for the Detection of Perineural Invasion by Cutaneous Squamous Cell Carcinoma. *Dermatol Surg*, 32, 2, pp. 177-183, *ISSN*: 1524-4725

Lott, DG.; Manz, R.; Koch, C. & Lorenz, RR. (2010). Aggressive behavior of nonmelanotic skin cancers in solid organ transplant recipients. *Transplantation*, 90, 683-687, *ISSN*: *0041-1337*

Machado Filho, CDAS.; Fagundes, DS.; Sender, F.; Paschoal, LHC.; Costa, MCC. & Carazzato SG. (1996). Neoplasias malignas cutâneas: estudo epidemiológico. *An Bras Dermatol*, 7, pp.479-484 ISSN 0365-0596, *ISSN*:0365-0596

MacKie, RM. & Quinn, AG. (2004). Non-melanoma skin cancer and other epidermal skin tumours. In: *Rook's Textbook of Dermatology*. Burns, T.; Breathnach, S.; Cox, N. & Griffiths, C. pp. 36.1-36.50, 7th Edition, Blackwell Publishing, ISBN 978-1405161695, Massachusetts

Malone, JP.; Fedok, FG.; Belchis, DA. & Maloney, ME.; (2000). Basal cell carcinoma metastatic to the parotid: report of a new case and review of the literature. *Ear Nose Throat J*, 79, pp. 511–519, *ISSN*: 0145-5613

Marks, R.; Gebauer, K.; Shumack, S.; Amies, M.; Bryden, J.; Fox, TL. & Owens, ML. (2001). Imiquimod 5% cream in the treatment of superficial basal cell carcinoma: results of a multicenter 6-week dose-response trial. *J Am Acad Dermatol*, 44, (5), pp. 807-813, *ISSN*:0190-9622

Marmur, ES.; Berkowitz, EZ.; Fuchs, BS.; Singer, GK. & Yoo, JY. (2010). Use of high frequency, high-resolution ultrasound before Mohs surgery. *Dermatol Surg*, 36, pp. 841-847, *ISSN*: 1524-4725

Mc Loone, NM.; Tolland, J.; Walsh, M. & Dolan, OM. (2006). Follow-up of basal cell carcinomas: an audit of current practice. *J Eur Acad Dermatol Venereol*, 20, pp. 698-701, *ISSN* (printed): 0926-9959. *ISSN* (electronic): 1468-3083

McGillis, ST. & Fein, H. (2004). Topical Treatment Strategies for Non-Melanoma Skin Cancer and Precursor Lesions. *Semin Cutan Med Surg*,23, pp. 174-183, *ISSN*: 1085-5629

Menzies, SW. (2002). Dermoscopy of pigmented basal cell carcinoma. *Clin Dermatol*, 20, pp. 268-269, *ISSN*: 0738-081X (Print) 1879-1131 (Electronic)

Mertz, KD.; Proske, D.; Kettelhack, N.; Kegel, C.; Keusch, G.; Schwarz, A.; Ambühl, PM.; Pfaltz, M. & Kempf, W. (2010). Basal cell carcinoma in a series of renal transplant recipients: epidemiology and clinicopathologic features. *Int J Dermatol*, 49, pp. 385-389, Print *ISSN*: 0011-9059. Online *ISSN*: 1365-4632

Miller, SJ. & Moresi, JM. (2008). Actinic keratosis, basal cell carcinoma and squamous cell carcinoma. In: *Dermatology*. Bolognia, JL.; Jorizzo, JL. & Rapini RP. pp. 1677-1696, Mosby, ISBN 978-1-4160-2999-1, London

Moesen, I.; Duncan, M. & Cates, C. (2010). Nitrous oxide cryotherapy for primary periocular basal cell carcinoma: outcome at 5 years follow-up. *Br J Ophthalmol*, Sep 9. [Epub ahead of print], *ISSN* 1468-2079

Morris, JG. & Joffe, R. (1983). Perineural spread of cutaneous basal and squamous cell carcinomas. The clinical appearance of spread into the trigeminal and facial nerves. *Arch Neurol*, 40, pp. 424–429, Print: *ISSN* 0003-9942. Online: *ISSN* 1538-3687

Mosterd, K.; Thissen, MR. & Nelemans, P. (2008). Fractionated 5-aminolaevulinic acid photodynamic therapy vs. surgical excision in the treatment of nodular basal cell carcinoma: results of a randomized controlled trial. *Br J Dermatol*, 159, pp. 864-870, *ISSN*: 1365-2133.

Mosterd, K.; Arits, AH.; Thissen, MR. & Kelleners-Smeets, NW. (2009). Histology-based treatment of basal cell carcinoma. *Acta Derm Venereol*, 89, pp. 454-458, *ISSN*:0001-5555 (Print); 0001-5555

Muller, FM.; Dawe, RS.; Moseley, H. & Fleming, CJ. (2009). Randomized comparison of Mohs micrographic surgery and surgical excision for small nodular basal cell carcinoma: tissue-sparing outcome. *Dermatol Surg*, 35, pp. 1349-1354, *ISSN*: 1524-4725

Murchison, AP.; Walrath, JD. & Washington, CV. (2011). Non-surgical treatments of primary, non-melanoma eyelid malignancies: a review. *Clin Experiment Ophthalmol*, 39, pp. 65-83, *ISSN*: 1442-9071

Navi, D. & Huntley, A. (2004). Imiquimod 5 percent cream and the treatment of cutaneous malignancy. *Dermatology Online Journal*, 15, 10, (1), 4, *ISSN 1087-2108*

Neville, JA.; Welch, E. & Leffell, DJ. (2007). Management of nonmelanoma skin cancer in 2007. *Nat Clin Pract Oncol*, 4, 8, pp. 462–469, *ISSN* (printed): 1743-4254. *ISSN* (electronic): 1743-4262

Nouri, K.; Ballard, CJ.; Patel, AR. & Brasie, RA. (2007). Basal cell carcinoma. In: *Skin Cancer*. Nouri K. pp. 61-85, Mc Graw Hill, ISBN 978-0071472562, New York

Odom, RB.; James, WD. & Berger, TG. (2000). Epidermal nevi, neoplasms, and cysts. In: *Andrew's Diseases of the Skin Clinical Dermatology*, 7. Ed., pp. 800-868, WB Saunders, ISBN 0-7216-5832-6, Philadelphia

Orsini, RC.; Catanzariti, A.; Saltrick, K.; Mendicino, RW. & Stokar, L. (2001). Basal cell carcinoma of the nail unit: a case report. *Foot Ankle Int*, 22, pp. 675-678, *ISSN*: 1071-1007

Oseroff, A. (2006). "PDT as a cytotoxic agent and biological response modifier: implications for cancer prevention and treatment in immunosuppressed and immunocompetent patients," *Journal of Investigative Dermatology*, 126, 3, pp. 542–544, *ISSN: 0022-202X*

Ozgediz, D.; Smith, EB.; Zheng, J.; Otero, J.; Tabatabai, ZL. & Corvera, CU. (2008). Basal cell carcinoma does metastasize. *Dermatol Online J*, 15, pp. 14-15, *ISSN*:1087-2108

Pfeiffer, P.; Hansen, O. & Rose, C. (1990). Systemic cytotoxic therapy of basal cell carcinoma. A review of the literature. *Eur J Cancer*, 26, pp. 73-77, *ISSN* 1359-6349

Pieh, S.; Kuchar, A.; Novak, P.; Kunstfeld, R.; Nagel, G. & Steinkogler, FJ. (1999). Long term results after surgical basal cell carcinoma excision in the eyelid region. *Br J Ophthalmol*, 83, pp. 85-88, *ISSN* 1468-2079

Pua, VS.; Huilgol, S. & Hill, D. (2009). Evaluation of the treatment of non-melanoma skin cancers by surgical excision. *Australas J Dermatol*, 50, pp. 171-175, *ISSN*:0004-8380

Raasch, B. (2009). Management of superficial basal cell carcinoma: focus on imiquimod. *Clinical, Cosmetic and Investigational Dermatology*, 2, pp. 65–75, *ISSN*: 11787015

Randle, HW. (1996). BCC. Identification and treatment of the high-risk patient. *Dermatol Surg*,22, pp. 255-261, *ISSN*: 1524-4725

Ratner, D.; Lowe, L.; Johnson, TM. & Fader, DJ. (2000). Perineural spread of basal cell carcinomas treated with Mohs micrographic surgery. *Cancer*, 88, pp. 1605-1613, *ISSN*: 1097-0142.

Repertinger, SK.; Stevens, T.; Markin, N.; Klepacz, H. & Sarma, DP. (2008). Fibroepithelioma of Pinkus with pleomorphic epithelial giant cell. *Dermatol Online J*, 15, 14, 12, 13, *ISSN*:1087-2108

Rhodes, LE.; de Rie, MA. & Enstr¨om, Y. (2004). "Photodynamic therapy using topical methyl aminolevulinate vs surgery for nodular basal cell carcinoma: results of a multicenter randomized prospective trial," *Archives of Dermatology*, 140, 1, pp. 17–23, *ISSN: 0003987X*

Rhodes, LE.; de Rie, MA. & Leifsdottir, R. (2007). Five-year follow-up of a randomized, prospective trial of topical methyl aminolevulinate photodynamic therapy vs surgery for nodular basal cell carcinoma. *Arch Dermatol*, 143, pp. 1131-1136, *ISSN: 0003987X*

Richard, R.; Jahan, T.; Alston, JL. & Umphlett, M. (2010). Basal cell carcinoma with metastasis to the lung in an African American man. *J Am Acad Dermatol*,63, pp. 87-89, *ISSN*:0190-9622

Richmond, JD. & Davie, RM. (1987). The significance of incomplete excision in patients with basal cell carcinoma. *Br J Plast Surg*, 40, pp. 63–67, *ISSN*: 0007-1226

Robinson, JK.; Hernandez, C.; Anderson, R. & Nickoloff, B. (2003). Topical and Light-based Treatments for Basal Cell Carcinoma. *Seminars in Cutaneous Medicine and Surgery*, 22, pp. 171-176, *ISSN*: 1085-5629

Robinson, JK. & Dahiya, M. (2003). Basal cell carcinoma with pulmonary and lymph node metastasis causing death. *Arch Dermatol*, 139, 5, pp. 643-648 *ISSN: 0003987X*

Rogers, CR. & Bentz, ML. (2011). An evidence-based approach to the treatment of nonmelanoma facial skin malignancies. *Plast Reconstr Surg,* 127, pp. 940-948, *ISSN*: 1529-4242

Rowe, DE.; Carroll, RJ. & Day, CL Jr. (1989). Mohs surgery is the treatment of choice for recurrent (previously treated) basal cell carcinoma. *J Dermatol Surg Oncol,* 15, pp. 424-431, *ISSN*: 0148-0812

Russo, GG. (2005). Actinic keratoses, basal cell carcinoma, and squamous cell carcinoma: uncommon treatments. *Clin Dermatol,* 23, pp. 581-586, *ISSN*: 0738-081X

Saladi, RN.; Singh, F.; Wei, H.; Lebwohl, MG. & Phelps, RG. (2004). Use of Ber-EP4 protein in recurrent metastatic basal cell carcinoma: a case report and review of the literature. *Int J Dermatol,* 43, pp. 600-603, Print *ISSN*: 0011-9059. Online *ISSN*: 1365-4632

Samarasinghe, V.; Madan, V. & Lear, JT. (2011). Focus on Basal cell carcinoma. *J Skin Cancer,* 2011: 328615, Epub 2010 Oct 24.

Santiago, F.; Serra, D.; Vieira, R. & Figueiredo, A. (2010). Incidence and factors associated with recurrence after incomplete excision of basal cell carcinomas: a study of 90 cases. *J Eur Acad Dermatol Venereol,* 24, 1421-4, *ISSN* (printed): 0926-9959. *ISSN* (electronic): 1468-3083

Scalvenzi, M.; Lembo, S.; Francio, MG. & Balato, A. (2008). Dermoscopic patterns of superficial basal cell carcinoma. *Int J Dermatol,* 47, pp. 1015-1018, Print *ISSN*: 0011-9059. Online *ISSN*: 1365-4632

Schwartz, RA. (2008). Basal cell carcinoma. In: *Skin Cancer Recognition and Management.* pp. 87-104, Blackwell, ISBN 978-1405159616, Massachusetts

Sherry, KR.; Reid, LA. & Wilmshurst, AD. (2010). A five year review of basal cell carcinoma excisions. *J Plast Reconstr Aesthet Surg,* 63, pp. 1485-1489, . *ISSN* (printed): 1748-6815

Shumack, S.; Robinson, J. & Kossard, S. (2002). Efficacy of topical 5% imiquimod cream for the treatment of nodular basal cell carcinoma: comparison of dosing regimens. *Arch Dermatol,* 138, 9, pp. 1165–1171, *ISSN* (printed): 0003-987X. *ISSN* (electronic): 0096-5359

Sikar Aktürk, A.; Kıran, R.; Odyakmaz Demirsoy, E.; Bayram Gürler, D. & Demir Yıldız, K. (2011). Basal Cell Carcinoma on the lower lip: Case report. *Turkiye Klinikleri J Dermatol,* 21, 1, pp.59-61, ISSN 1300-0330

Silverman, MK.; Kopf, AW. & Gladstein, AH. (1992). Recurrence rates of treated basal cell carcinomas. Part 4: X–ray therapy. *J Dermatol Surg Oncol,* 18, pp. 549–554, *ISSN*: 0148-0812

Snipes, CJ.; Sniezek, PJ. & Walling, HW. (2006). Basal cell carcinoma responding to systemic 5-fluorouracil. *J Am Acad Dermatol,* 54, pp. 1104-1106, *ISSN*:0190-9622

Snow, SN.; Sahl, W. & Lo, JS. (1994). Metastatic basal cell carcinoma. Report of five cases. *Cancer,* 73, pp. 328–335, *ISSN*: 1097-0142

Soler, AM.; Warloe, T. & Berner, A. (2001). A follow-up study of recurrence and cosmesis in completely responding superficial and nodular basal cell carcinomas treated with methyl 5-aminolaevulinate-based photodynamic therapy alone and with prior curettage. *Br J Dermatol,* 145, pp. 467–471, *ISSN*: 1365-2133

Soleymani, AD.; Scheinfeld, N.; Vasil, K.; & Bechtel, MA. (2008). Metastatic Basal Cell Carcinoma Presenting as Unilateral Axillary Lymphadenopathy. *J Am Acad Dermatol,* 59, 2 Suppl 1, pp. 1-3, *ISSN*:0190-9622

Spates, ST.; Mellette, JR. & Fitzpatrick, J. (2003). Metastatic basal cell carcinoma. *Dermatol Surg*,29, pp. 650-652, *ISSN*: 1524-4725

Su, SY.; Giorlando, F.; Ek, EW. & Dieu, T. (2007). Incomplete excision of basal cell carcinoma: a prospective trial. *Plast Reconstr Surg*, 120, pp. 1240-8, *ISSN*: 1529-4242

Szeimies, RM.; Ibbotson, S. & Murrell, DF. (2008). A clinical study comparing methyl aminolevulinate photodynamic therapy and surgery in small superficial basal cell carcinoma (8-20 mm), with a 12-month follow-up. *J Eur Acad Dermatol Venereol*, 22, pp. 1302-1311, *ISSN* (electronic): 1468-3083

Tang, JY.; Xiao, TZ.; Oda, Y.; Chang, KS.; Shpall, E.; Wu, A.; So, PL.; Hebert, J.; Bikle, D. & Epstein, EH Jr. (2011). Vitamin d3 inhibits hedgehog signaling and proliferation in murine Basal cell carcinomas. *Cancer Prev Res (Phila)*, 4, 5, pp. 744-751, *ISSN*: 1940-6207 (Print) 1940-6215 (Electronic)

Telfer, NR.; Colver, GB. & Bowers, PW. (1999). Guidelines for the management of basal cell carcinoma. British Association of Dermatologists. *Br J Dermatol*, 141, 3, pp. 415–423, *ISSN*: 1365-2133

Telfer, NR.; Colver, GB. & Morton, CA. (2008). Guidelines for the management of basal cell carcinoma. *Br J Dermatol*, 159, pp. 35-48, *ISSN*: 1365-2133

Ting, PT.; Kasper, R. & Arlette, JP. (2005). Metastatic basal cell carcinoma: report of two cases and literature review. *J Cutan Med Surg*, 9, pp. 10-15, *SSN* (printed): 1203-4754. *ISSN* (electronic): 1615-7109.

Torres, A.; Niemeyer, A. & Berkes, B. (2004). Treatment of basal cell carcinoma using imiquimod 5% cream as an adjuvant therapy to Mohs micrographic surgery. *J Eur Acad Dermatol Venereol*, 30, 12 Pt 1, 1462-1469, *SSN* (printed): 0926-9959. *ISSN* (electronic): 1468-3083

Tsuji, T.; Otake, N. & Nishimura, M. (1993). Cryosurgery and topical fluorouracil: a treatment method for widespread basal cell epithelioma in basal cell nevus syndrome. *J Dermatol*, 20, pp. 507–513, *ISSN*: 1346-8138

Tucker, SB.; Polasek, JW.; Perri, AJ. & Goldsmith, EA. (2006). Long-term follow-up of basal cell carcinomas treated with perilesional interferon alfa 2b as monotherapy. *J Am Acad Dermatol*, 54, 6, pp. 1033–1038, *ISSN*:0190-9622

Tzellos, T.; Kyrgidis, A.; Vahtsevanos, K.; Triaridis, S.; Printza, A.; Klagas, I.; Zvintzou, E.; Kritis, A.; Karakiulakis, G. & Papakonstantinou, E. (2011). Nodular basal cell carcinoma is associated with increased hyaluronan homeostasis. *J Eur Acad Dermatol Venereol*, 25, 6, pp. 679-687, *ISSN* (printed): 0926-9959. *ISSN* (electronic): 1468-3083

Varga, E.; Korom, I.; Raskó, Z.; Kis, E.; Varga, J.; Oláh, J. & Kemény, L. (2011). Neglected Basal cell carcinomas in the 21st century. *J Skin Cancer*, 2011: 392151

Von Domarus, H. & Stevens, PJ. (1984). Metastatic basal cell carcinoma. Report of five cases and review of 170 cases in the literature. *J Am Acad Dermatol*, 10, 6, pp. 1043-1060, *ISSN*:0190-9622

Wadhera, A.; Fazio, M.; Bricca, G. & Stanton, O. (2006). Metastatic basal cell carcinoma: a case report and literature review. How accurate is our incidence data?. *Dermatol Online J*, 12, pp. 7, *ISSN*:1087-2108 (Electronic) ; 1087-2108 (Linking)

Walling, HW.; Fosko, SW.; Geraminejad, PA.; Whitaker, DC. & Arpey, CJ. (2004). Aggressive basal cell carcinoma: Presentation, pathogenesis, and management. *Cancer*

Metastasis, 23, 3-4, pp. 389-402, *ISSN* (printed): 0167-7659. *ISSN* (electronic): 1573-7233

Wetzig, T.; Maschke, J.; Kendler, M. & Simon, JC. (2009). Treatment of basal cell carcinoma. *J Dtsch Dermatol Ges,* 7, pp. 1075-1082, *ISSN*:1610-0379 (Print); 1610-0387 (Electronic); 1610-0379

Wetzig, T.; Woitek, M.; Eichhorn, K.; Simon, JC. & Paasch, U. (2010). Surgical excision of basal cell carcinoma with complete margin control: outcome at 5-year follow-up. *Dermatology,* 220, pp. 363-369, *ISSN* 1018-8665

Wong, CS.; Strange, RC. & Lear, JT. (2003). Basal cell carcinoma. *British Medical Journal,* 327, pp. 794-798, *ISSN*: *09598138*

Wood, LD. & Ammirati, CT. (2011). An overview of mohs micrographic surgery for the treatment of basal cell carcinoma. *Dermatol Clin,* 29, pp. 153-160, *ISSN*: 0738-081X (Print) 1879-1131 (Electronic)

Wu, JK.; Oh, C.; Strutton, G. & Siller G. (2006). An open-label, pilot study examining the efficacy of curettage followed by imiquimod 5% cream for the treatment of primary nodular basal cell carcinoma. *Australas J Dermatol,* 47, pp. 46-48, *ISSN*:0004-8380

Youssef, KK.; Van Keymeulen, A.; Lapouge, G.; Beck, B.; Michaux, C. & Achouri, Y. (2010). Identification of the cell lineage at the origin of basal cell carcinoma. *Nat Cell Biol.* 12, pp. 299-305, ISSN 1097-6256

4

An Overview on Basal Cell Carcinoma

Gulden Avci
Canakkale Onsekiz Mart University, Faculty of Medicine
Turkey

1. Introduction

Basal cell carcinoma (BCC), first described by Jacob in the early 1800(1), is the most common cancer in the general population, accounting for 80% of nonmelanoma skin cancer (2). Worldwide incidence is increasing by about 10% per annum, so the prevalence of BCC will soon equal that of all other cancers combined(3). The average lifetime risk for white skinned individuals to develop BCC is approximately 30 %(4). BCC is uncommon in dark skinned races. Studies have estimated that 1.2% to 4.6% of BCCs arise in black patients (5). BCC is more common in men than in women (ratio of approximately 2:1). BCC most commonly occurs in older than 50 years old (6). Interestingly, women younger than 40 years of age have been found to slightly outnumber men in this age group (7). The increased incidence rates could be attributed to changes in sunbathing behavior in the young and the middleaged, which has changed during the 20th century. Particularly after the Second World War, more people had leisure time for outdoor activities. Also, women's clothing changed allowing larger parts of the body to be exposed to the sun (8).

2. Etiology

The etiology of BCC is still unclear but appears to be of multifactorial origin, resulting from a complex interaction of both intrinsic and extrinsic factors(Table 1).

Extrinsic factors	**Intrinsic factors**
intermittent'' sun exposure during childhood or teenage years	Increasing age
ingestion of arsenic acid (medicine, pesticides),	Positive family history
ionizing radiation	gender (male predominantly)
X-ray and grenz-ray exposure	Fitzpatrick skin type I-type2
low vitamin intake	Red or blond hair
high dietary energy, especially from fats	light eye color (blue or green eyes)
topical nitrogen mustard administration	immunosuppression
thermal burns	Genodermatoses (albinism, xeroderma pigmentosa, Rasmussen syndrome, Rombo syndrome, Bazex–Christol–Dupre syndrome, albinism and Darier's disease, and the naevoid BCC syndrome (Gorlin's syndrome))
Psoralen and UVA (PUVA) treatment	posttransplantation
scars, draining sinuses, ulcers, burn sites and foci of chronic inflammation	

Table 1. Risk factors for basal cell carcinoma.

UV radiation (UVR), and especially UVB, is responsible for the majority of cutaneous damage and is believed to be the primary established risk factor in the development of BCC (9,10). The role of "intermittent" sun exposure during childhood or teenage years (periods that are supposed to be critical for tumor development) appears to be of particular importance and has been shown to be a strong risk factor for BCC. The infrequent, intense and intermittent sun exposure during childhood and adolescence, especially before the age of 20, increases the risk of BCC more than if a similar dose was delivered more continuously over the same time period (11). Increased risk of nodular, but not superficial BCC, has been reported in association with occupational sun exposure, Moreover, a strong association has been shown between BCC and skin lesions that are "objective" markers of cumulative sun exposure (whether long-term or intense intermittent), such as actinic keratoses and solar lentigines, which result from a combined effect of sun exposure and skin pigmentation characteristics (12, 13, 14). UVR especially prior to the age of 20 years is suggested to initiate a process of basal cell carcinogenesis (15). UVR has two major effects that influence BCC development, namely DNA damage and immunosuppression (16). Exposure to UVR, specifically UVB, induces covalent bonds in DNA between adjacent pyrimidines, generating photoproducts such as cyclodipyrimidine dimers (T /T) and pyrimidine lesions which are mutagenic if not repaired. Unlike UVB, UVA may have more indirect effects in DNA through ROS (17). UVR is also a local immunosuppressant in skin, giving rise to the suggestion that this may compromise local antitumour activity. Exposure to UVR results in a cascade of events including a T-lymphocyte-mediated immunosupression (18). Burning and tanning response of skin (skin type) is important in determining BCC risk. BCCs are more common in males and those with skin types 1 and 2 demonstrate an increased susceptibility with relative risks between 4.0. and 2.1 (19, 20).

In sporadic BCC, DNA repair capacity below the upper 30th percentile was associated with a 2-3-fold increase in BCC relative risk. However, some studies have reported increased repair in BCC patients and so batch variability and the effects of age, family history of skin cancer and current sun exposure may confound results (21).

The incidence rates of BCC are increasing each year. These trends may be due to increases in both acute and prolonged sun exposure (due to altered life style and pro-tanning behavior), and the depletion of stratospheric ozone, together with the increasing aging of the general population (22). Similar to melanoma and in contrast to SCC, sporadic BCC may occur in individuals with intermittent extreme UV exposure behavior (11, 23).

Other extrinsic risk factors, beyond UVR, predisposing to BCC, include ingestion of arsenic acid (medicine, pesticides), ionizing radiation, X-ray and grenz-ray exposure, low vitamin intake, high dietary energy, especially from fats, topical nitrogen mustard administration and thermal burns. Psoralen and UVA (PUVA) treatment, classically for psoriasis, carries a modest increased risk. Constitutional factors include gender, age, immunosuppression and genetic predisposition (a family history of BCC, genetically inherited nucleotide excision repair defects such as xeroderma pigmentosum) . Also, pigmentary traits, such as fair skin, blond or red hair, light eye color, tendency to sunburn and poor tanning ability (skin Type I), have all been associated with a higher risk of BCC (22-24). Fitzpatrick skin type I (always burns, never tans), male gender, red or blond hair and blue or green eyes have been shown to be associated with increased risk of BCC development. Several genodermatoses are associated with the development of BCC, including albinism, xeroderma pigmentosa, Rasmussen syndrome, Rombo syndrome, Bazex–Christol–Dupre syndrome, albinism and

Darier's disease, and the naevoid BCC syndrome (Gorlin's syndrome) (25). These syndromes variably either decrease epidermal pigmentation and thus increase the risk of UV light-induced oncogenic transformation or promote genotypic instability in the epidermis.(26) Nevoid BCC syndrome (NBCCS) is linked to chromosome 9q22, which harbours the PTCH gene where activating germline mutations have been found in BCC tissue (27, 28). Somatic PTCH mutation has also been described in sporadic BCC (29, 30). Dysregulation of the PTCH pathway is thought to be a critical event in BCC development. The tumour suppressor gene (TSG) p53, involved in genome surveillance through the regulation of cell proliferation and death, is frequently inactivated in BCC (31, 32) with up to 56% of tumours displaying mutation in the conserved region of one p53 allele. Indeed, it has been suggested that p53 mutation is a crucial but late event in BCC progression (33).

BCC may, like squamous cell carcinoma, arise in the setting of scars, draining sinuses, ulcers, burn sites and foci of chronic inflammation(15). The incidence of BCC arising from chronic wounds is low, and as few as 2.4% of malignancies develop from chronic leg ulcers(34). The role of immune compromise in provoking an increased risk of BCC may be due to impairment of the immune surveillance of oncogenic viruses. Immunosuppressive therapy also increases risk (ten-16 fold in renal transplant recipients) (35). BCC is the second most common cancer among solid organ transplant recipient(SOTR). The peak incidence rate was 5 years posttransplantation for patients older than 50 and 8 to 10 years for younger patients. Of the various organs transplanted, liver engraftment may bestow greater risk for BCC than others. BCCs in SOTR more often affected younger males and were more likely to present in sun-protected or bizarre locations, such as genitalia, external auditory meatus, and axilla. Lesions developed sooner after heart transplantation (5.7 years) than after renal transplantation (8.1 years). Renal transplant recipients with BCCs were more often younger and male compared to controls. Lesions were more commonly multifocal but not more likely to recur or metastasize. The mean time to tumor development was 10.5 years (36, 37).

3. Clinicopathologic aspects of BCC

The typical BCC is a pearly pink or flesh colored papule with telangiectasia. Lesions may be translucent or slightly erythematous with a rolled border, occasionally accompanied by bleeding, scaling or crusting(Fig. 1). Aggressive growth tumors tend to show more frequent ulceration and large, untended neoplasms can be locally destructive of eyes, ears and nares (38). BCCs are usually slow-growing tumors that only rarely metastasize (39). Growth of BCCs is usually localized to the area of origin; however, some BCCs tend to infiltrate tissues in a three-dimensional fashion through the irregular growth of finger-like projections, which may not be obvious on visual inspection (40, 41). If left untreated, or inadequately treated, the BCC can cause extensive tissue destruction, particularly on the face(Fig. 2). The clinical course of BCC is unpredictable; it may remain small for years, or it may grow rapidly or proceed by successive spurts of extension of tumor and partial regression (42). Thus, early prompt treatment is essential to minimize the morbidity of both cancer and treatment. Eighty percent of BCCs appear on the head and neck compared to 15% on the trunk and 5% on the extremities "larger lesions" are also more likely to be located in areas of the body other than the face where patients do not notice or complain about them as early (43).

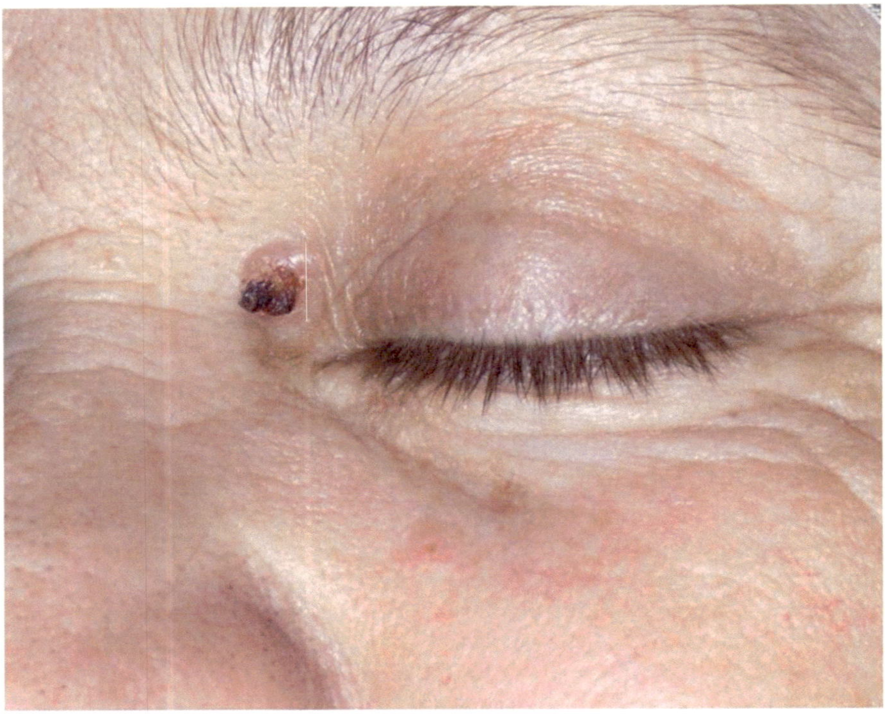

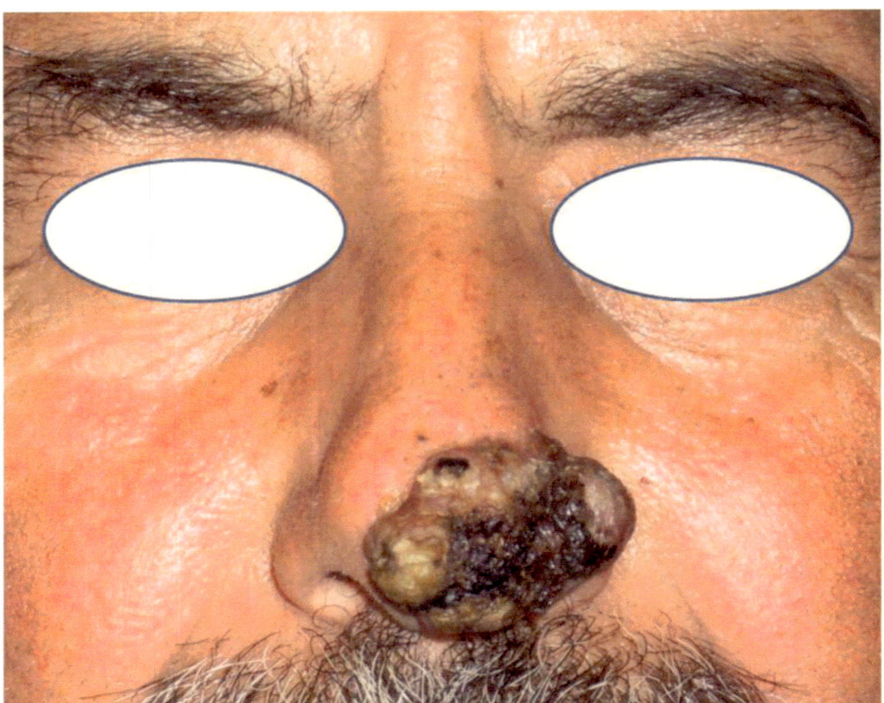

A BCC can usually be diagnosed on the clinical aspect, but histological confirmation is necessary to determine the best treatment option. Although 26 histological subtypes have been described(44), BCC subtypes were categorized based upon the histologic classifications of Lang and Maize(45), Sexton and colleagues(46) and Kirkham(47): (1) those with nonaggressive growth patterns (superficial, nodular, and adnexal, such as follicular) or (2) those with aggressive growth patterns (keratinizing, micronodular, infiltrating, sclerosing, and perineural) or (3) both.

The three most common tumor subtypes are nodular (nBCC), superficial (sBCC), and morpheaform. In a large, retrospective analysis of 13,457 cases of BCC diagnosed at a single center from 1967 to 1996, 79% of BCCs were nodular, 15% were superficial, and 6% were morpheaform In addition, nodular and morpheaform types were most commonly observed on the head region (90% and 95%, respectively), whereas 46% of superficial types were observed on the trunk region. (48)

3.1 Nonaggresive BCC

Nodular BCC is the most common variety and is usually composed of one or a few small, waxy, semitranslucent a flesh-to-pearl-colored papule with a characteristic rolled border that sometimes form around a central depression. Central ulceration and overlying telangiectases are also cardinal features(Fig. 3) (49).

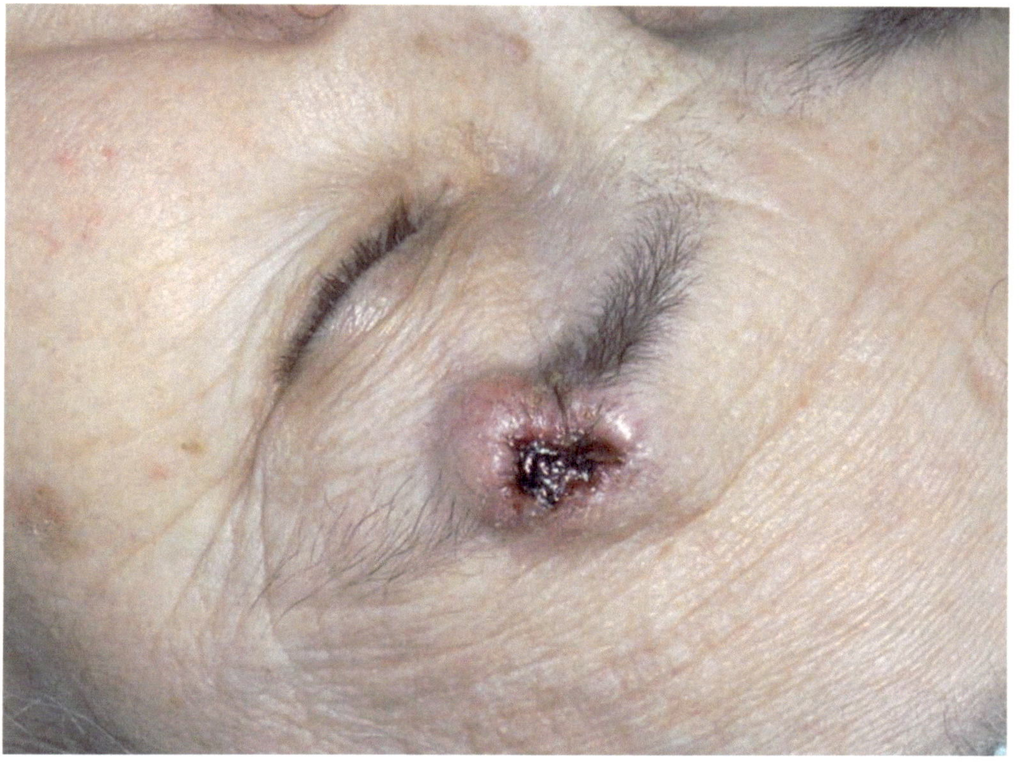

Superficial BCC (sBCC) is often larger than other subtypes and occurs mainly on the trunk where they can be multiple. Superficial BCC may mimic psoriasis, fungus, or eczema. The superficial variant of BCC presents as an enlarging erythematous plaque with mild scale and a scalloped border(Fig. 4).

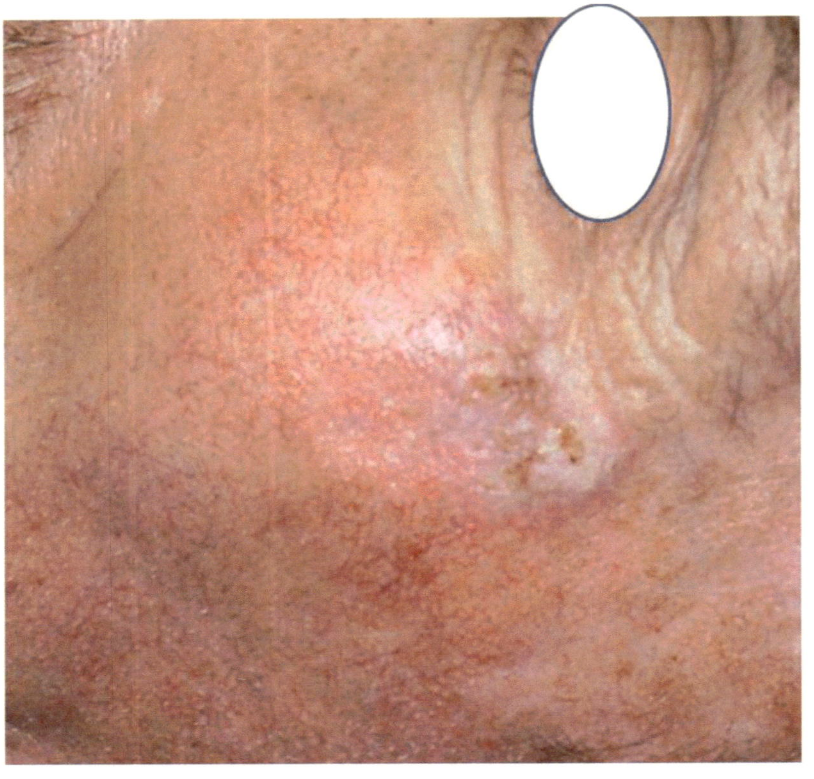

Pigmented HNBCC are seen more commonly in darkskinned individuals and can mimic a mole or even a melanoma. BCCs may also demonstrate hyperpigmenation, leading to confusion with melanoma in some cases(Fig. 5).
Cystic HNBCC are filled with fluid and may mimic benign cystic lesions, especially around the eye(50).

3.2 Aggressive BCC

This subgroup included BCCs with keratinizing, micronodular, infiltrating, sclerosing, and basosquamous carcinoma (51).
A scar-like or *morpheaform* variant of BCC may appear as depressed, indurated plaque with ill-defined margins.
BCCs with follicular pattern demonstrate basaloid nodular islands of tumor cells in association with a hair follicle; in addition, the tumor epithelium and surrounding stroma form structures reminiscent of follicular germs or contain horn cyst formation resembling a follicular structure or both.

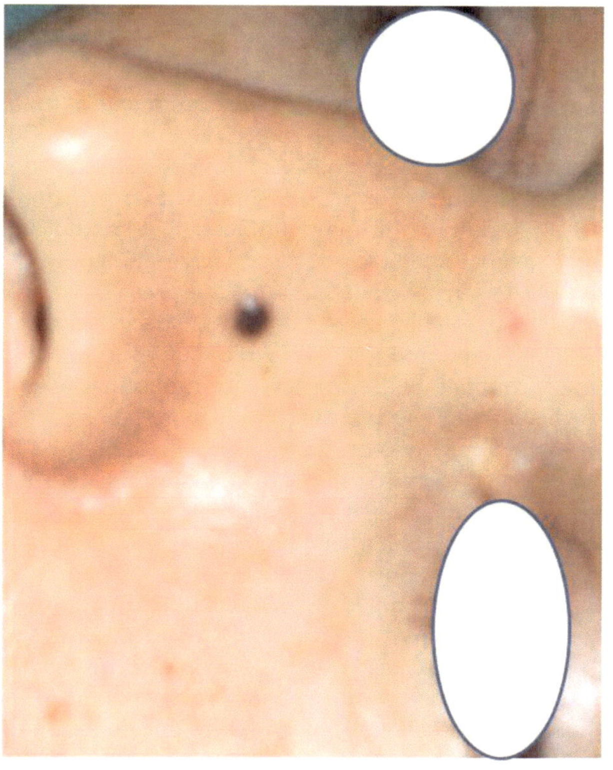

Keratinizing BCCs show nodules of basaloid tumor cells which have a central foci of large horn cysts or pronounced squamous differentiation with keratinization or both; in addition to the undifferentiated basaloid tumor cells, parakeratotic tumor cells with elongated nuclei and slightly eosinophilic cytoplasm may also be present as strands, as concentric whorls, or as cells around the horn cysts.

Basosquamous carcinoma is a subtype of BCC with aggressive behavior and higher tendency for recurrence and metastases. Most authors recognize that basosquamous carcinoma has a nonspecific clinical presentation and the diagnosis is made only after biopsy. The majority of lesions arise on the head and neck (80%) with the central face and perinasal areas being the most common locations (30%). The location of tumors is similar to other types of BCC. The term "basosquamous carcinoma" usually implies a BCC with areas of lineage differentiation into squamous cell carcinoma (52). This tumor has areas of BCC and squamous cell carcinoma plus a transition zone between them. The reported incidence of basosquamous carcinoma ranges from 1.2% to 2.7%. Published recurrence rates are 12% to 51% for surgical excision and 4% for Mohs micrographic surgery. The incidence of metastasis is at least 5%. The aggressive biological behavior and clinical course distinguish basosquamous carcinoma from other forms of BCC. Pulmonary metastases occurred in 7.4% of basosquamous carcinomas compared with 0.87% of squamous cell carcinomas. The incidence of perineural invasion was 7.9%. There are no clinical features to distinguish basosquamous carcinoma and the diagnosis is made only after biopsy. It presents in the same locations and with similar clinical characteristics as other BCCs (53).

3.3 BCC with mixed histology

BCC with mixed histology (BCC-MH) is a cutaneous neoplasm which demonstrates two or more pathologic patterns of tumor within the same malignancy, such as superficial BCC in the papillary dermis and sclerosing BCC in the deeper reticular dermis (1-6). The incidence of BCCs with mixed histology is varied between 11% and 43% (54). BCC with mixed histology is most commonly found on the nose, followed by the ear, cheek, and scalp. This is not surprising as the most frequently reported site for either primary or recurrent BCCs is the nose (55, 56). BCCs with mixed histology (almost 40%) should be treated according to their most aggressive histopathological subtype. Shave/punch biopsy specimens fail to diagnose one of both subtypes in approximately 20% of cases (1).

The different histomorphologic subgroups have their specific clinical correlates. On rare occasions, a lesion manifests tenderness or pain which can be a clue to perineural infiltration in the aggressive growth varieties. Sensorimotor compromise has been reported particularly in lesions of the preauricular and cheek areas (57). Tumor aggressiveness seems to correlate with the presence of perineural invasion that has an incidence of 1% in BCC. Perineural spread is a well-documented feature of cutaneous tumors and may portend a more aggressive course: perineural invasion is associated with larger, more aggressive tumors, and the risk of 5-year recurrence is higher (58). The choice and the selection of the most appropriate therapy depend on many factors, including the size of the tumor, location, whether the tumor is primary or recurrent, histology, and individual patient factors.

Documentation of the specific anatomical location, size in millimeters, and appearance of the cutaneous neoplasm is helpful, as it may be required for later staging. Appearance includes such characteristics as color, margins, symmetry, diameter, and the presence of ulceration. Such features include size greater than 2 cm, location on the central face or ears, long duration, perineural or perivascular invasion, and poorly defined margins. Histologically, morpheaform, metatypical, and infiltrative growth patterns associate with poorer clinical outcomes (59). The ABCD (asymmetry, border, color, and diameter) mnemonic used in melanoma is helpful here too. Many surgeons find photographic documentation of lesions an accurate and speedy means of mapping lesions. Metastatic spread of BCC is very rare, but it is not impossible. Accordingly, palpation of the regional lymph nodes is indeed a mandatory part of the complete workup (60, 61).

4. Metastatic disease

BCCs very rarely metastasize, occurring in 0.0025% to 0.55% of cases (62). Metastatic BCC generally tends to occur on a background of large neglected tumors on the head and neck, mainly in men Metastases most are said to more closely correlate to the size and depth and less so to the histologic subtype of the original tumor. The incidence of metastases and/or death is said to correlate to large tumors greater than 3 cm in diameter in which setting patients are said to have a 1–2% risk of metastases that increases to up to 20–25% in lesions greater than 5 cm and up to 50% in lesions greater than 10cm in diameter. A 'giant' BCC is designated as one that is greater than 5 cm in diameter and has a significant risk of morbidity and mortality. A BCC arising in a young person (ie less than 35 years of age) may have an aggressive clinical course (63, 64).

When metastatic spread occurs, regional lymph nodes are affected first followed by bone, lung, liver and abdominal viscera.. An BCC that metastasizes has an extremely poor prognosis;, the median survival of patients with metastatic BCC is about 10 months. There is less than 20% survival at 1 year and approximately 10% survival at 5 years (65). Occasionally surgical resection of metastatic disease is possible; cases should be referred to specialist centers for full assessment (66).

5. Other malignancies

The risk of developing a squamous cell carcinoma is increased slightly after developing a BCC (6% risk at 3 years) and there is also a higher risk of developing a malignant melanoma. The relationship of development of other malignancy after development of a BCC is uncertain - some studies have shown a small increased risk with cancer of the lung, thyroid, mouth, breast and cervix and non-Hodgkin's lymphoma, whilst others have shown no association (67).

6. Treatment

The choice for a treatment modality should depend on the site, the size and whether the BCC shows indolent (superficial or nodular BCC) or aggressive growth (infiltrative BCC or basosquamous carcinoma) (5, 8). Careful selection is essential and depends upon individual factors. A biopsy of the lesion prior to definitive treatment can help guide choice. Essentially, the method chosen should take into account the prognostic factors for the tumour under consideration, local facilities available, operator expertise and any comorbidity. Several different modalities are used in the treatment of BCC (1, 50) (Table 2).

Anatomical location	central face or ears
Tumour size	greater than 2 cm
Histological type	morpheaform, metatypical, and infiltrative
Perineural/ perivascular invasion	portend a more aggressive course
Recurrence	scar tissue can cover residual tumour,
Treatment failure	A decrease in resection margin increases the recurrence rate. The optimal resection margin in terms of recurrence is 5 mm
Immunocompromised patients	more aggressive biologic behavior, higher recurrence rate

Table 2. Prognostic factors for BCC

Invasive	**Non -invasive**
Excision	Photodynamic therapy
Mohs' micrographic surgery	Radiotherapy
Curettage and cautery	Chemotherapy :• 5-fluorouracil • imiquimod
Cryosurgery	

Table 3. Treatment options for basal cell carcinoma.

7. Surgery

This method requires that normal tissue surrounding the tumor margins be removed in addition to diseased tissue to ensure that the tumor has been fully excised. BCC lesions are resected with a preplanned size of surgical margin depending on the surgeon preference, the location, and the size of the lesion. The goal is to safely predict appropriate margins of resection of BCC lesions while sacrificing a minimum amount of healthy surrounding skin. Although surgical excision is a common method for treating BCC, there are important safety and quality of life, Patient age and health status (e.g. immunocompromized) may increase associated risks with a surgical procedure including bleeding and infection. In addition, some patients are afraid of surgery, particularly when treating larger.

An advantage of surgical treatments is the histological examination of tumor margins to establish clearance. One disadvantage of surgical excision is incomplete margin control. The incidence of incomplete excision of BCC has varied, with reports ranging from 4.7% to 10.8% of treated patients (68, 69). The success of surgical excision can vary depending on the experience of the surgeon, histologic subtype, and excision margin (70). In a retrospective cohort analysis of 1983 BCC cases, significant risk factors for incomplete excision included lesions located on the head and neck ($P < 0.001$), surgeons performing < 51 procedures during the 2- year study period ($P < 0.001$), and patients with aggressive histologic BCC subtypes (e.g. morpheaform and infiltrative) ($P < 0.01$). The study further indicated that curettage before surgical excision of BCC decreased the incomplete excision rate by up to 24% ($P = 0.03$) (71).

A decrease in resection margin increases the recurrence rate. Relative risk of recurrence increases steadily. The relative risks (hazard ratio) for 4-, 3-, and 2-mm margins are 4.2, 6.5, and 10, respectively. It is clear that smaller margins are inherently riskier than larger ones, even if the difference is 1 mm. the reported mean recurrence rates decrease linearly with increasing size of margins until it reaches 5 mm. The optimal resection margin in terms of recurrence is 5 mm.(72)

Consistently, relative risk is inversely proportional to the size of the surgical margin. Using this criterion alone, the best margin in terms of relative recurrence is a 5-mm margin. However, the anatomical constraints require prejudice in choosing the resection margins, especially for lesions of the face. Thus, for those surgeons who desire a minimum 95 percent cure rate, these data indicate that a 3-mm surgical margin can be safely used for BCC lesions 2 cm or smaller. Furthermore, a positive pathologic margin has a mean recurrence rate of 27 percent and thus does not necessarily indicate that a BCC will recur. Thus, when faced with a positive surgical margin, a case-by-case consideration of the risks of observation versus reresection should be applied when determining the next step in management (72).

A study using MMS for excising primary (ie previously untreated BCC) found that for small (<20 mm) well defined tumours 3 mm surgical margins gave tumour clearance rates of 85%, whereas 4–5 mm margins gave clearance rates of 95%. Large and morphoeic BCCs require wider margins to achieve complete histological resection (13–15 mm surgical margins for 95% clearance) (73).

7.1 Mohs micrographic surgery

Mohs micrographic surgery (MMS) is a specialized surgical procedure that is commonly used for patients who present with large (> 2 cm) tumors, high-risk morphea-type BCC tumors, recurrent tumors, or tumors located in cosmetically sensitive locations such as the face (74). But Mohs' micrographic surgery (MMS) is a specialised technique that uses horizontal frozen sectioning to examine serial sections of tissue until all margins are free of tumour. MMS allows for greater tissue conservation and margin control compared with other surgical procedures. This technique histologically maps the margins of the tumor to more accurately delineate the pattern of tumor infiltration into tissue, while sparing healthy tissue. MMS gives high cure rates for tumours in high-risk sites with maximal conservation of uninvolved tissue. The suggested overall 5-year cure rates for primary and recurrent BCC are 99% and 94.4%, respectively (75, 76).

7.2 Curettage and electrodesiccation

Electrodesiccation and curettage (ED & C) is the most common method used by dermatologists to treat primary nBCC and sBCC tumors < 1.5 cm in diameter. After the tumor is scraped with a curette, the area is then treated with electrosurgery (electrodesiccation or coagulation) to control bleeding and eradicate cancer cells remaining around the wound margins and circumference. Typically two or three treatment cycles are recommended to completely remove the tumor (77). Recurrence rates are varied between 3% to 19%im 5 years (78). Recurrence was higher in nasal, paranasal, and forehead areas (78). Although ED & C appears to have a higher risk for disease recurrence compared with surgical excision, a nonrandomized retrospective chart review suggested that the two treatment modalities are not significantly different (79). If the dermis and the fatty layer is penetrated with ED & C, surgical excision should be performed.Although multiple cycles of ED & C are recommended, there have been reports that single-cycle therapy may reduce the risk of scarri(74). However, a reduction in ED & C treatment cycles may lead to higher recurrence rates. 32(80) Atrophic or hypertropic scar can be develop after ED & C (78). Problematic wounds, with subsequent poor cosmesis, are occasional sequelae.

7.3 Cryosurgery

Cryosurgery is a cytodestructive technique that involves using a liquid nitrogen spray or probe to induce cell necrosis by exposing tissue to low temperatures. Cryosurgery is commonly reserved for tumors with welldefine borders, and two freeze–thaw cycles with a tissue temperature of - 50 °C are recommended. 6. (74) two freeze–thaw cycles of 30 s each are still recommended in the treatment of facial BCC. A systematic review of recurrence rates of studies (≥ 50 patients) published between 1970 and 1997 indicated that cryotherapy in the treatment of primary BCC resulted in a cumulative 5-year recurrence rate of 4% to 17%(81). For treatment of recurrent BCC, the recurrence rate has ranged from 4% (for 56 tumors) to 12% (for 164 tumors), with variable follow-up periods reported (82, 83). Cryosurgery is associated with many adverse events. Shortterm adverse events include perioperative and postoperative pain, tenderness, bulla or vesicle formation, erythema, sloughing of necrotic tissue or eschar formation, and localized edema (84). This procedure can also result in scarring including hypertrophic scarring, local hypopigmentation, and/or peripheral hyperpigmentation (84). When aggressive cryosurgery is used, tumor recurrence may become extensive before diagnosis because of the tumor's concealment by a fibrous scar (74). Cryosurgery should be avoided in areas of hair growth (e.g. scalp or beard area) and in patients with conditions sensitive to temperature, including Raynaud's syndrome, cold panniculitis, and cryoglobulinemia.

8. Photodynamic therapy

Photodynamic therapy (PDT), which uses the intrinsic cellular haem biosynthetic pathway and photo illumination to initiate tumour cell destruction, is a relatively new treatment for superficial BCCs, which is increasingly available for superficial non-melanoma skin cancers.

After topical application, precursor molecules are selectively concentrated in tumour tissue where they undergo further metabolism. After irradiation by visible light of a certain wavelength, these molecules become excited and jump to a higher energy level. Upon release of this energy, reactive oxygen species are released; these cause cellular destruction, and so resolution of the tumour - without scarring. (It is thought that, fundamentally, holes are punched into cellular organelles, especially mitochondria, so the cells can no longer function.). This procedure causes cell death in two ways: through cellular damage and apoptosis. Several studies have indicated that sBCC lesions do not clear with single-treatment PDT The best clearance rate (96% median follow up, 27 months).) is achieved with two exposures 1 week apart. PDT offers patients with large and/or multiple superficial BCCs particular benefits as it gives a low rate of adverse events with good cosmetic results by selectively targeting tumour cells (3).
Although one advantage of PDT is that multiple BCC tumors can be treated simultaneously, PDT is a relatively inconvenient treatment option. Treatment involves a two stage process requiring several office visits. After the topical agent is applied, patients must wait several hours before the light-application phase of the treatment can be initiated. This second-stage of treatment must be performed within a certain time frame after agent application. Furthermore, because single PDT treatments demonstrate poor efficacy in BCC, multiple visits to a healthcare provider's office are required. Increased photosensitivity during the first-stage of treatment provides additional inconvenience because patients must avoid sunlight and bright indoor lighting to reduce the risk of stinging and/or burning sensations from photosensitized skin. Treatment with PDT is typically associated with localized adverse events, including stinging or burning, erythema, and edema (85). Photosensitivity is also associated with this treatment regimen. After application of topical agents, patients should avoid exposure to sunlight or bright indoor light until after controlled exposure to the light source that completes treatment. Treatment with PDT is contraindicated in patients with porphyria, known allergies to porphyrins, and patients with photosensitivity to wave lengths of applied light sources. Further development of PDT for BCC will likely make this a more practical and useful modality (86).

9. Radiotherapy

Radiotherapy is an effective treatment for many BCCs. It has been particularly useful in the treatment of elderly patients and for larger tumors or tumors in difficult-to treat locations. Lower risk areas, such as the trunk and extremities, as well as the genitalia, hands, and feet are usually not treated with this modality. Radiation therapy may be a very useful modality as adjunct treatment for BCC when margins are positive after excision and for extensive perineural or large nerve involvement. The total dose and treatment regimen (e.g. number of fractionated doses) depends on many factors including tumor location, size, type, and depth. A study of BCC irradiated by a 'standardized' X-ray therapy schedule indicated an overall 5-year recurrence rate of 7.4% for primary (n = 862) and 9.5% for recurrent (n = 211) BCC. Radiation therapy is not recommended in younger patients (e.g. < 50 years of age) as less favorable cosmetic outcomes (e.g. late-onset changes of cutaneous atrophy and telangiectasia) may result over time, and there is a risk of developing additional nonmelanoma skin cancers in the radiation field (usually after 10–20 years) (87). Radiation therapy is contraindicated in certain genetic disorders, which predisposes patients to skin cancers (e.g. patients with Gorlin's syndrome, xeroderma pigmentosum, or connective tissue diseases, such as lupus and scleroderma)(88).

10. Chemotherapy of BCC

10.1 Topical 5-Fluorouracil

Topical 5-fluorouracil cream is useful for low-risk tumours on the trunk and limbs, but there is a high incidence of local side effects. 5-Fluorouracil (5-FU) is a chemical ablative agent that inhibits DNA synthesis, prevents cell proliferation, and causes tumor necrosis. Solution and cream formulations of 5% 5- FU administered twice daily for at least 6 weeks have been approved by the FDA in the treatment of sBCC when conventional methods are impractical (e.g. difficult treatment site). 47However, therapy may be required for as long as 10–12 weeks. Because limited data are available, the actual clearance rate for the topical treatment of sBCC with 5-FU is currently unknown. Application of 5-FU causes severe local skin reactions, including pain and burning, pruritus, irritation, inflammation, swelling, tenderness, hyperpigmentation, and scarring. (48)

10.2 Imiquimod

Imiquimod is a member of a newer class of agents called immune-response modifiers. Imiquimod is currently approved by the FDA in the treatment of external genital and perianal warts and actinic keratosis on the face or scalp. The mechanism of action of imiquimod is thought to occur through the activation of macrophages and other cells via binding to cellsurface receptors, such as Toll-like receptor (89). This binding activity induces proinflammatory cytokine secretion (e.g.interferon- α and tumor necrosis factor-α) favoring a type 1 helper T-cell-mediated immune response because of the generation of cytotoxic effector cells Investigators noted a significant correlation between the histologic clearance rate and severity of local skin reactions (i.e. erythema, erosion, and scabbing/crusting) commonly experienced during treatment with imiquimod 5% cream. The data suggested that as the severity of these three local skin reactions increased, there was a greater trend in histologic clearance of sBCC (48).

In addition to sBCC, imiquimod also has demonstrated efficacy in the treatment of nBCC.50,56 (90, 91) Treatment with imiquimod once daily, seven times per week, for either 6 or 12 weeks resulted in nBCC histologic clearance rates of 71% to 76% (90).

Because imiquimod promotes an inflammatory reaction to treat the tumor, treatment is generally associated with mild to- moderate local skin reactions, with severity related to frequency of application (92, 93). In a phase II study, the most common local skin reactions were erythema, crusting, flaking, and erosion (92). However, these dose-related side-effects were generally well tolerated, and none of the patients discontinued because of local skin reactions.

In addition to monotherapy, imiquimod 5% cream may also be useful as adjunctive therapy in the treatment of BCC. Treatment with imiquimod significantly reduced the size of the target tumor and thereby resulted in a smaller cosmetic defect from the MMS excision compared with vehicle. Adjunctive therapy with imiquimod reduced the frequency of residual tumor with ED & C compared with ED & C alone and also appeared to improve cosmetic appearance. These studies suggest that imiquimod 5% cream may be useful as adjunctive therapy in the treatment of nBCC (48).

11. Issues in the treatment of BCC

BCC treatments have many advantages and disadvantages, which depend on many factors, including tumor type, tumor location, cosmetic considerations, and physician and patient convenience. Surgical procedures such as MMS and surgical excision have the lowest 5-year recurrence rates (Table 4). However, effective clearance of BCC tumors with surgical procedures is highly dependent on tumor margins and the skill of the healthcare provider. Thissen *et al.* (81) recommend that surgical excision is preferred over common procedures such as cryosurgery and ED & C, provided surgery is not contraindicated. With PDT, there is limited tissue penetration (i.e. depth), a critical requirement when treating invasive tumors. Mohs micrographic surgery is recommended for larger BCC tumors in high-risk areas of the face and head and for tumors with aggressive growth patterns (81).

Treatment option	Description	5-year recurrence rate, %
Surgical excision	Surgical excision of diseased and surrounding healthy tissue	Complete excision: 3–14 Incomplete excision: 26–42
Curettage and electrodesiccation	Multiple cycles of diseased tissue excision and electrodesiccation to control bleeding and eradicate cancer cells in surrounding margins	3–19
Mohs micrographic surgery	Specialized surgical procedure to maximize excision of diseased tissue and minimize loss of healthy tissue	Primary BCC: 1 Recurrent BCC: 6–10
Cryosurgery	Multiple cycles of cytodestruction (i.e. cell necrosis) of diseased tissue with liquid nitrogen	4–17
Radiation	X-rays or high-energy particles administered in fractionated doses to kill tumor cells	7–10
PDT	Multiple cycles of 2-stage process (photosensitization via topical agent and light exposure) creates cytotoxic reaction in tumor cell	Single cycle: 21–50* Double cycle: 4†

BCC = basal cell carcinoma; PDT = photodynamic therapy; ALA = aminolevulinic acid.
* Projected overall cure rate based on median follow up of 19–35 months.
† Study of 26 lesions with median follow up of 27 months. Data and table from 48th reference.

Table 4. Treatment options and recurrence rates of BCC

12. Recurrency of BCC

The likelihood of BCC recurrence may be influenced by one or more factors(Table 2). In addition to fthe tumor's treatment, the cancer's biologic behavior and the patient's immune status are related to the incidence of tumor recurrence. For example, in immunosuppressed individuals, BCCs not only demonstrate more aggressive biologic behavior but also have a significantly higher recurrence rate as compared with this malignancy in patients who have an intact immune system (94).

The histologic subtype of BCC influences the biologic behavior of the tumor. Recurrent BCCs are commonly associated with a primary cancer that has an aggressive histologic subtype (95-98).

Also, BCCs with aggressive histologic patterns require more aggressive treatment; in addition, when the Mohs micrographic surgical technique is used, a greater number of stages are required to achieve tumor free margins as compared with BCCs without aggressive tumor growth patterns (99).

Inadequate treatment of BCCMH may represent an unsuspected etiology for recurrent skin cancer. For example, an unexpected aggressive pathologic pattern of BCC may not be detected after a superficial biopsy. Subsequently, the cancer may recur if the initial treatment for the diagnosed nonaggressive tumor subtype is inadequate for the undiscovered aggressive carcinoma. Clinical recurrence of cancer results when there has been persistence of the original tumor secondary to inadequate eradication (54). The recurrence rate for BCC lesions with positive margins calculated from the aggregated data is 27 percent (72). The reported percent of BCC recurrence varies depending on the treatment modality (54).

Recurrent BCC (rBCC) is known to be a high-risk tumour with a worse prognosis than primary BCC (50, 59, 76, 100). This may be due to the fact that scar tissue can cover residual tumour fields or because the appearance of basaloid tumour cells in recurrent tumours is frequently squamified, lacy and morpheaform, which may be easily missed in scar tissue (76). The only RCT investigating treatment modalities in rBCC showed that after 5 years of follow-up MMS is the preferred treatment for facial rBCC because of statistically significant lower recurrence rates (101).

Besides tumour characteristics, patient characteristics are of importance when choosing a treatment for an individual. In a few cases where surgery is impossible or undesirable, it may be advantageous to treat a patient with a different, possibly less effective, treatment. Particular management difficulties are posed by recurrent tumours. In general, they are best treated by Mohs' micrographic surgery in high-risk sites and excision elsewhere.

13. References

[1] Crowson AN. Basal cell carcinoma: biology, morphology and clinical implications. Mod Pathol 2006;19(Suppl):127-47

[2] Rubin AI, Chen EH, Ratner D. Basal-cell carcinoma. N Engl J Med 2005;353:2262-9.

[3] Brooke RCC. Basal cell carcinoma *Clin Med* 2005;5:551–4

[4] Dessinioti C, Antoniou C, Katsambas A, Stratigos AJ. Basal Cell Carcinoma: What's New Under the Sun. Photochemistry and Photobiology, 2010, 86: 481–491

[5] Richard R. Jahan-Tigh, Jennifer L. Alston, Melissa Umphlett. Basal cell carcinoma with metastasis to the lung in an African American man. J Am Acad Dermatol 2010 ;63:e87-9.

[6] Harris, R, Griffith K, Moon TE. Trends in the incidence of non-melanoma skin cancers in southeastern Arizona, 1985–86. J. Am. Acad. Dermatol. 2001;45: 528–36.

[7] Hoey SE, Devereux CEJ, Murray L, Catney D, Gavin A, Kumar S, Donnelly D, Dolan OM. () Skin cancer trends in Northern Ireland and consequences for provision of dermatology services. Br. J. Dermatol. 2007; 156:1301–7.

[8] De Vries, E, Louwman M, Bastiaens M, de Gruijl F, Coebergh JW. Rapid and continuous increases in incidence rates of basal cell carcinoma in the southeast Netherlands since 1973. J. Invest. Dermatol. 2004:123;634–8.

[9] Gallagher RP, Lee TK. Adverse effects of ultraviolet radiation: A brief review. Prog. Biophys. Mol. Biol. 2006: 96; 252–261.

[10] Oberyszyn, TM. Non-melanoma skin cancer: Importance of gender, immunosuppressive status and vitamin D. Cancer Lett. 2008;261: 127-136

[11] Kricker, A, Armstrong BK, English DR, Heenan PJ. Does intermittent sun exposure cause basal cell carcinoma: A case-control study in Western Australia. Int. J. Cancer 1995: 60; 489-94.

[12] Walther, U, Kron M, Sander S, Sebastian G, Sander R, Peter RU, Meurer M, Krahn G, Kakel P. Risk and protective factors for sporadic basal cell carcinoma: Results of a two-centre case-control study in southern Germany. Clinical elastosis may be a protective factor. Br. J. Dermatol. 2004;151: 170-8.

[13] Corona, R, Dogliotti E, D'Errico M, Sera F, Iavarone I, Baliva G, Chinni LM, Gobello T, Mazzanti C, Puddu P, Pasquini P. Risk factors for basal cell carcinoma in a Mediterranean population: Role of recreational sun exposure early in life. Arch. Dermatol. 2001;137: 1162-8.

[14] Neale, RE, Davis M, Pandeya N, Whiteman DC, Green AC. Basal cell carcinoma on the trunk is associated with excessive sun exposure. J. Am. Acad. Dermatol. 2007; 56: 380-6.

[15] Goldberg, LH. Basal cell carcinoma. Lancet 1996: 347; 663-7.

[16] Grossman D, Leffell DJ. The molecular basis of nonmelanoma skin cancer. New understanding. Arch. Dermatol. 1997:133; 1263-70.

[17] Madan V, Hoban P, Strange RC, Fryer AA, Lear JT. Genetics and risk factors for basal cell carcinoma British Journal of Dermatology 2006; 154 (Suppl. 1): 5-7.

[18] de Laat JMT, de Gruijl FR. The role of UVA in the aetiology of non-melanoma skin cancer. In: Skin Cancer (Leigh IM, Newton-Bishop JA, Kripke ML, eds), 1st edn. New York: Cold Spring Harbor Laboratory Press 1996; 173-92.

[19] Kricker A, Armstrong BK, English DR, Heenan PJ. Pigmentary and cutaneous risk factors for non-melanocytic skin cancer—a case-control study. Int J Cancer 1991; 48: 650-2.

[20] Lear JT, Tan BB, Smith AG et al. Risk factors for basal cell carcinoma in the United Kingdom: a matched case control study in 806 patients. J Royal Soc Med 1997; 90: 371-4.

[21] Hall J, English DR, Artuso M et al. DNA repair capacity as a risk factor for non-melanocytic skin cancer—a molecular epidemiology study. Int J Cancer 1994; 58: 179-84.

[22] Trakatelli, M, Ulrich C, del Marmol V, Euvrand S, Stockfleth E, Abeni D. Epidemiology of nonmelanoma skin cancer (NMSC) in Europe: Accurate and comparable data are needed for effective public health monitoring and interventions. Br. J. Dermatol. 2007;156(Suppl. 3):1-7.

[23] Zanetti, R., S. Rosso, C. Martinez, C. Navarro, S. Schraub, H.Sancho-Garnier, S. Franscheschi, L. Gafa, E. Perea, M. J. Torno, R. Laurent, C. Schrameck, M. Cristofolini, R. Tumino and J. Wechsler. The multicenter south European study 'Helios'I: Skin characteristics and sunburns in basal cell and squamous cell carcinomas of the skin. Br. J. Cancer 1996; 73: 1440-6.

[24] Green, A, Battistutta D, Hart V, Leslie D, Weedon D. Skin cancer in a subtropical Australian population: Incidence and lack of association with occupation. The Nambour Study Group. Am. J. Epidemiol. 1996; 144: 1034-40.

[25] Carter DM, Lin AN. Basal cell carcinoma. In: Fitzpatrick TM, Eisen AZ, Wolff K, et al (eds). Dermatology in General Medicine, 4th edn. McGraw-Hill: New York, 1993, pp 840-847.

[26] Crowson AN, Magro CM, Kadin M, et al. Differential expression of bcl-2 oncogene in human basal cell carcinoma. Hum Pathol 1996;27:355–9.

[27] Hahn H, Wicking C, Zaphiropoulos PG et al. Mutations of the human holmolog of Drosophila patched in the nevoid basal cell carcinoma syndrome. Cell 1996; 85: 841–51.

[28] Johnson RL, Rothman AL, Xie J et al. Human homolog of patched, a candidate gene for the basal cell nevus syndrome. Science 1996;272: 1668–71.

[29] Azsterbaum M, Rothman A, Johnson RL et al. Identification of mutations in the human PATCHED gene in sporadic basal cell carcinomas and in patients with the basal cell nevus syndrome. J Invest Dermatol 1998; 110: 885–8.

[30] Gailani MR, Stahle-Backdahl M, Leffell DJ et al. The role of the human homologue of drosophila patched in sporadic basal cell carcinomas. Nat Genet 1996; 14: 79–81.

[31] Rady P, Scinicariello F, Wagner RF, Tyring SK. P53 mutations in basal cell carcinomas. Cancer Res 1992; 52: 3084–6.

[32] Ziegler A, Leffell DJ, Kunala S et al. Mutation hotspots due to sunlight in the p53 gene of nonmelanoma skin cancers. Proc Natl Acad Sci USA 1993; 90: 4216–20.

[33] Van der Riet P, Karp D, Farmer E et al. Progression of basal cell carcinoma through loss of chromosome 9q and inactivation of a single p53 allele. Cancer Res 1994; 54: 25–7.

[34] Schnirring-Judge M, Belpedio D. Malignant Transformation of a Chronic Venous Stasis Ulcer to Basal Cell Carcinoma in a Diabetic Patient: Case Study and Review of the Pathophysiology. The Journal of Foot & Ankle Surgery 2010;49: 75–9.

[35] Hartevelt MM, Bavinck JN, Kootte AM, Vermeer BJ, Vandenbroucke JP. Incidence of skin cancer after renal transplantation inThe Netherlands. Transplantation 1990;49: 506–9.

[36] Lindelof B. The epidemiology of skin cancer in organ transplant recipients. In: Otley CC, Stasko T, editors. Skin disease in organ transplantation. New York: Cambridge University Press; 2008. p. 142-6.

[37] Perera GK, Child FJ, Heaton N, O'Grady J, Higgins EM. Skin lesions in adult liver transplant recipients: a study of 100 consecutive patients. Br J Dermatol 2006;154:868-72.

[38] Boyd AS. Tumors of the epidermis. In: Barnhill R, Crowson AN (eds). Textbook of Dermatopathology, 2nd edn. McGraw-Hill Co: New York, 2004, pp 575-634.

[39] Lo JS, Snow SN, Reizner GT, Mohs FE, Larson PO, Hruza GJ. Metastatic basal cell carcinoma: Report of twelve cases with a review of the literature. J Am Acad Dermatol. 1991;24: 715–9.

[40] Miller SJ. Biology of basal cell carcinoma (part 1). J Am Acad Dermatol. 1991;24:1–13

[41] Breuninger H, Dietz K. Prediction of subclinical tumor infiltration in basal cell carcinoma. J Dermatol Surg Oncol.1991;17:574–8.

[42] Franchimont C. Episodic progression and regression of basal cell carcinomas. Br J Dermatol. 1982;106:305–10.

[43] Benjamin Stoff , Catherine Salisbury, Douglas Parker, Fiona O'Reilly Zwald. Dermatopathology of skin cancer in solid organ transplant recipients Transplantation Reviews 2010;24: 172–89.

[44] Klara Mosterd, Aimee H.M.M. Arits, Monique R.T. Thisen and Nicole W.J. Keleners-Smets Histology-based Treatment of Basal Cell Carcinoma .Acta Derm Venereol 2009; 89: 454–8.

[45] Lang PG Jr, Maize JC. Histologic evolution of recurrent basal cell carcinoma and treatment implications. J Am Acad Dermatol 1986;14:186–96.

[46] Sexton M, Jones DB, Maloney ME. Histologic pattern analysis of basal cell carcinoma. Study of a series of 1039 consecutive neoplasms. J Am Acad Dermatol 1990;23:1118–26.

[47] Kirkham N. Tumors and cysts of the epidermis.In: Elder E, Elenitsa SR, Jaworsky C, Johnson B Jr, editors. Lever's histopathology of the skin, 8th ed. Philadelphia: Lippincott-Raven Publishers, 1997. p. 685–746

[48] Ceilley RI, Del Rosso. Current modalities and new advances in the treatment of basal cell carcinoma Int J Dermatol 2006; 45: 489 –98.

[49] Hendrix JD Jr, Parlette HL. Micronodular basal cell carcinoma: a deceptive histologic subtype with frequent clinically undetected tumor extension. Arch Dermatol 1996;132:295-8.

[50] Smeets NW, Kuijpers DI, Nelemans P, Ostertag JU, Verhaegh ME, Krekels GA, et al. Mohs' micrographic surgery for treatment of basal cell carcinoma of the face – results of a retrospective study and review of the literature.Br J Dermatol 2004; 151: 141–7.

[51] Wade JJ. Why classify basal cell carcinomas? Histopathology 1998; 32: 393–8.

[52] Garcia C, Poletti E, Crowson AN. Basosquamous carcinoma J Am Acad Dermatol 2009;60:137-43.

[53] Lopes de FJ. Basal cell carcinoma of the skin with areas of squamous cell carcinoma: a basosquamous cell carcinoma? J Clin Pathol 1985;38:1273-7.

[54] Cohen R, Schulze KE, Nelson BR. Basal Cell Carcinoma with Mixed Histology:A Possible Pathogenesis for Recurrent Skin Cancer PHILIP _ Dermatol Surg 2006;32:542–51

[55] Dixon AY, Lee SH, McGregor DH. Factors predictive of recurrence of basal cell carcinoma. Am J Dermatol 1989;11:222–32.

[56] Bialy TL, Whalen J, Veledar E, Lafreniere D, Spiro J, Chartier T, Chen SC. Mohs micrographic surgery vs traditional surgical excision: a cost comparison analysis. Arch Dermatol 2004;140: 736–42.

[57] Niazi ZBM, Lamberty BGH. Perineural infiltration in basal cell carcinomas. Br J Plast Surg 1993;6:156–7.

[58] Ratner D, Lowe L, Johnson TM, et al. Perineural spread of basal cell carcinomas treated with Mohs micrographic surgery. Cancer 2000;88:1605-16.

[59] Telfer NR, Colver GB, Morton CA. Guidelines for the management of basal cell carcinoma. Br J Dermatol 2008;159:35-48.

[60] Zbar RI, Canady JW. Nonmelanoma Facial Skin Malignancy *Plast. Reconstr. Surg.* 2008;121(1 Suppl):1-9.

[61] von Domarus, H, Stevens, PJ. Metastatic basal cell carcinoma: Report of five cases and review of 170 cases in the literature. *J. Am. Acad. Dermatol.* 1984 ;10:1043-60.

[62] Rubin AI, Chen EH, Ratner D. Basal-cell carcinoma. N Engl J Med 2005;353:2262-9.

[63] Sahl WJ. Basal cell carcinoma: Influence of tumor size on mortality and morbidity. Int J Dermatol 1995;34: 319–21.

[64] Randle HW. Basal cell carcinoma: identification and treatment of the high-risk patient. Dermatol Surg 1996;22:255–61.

[65] Mall J, Ostertag H, MallW, et al. Pulmonary metastasis from a basal-cellcarcinoma of the retroauricular region. Thorac Cardiovasc Surg 1997;45:258-60.

[66] Lo JS, Snow SN, Reizner GT, Mohs FE *et al.* Metastatic basal cell carcinoma: report of twelve cases with a review of the literature. J Am Acad Dermatol 1991;24(5 Pt 1):715–9.

[67] Wong CS, Strange RC, Lear JT. Basal cell carcinoma. Review. BMJ 2003;327:794–8.
[68] Bogdanov-Berezovsky A, Cohen A, Glesinger R, et al. Clinical and pathological findings in reexcision of incompletely excised basal cell carcinomas. Ann Plast Surg 2001; 47: 299–302.
[69] Dieu T, Macleod AM. Incomplete excision of basal cell carcinomas: a retrospective audit. *ANZ J Surg* 2002; 72: 219–21.
[70] Kumar P, Orton CI, McWilliam LJ, *et al.* Incidence of incomplete excision in surgically treated basal cell carcinoma: a retrospective clinical audit. Br J Plast Surg 2000; 53: 563–6.
[71] Chiller K, Passaro D, McCalmont T, et al. Efficacy of curettage before excision in clearing surgical margins of nonmelanoma skin cancer. Arch Dermatol 2000; 136: 1327–32.
[72] Gulleth Y, Goldberg N, Silverman RP, Gastman BR. What Is the Best Surgical Margin for a Basal Cell Carcinoma: A Meta-Analysis of the Literature, Plast. Reconstr. Surg. 2010;126:1222-31.
[73] Wolf DJ, Zitelli JA. Surgical margins for basal cell carcinoma. Arch Dermatol 1987; 123:340–4.
[74] Leffell DJ, Carucci JA. Management of skin cancer. In: DeVita VT Jr, Hellman S, Rosenberg SA, eds. Cancer: Principles and Practice of Oncology, Vol. 2, 6th edn. Philadelphia, PA: Lippincott. Williams & Wilkins, 2001: 1976–2002.
[75] Rowe DE, Carroll RJ, Day CL Jr. Long-term recurrence rates in previously untreated (primary) basal cell carcinoma: implications for patient follow-up. Review. J Dermatol Surg Oncol 1989;15:315–28.
[76] Rowe DE, Carroll RJ, Day CL Jr. Mohs surgery is the treatment of choice for recurrent (previously treated) basal cell carcinoma. J Dermatol Surg Oncol 1989;15: 424–31.
[77] Salasche SJ. Status of curettage and desiccation in the treatment of primary basal cell carcinoma. J Am Acad Dermatol 1984; 10: 285–7.
[78] Silverman MK, Kopf AW, Grin CM et al. Recurrence rates of treated basal cell carcinomas. Part 2: Curettageelectrodesiccation. J Dermatol Surg Oncol 1991; 17: 720- 6.
[79] Werlinger KD, Upton G, Moore AY. Recurrence rates of primary nonmelanoma skin cancers treated by surgical excision compared to electrodesiccation-curettage in a private dermatological practice. Dermatol Surg 2002; 28: 1138–1142; discussion 1142.
[80] Robins P, Albom MJ. Recurrent basal cell carcinomas in young women. J Dermatol Surg 1975; 1: 49–51.
[81] Thissen MR, Neumann MH, Schouten LJ. A systematic review of treatment modalities for primary basal cell carcinomas. Arch Dermatol 1999; 135: 1177–83.
[82] Kuflik EG, Gage AA. Recurrent basal cell carcinoma treated with cryosurgery. J Am Acad Dermatol 1997; 37: 82–4.
[83] Kuflik EG, Cage AA. Cryosurgical Treatment for Skin Cancer. New York: Igaku-Shoin, 1990: 243–54.
[84] Zouboulis CC. Cryosurgery in dermatology. Eur J Dermatol 1998; 8: 466–74.
[85] Wang I, Bendsoe N, Klinteberg CA et al. Photodynamic therapy vs. cryosurgery of basal cell carcinomas: results of a phase III clinical trial. Br J Dermatol 2001; 144: 832–40.

[86] Rhodes LE, de Rie M, Enstrom Y et al. Photodynamic therapy using topical methyl aminolevulinate vs surgery for nodular basal cell carcinoma: results of a multicenter randomized prospective trial. Arch Dermatol 2004; 140: 17–23.

[87] Silverman MK, Kopf AW, Gladstein AH, et al. Recurrence rates of treated basal cell carcinomas. Part 4: X-ray therapy. J Dermatol Surg Oncol. 1992; 18: 549–54.

[88] Martin H, Strong E, Spiro RH. Radiation-induced skin cancer of the head and neck. Cancer 1970; 25: 61–71.

[89] Stanley MA. Imiquimod and the imidazoquinolones. mechanism of action and therapeutic potential. Clin Exp Dermatol 2002; 27: 571–7.

[90] Shumack S, Robinson J, Kossard S, et al. Efficacy of topical 5% imiquimod cream for the treatment of nodular basal cell carcinoma: comparison of dosing regimens. Arch Dermatol 2002; 138: 1165–71.

[91] Sterry W, Ruzicka T, Herrera E, et al. Imiquimod 5% cream for the treatment of superficial and nodular basal cell carcinoma: randomized studies comparing low-frequency dosing with and without occlusion. Br J Dermatol 2002; 147: 1227–36.

[92] Marks R, Gebauer K, Shumack S, et al. Imiquimod 5% cream in the treatment of superficial basal cell carcinoma: results of a multicenter 6-week dose-response trial. J Am Acad Dermatol 2001; 44: 807–13.

[93] Geisse JK, Rich P, Pandya A, et al. Imiquimod 5% cream for the treatment of superficial basal cell carcinoma: a doubleblind, randomized, vehicle-controlled study. J Am Acad Dermatol 2002; 47: 390–98.

[94] Mehrany K, Weenig RH, Pittelkow MR, Roenigk RK, Otley CC. High recurrence rates of basal cell carcinoma after Mohs surgery in patients with chronic lymphocytic leukemia. Arch Dermatol 2004;140: 985–8.

[95] Jacobs GH, Rippey JJ, Altini M. Prediction of aggressive behavior in basal cell carcinoma. Cancer 1982;49:533–7.

[96] Dixon AY, Lee SH, McGregor DH. Histologic evolution of basal cell carcinoma. Am J Dermatopathol 1991;13:241–7.

[97] Dixon AY, Lee SH, McGregor DH. Histologic features predictive of basal cell carcinoma recurrence: results of a multivariate analysis. J Cutan Pathol 1993;20:137–42.

[98] Wrone DA, Swetter SM, Egbert BM, Smoller BR, Khavari PA. Increased proportion of aggressive-growth basal cell carcinoma in the veterans affiars population of Palo Alto, California. J Am Acad Dermatol 1996;35:907–10.

[99] Orengo IF, Salasche SJ, Fewkes J, Khan J, Thornby J, Rubin F. Correlation of histologic subtypes of primary basal cell carcinoma and number of Mohs stages required to achieve a tumor-free plane. J Am Acad Dermatol 1997;37:395–7.

[100] Silverman MK, Kopf AW, Grin CM, Bart RS, Levenstein MJ. Recurrence rates of treated basal cell carcinomas. Part 1: overview. J Dermatol Surg Oncol 1991; 17: 713–8.

[101] Mosterd K, Krekels GA, Nieman FH, Ostertag JU, Essers BA, Dirksen CD, et al. Surgical excision versus Mohs' micrographic surgery for primary and recurrent basal-cell carcinoma of the face: a prospective randomised controlled trial with 5-years' follow-up. Lancet Oncol 2008; 9: 1149–56.

Part 2

Diagnosis and Treatment

5

Determination of Melanoma Lateral and Depth Margins: Potential for Treatment Planning and Five-Year Survival Rate

Tianyi Wang, Jinze Qiu and Thomas E. Milner
The University of Texas at Austin
USA

1. Introduction

Cutaneous malignant melanoma (CMM) is a serious type of cancer accounting for 75% of all deaths associated with skin cancer (Jerant et al., 2000). CMM incidence has dramatically increased in the past few decades and, recently, approximately 160,000 new cases of CMMs are diagnosed worldwide each year (Ries et al., 2003). In 2010, the American Cancer Society estimated that 68,130 cases of melanoma (38,870 males; 29,260 females) and 8,700 melanoma deaths (5,670 males; 3,030 females) were expected in the United States (American Cancer Society (ACS), 2010). In the United States, the lifetime risk for developing CMM has increased from 1 in 1500 in 1930 to 1 in 50 in 2010 (ACS, 2010; King, 2004).

Proper staging of CMM is crucial for defining prognosis and for determining the optimal treatment approach. Several cancer staging systems are being used worldwide. One of the most common staging systems is the tumor-node-metastasis (TNM) classification established by the American Joint Committee on Cancer (AJCC) (Balch et al., 2001). The TNM system classifies CMM in three categories: (1) the size and extent of the primary tumor (T), (2) the involvement of regional lymph nodes (N) and, (3) the presence or absence of distant metastasis (M), determining CMM clinical Stage I, II, III, or IV. To remain current and relevant to clinical practice, the TNM classification is updated periodically based on advances in understanding of cancer prognosis. The latest revision of TNM (presented in the 7th edition of the AJCC Cancer Staging Manual) is applied for cases diagnosed on or after January 1, 2010 (Edge et al., 2010). The CMM invasion depth known as the Breslow thickness (Breslow, 1970) in T category is the single most important factor for CMM staging and closely related to survival rate (Mihm et al., 1988). The five-year survival rate is 95%-100% if CMM thickness is less than 1 mm, while the survival rate is reduced to 50% if the tumor thickness is greater than 4 mm (Figure 1).

Current surgical treatment for primary CMM has often been an excision with a margin determined by CMM thickness (Table 1). Since the risk of local recurrence is dependent on CMM thickness, a narrow margin of 5 mm is recommended for *in situ* CMMs, 1 cm for tumors thinner than 1 mm, 1-2 cm for tumors between 1.01 and 2 mm, and 2 cm for tumors thicker than 2.01 mm (Sladden et al., 2009). Because sentinel lymph node highly correlates with the metastatic status of CMM, a sentinel lymph node dissection (SLND) procedure is also performed on patients with intermediate thickness (1-4 mm) lesions (Balch & Ross,

1999; Kanzler & Mraz-Gernhard, 2001). Therefore, detection of CMM thickness is clinically significant and essential for five-year survival rate and surgical margin determination.

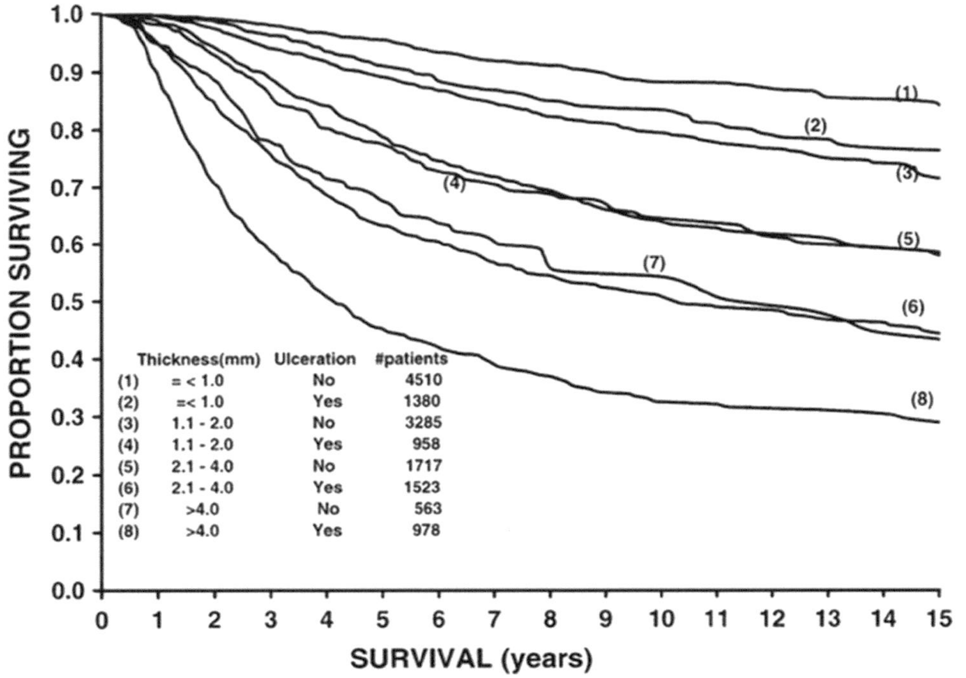

Fig. 1. CMM thickness and survival rate. Image adopted from Rubin., 2010.

T Category Classification	Breslow Thickness (mm)	Ulceration Status /Mitoses	Excision Margin (cm)
TX		Primary tumor cannot be assessed	
T0		No evidence of primary tumor	
Tis		Melanoma *in situ*	0.5
T1	≤ 1.0	Without ulceration or mitosis < 1 mm^2 With ulceration or mitosis > 1 mm^2	1
T2	1.01-2.0	Without ulceration With ulceration	1-2
T3	2.01-4.0	Without ulceration With ulceration	2
T4	> 4.0	Without ulceration With ulceration	2

Table 1. CMM classification in T category and current U.S. guidelines for excision margins.

The current gold standard for CMM diagnosis and tumor thickness measurement is achieved by taking a small biopsy for standard histology (Gambichler et al., 2006). Biopsy and histology allows the visualization of structures in a vertical section of the skin (i.e., from the epidermis through to the reticular dermis or even subcutaneous tissue). However, this procedure is invasive, time consuming and the sensitivity/specificity of CMM detection is highly dependent on location of biopsy. A real clinical need is recognized for non-invasive imaging techniques for *in vivo* evaluation of CMM. Currently, magnetic resonance imaging (MRI), computed tomography (CT), positron emission tomography (PET), high-frequency ultrasound (HFUS), optical coherence tomography (OCT), photoacoustic imaging (PAI), pulsed photothermal radiometry (PPTR), scanning confocal microscopy (SCM), multi-photon luminescence microscopy (MPLM), second harmonic generation (SHG), dermoscopy, multispectral imaging (MSI), diffuse reflectance spectroscopy (DRS) and Raman spectroscopy (RS) or some combination of these are being investigated for non-invasive diagnosis of CMM. Although MRI, CT and PET have the ability to identify nodal and distant metastasis, their routine use for localized CMM investigation is not indicated due to insufficient spatial resolution (King, 2004). Dermoscopy, MSI, DRS and RS are able to identify intrinsic differences between CMM, dysplastic nevi and normal skin but without providing the depth profile of CMM. SCM, MPLM and SHG provide the highest spatial resolution among all these imaging techniques and can also identify the morphological differences in CMM compared with dysplastic nevi. Moreover, SCM, MPLM and SHG have been successfully used to preoperatively delineate CMM lateral margins. However, the penetration depth of SCM, MPLM and SHG limits their use to detect depth margins of intermediate (1-4 mm) and more advanced (>4 mm) CMMs. HFUS, OCT, PAI and PPTR have spatial resolutions and penetration depths between MRI/CT/PET and SCM/MPLM/SHG, which underlines their potential applicability to not only diagnose CMM but also to detect lateral and depth margins.

This chapter examines the evidence for use of non-invasive imaging techniques, in particular, MRI, CT, PET, HFUS, OCT, PAI, PPTR, SCM, MPLM and SHG, in CMM diagnosis as well as tumor lateral and depth margin detection for preoperative CMM staging and surgical margin definition. Comparison between these imaging techniques in terms of spatial resolution, penetration depth, sensitivity/specificity, correlation with histology and temporal monitoring (possibility to monitor CMM changes at multiple time points) are described and, recommendations for future studies are indicated.

2. CMM imaging techniques

2.1 Magnetic Resonance Imaging (MRI)

Atomic nuclei in a magnetic field oscillate in the direction of the field at a specific frequency directly related to the field strength and the magnetic properties of the nuclei. If a pulse of current of the same frequency is applied to the coil surrounding the nuclei, an oscillating magnetic field is produced that creates a radio frequency within the coil. Magnetic field energy is absorbed by the nuclei and re-emitted as a radio-frequency signal immediately after the applied pulse. The re-emitted radio frequency energy is measured by the surface coil and reconstructed to form an MRI image (Baddeley, 1984). MRI has been widely employed in clinical oncology and introduced to examine cutaneous melanocytic and other types of skin lesions since 1989 (Zemtsov et al., 1989) due to good contrast between tumor regions and soft tissues (Totty et al., 1986; Weeks et al., 1985). The application of MRI to dermatology has become practical with the development and application of specialized surface coils that allow higher resolution imaging than standard MRI coils (Bittoun et al., 1990; Hyde et al., 1987; Marghoob et al., 2003; Querleux et al., 1988, 1995; Rajeswari et al.,

2003; Richard et al., 1991; Zemtsov et al., 1989). Although imaging thin cutaneous tumors (i.e., <1 mm) is not possible due to insufficient resolution, MRI was utilized to evaluate advanced skin tumors, particularly to determine the depth of malignant tumors and the degree of invasion. el Gammal et al combined a strong homogeneous magnetic field of 9.4 T with gradient fields of 11.7 G/cm and an imaging unit to obtain a voxel resolution of $40 \times 40 \times 300\ \mu m^3$, allowing differentiation between normal skin and skin tumors including CMMs (Figure 2) (el Gammal et al., 1996). Using this approach, a primary nodular melanoma with Breslow thickness of 1.65 mm was imaged. The tumor is visible in the image (Figure 2d) in the upper left part of the histological section. Skin layer, sub-layers and tumor were visualized by MRI (Figure 2c) with different signal contrast. An excellent correlation between MRI image and corresponding histological features was achieved.

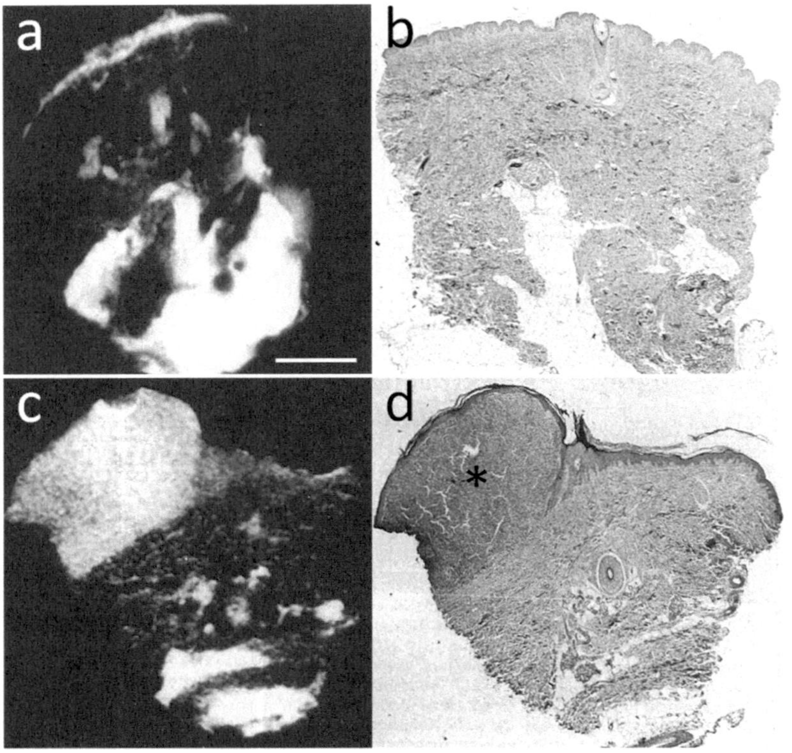

Fig. 2. (a,b) MRI and corresponding histology images, respectively, of normal skin from the upper leg of a 25-year-old man. (c,d) MRI and corresponding histology images, respectively, of primary nodular melanoma from the leg of a 31-year-old woman. (*) indicates the tumor location in (d) . Breslow thickness of the tumor was 1.65 mm. Scale bar is 1 mm. Image modified from el Gammal et al., 1996.

Ono et al applied MRI to the diagnosis of malignant skin tumors and reported selected cases (Ono & Kaneko, 1995). A more advanced CMM with lateral dimensions of $36 \times 26\ mm^2$ was imaged (Figure 3). The MRI image (Figure 3a) was found to reflect precisely the actual morphology and tumor depth (Figure 3b). The reconstructed 3-D MRI image (Figure 3c) yielded accurate information regarding the relationship between tumor and its surrounding tissue and also provided a 3-D view of the state of infiltration, useful for deciding on a resection area prior to surgery. MRI has also been used to image nodal and distant metastasis in a murine model (Foster et al., 2008) as well as different organs in humans (King, 2004). However, the availability and cost of MRI is a limiting factor. Therefore, although MRI is useful for advanced CMM thickness measurement and individual metastasis characterization, at present this approach is not a first-line investigation tool.

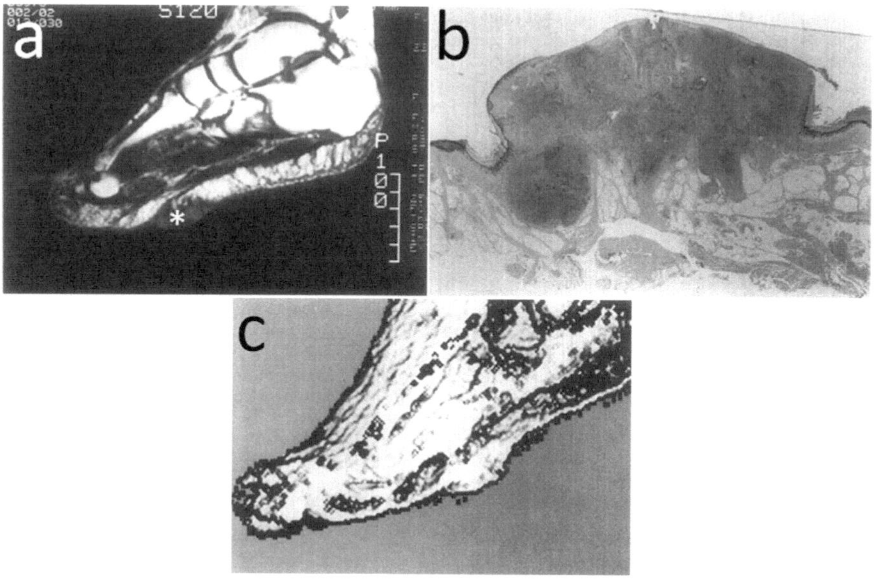

Fig. 3. CMM on the left sole of a 67-year-old woman. (a) MRI image longitudinally sectioning the tumor demonstrated an irregularly convex and concave region at the thick base of the tumor. (b) Histological section of the tumor. (c) A reconstructed 3-D image prepared from MRI slices. (*) indicates the tumor location in (a). Image modified from Ono & Kaneko, 1995.

2.2 Computed Tomography (CT) and Positron Emission Tomography (PET)

CT produces images with contrast given by the attenuation of X-ray photons by differing body tissues, in a manner similar to conventional radiography (Baddeley, 1984). Because CT has comparable or lower resolution than MRI (Link et al., 2003), it is not indicated to diagnose patients with primary CMMs but rather metastasis. The identification of CMM metastasis is dependent on the morphologic alteration of tissue malignancy and, therefore, CT is insensitive at detecting small tumor masses. Chest CT is sensitive to detect nodules (<1 cm), calcification within a nodule and to distinguish solitary from multiple pulmonary lesions (Armstrong et al., 2001; Halton, 1992). Although these findings are often non-specific for malignancy, they can provide a baseline scan allowing serial assessment of changes. Heaston et al showed that chest CT detected CMM metastasis in 19% of patients with normal chest X-ray (Heaston et al., 1983).

PET, a whole-body imaging technique, is widely used in the diagnosis of metastatic cancer. In a PET imaging procedure, an isotopic tracer is injected and used to label cancer cells.

Fluoro-deoxy-glucose (FDG) is one of the most widely applied PET tracers used to survey cell metabolism (Gritters et al., 1993; Strobel et al., 2007; Wagner et al., 1999). Because metabolic characterization of tumor cells usually exceeds physiological metabolic activity, excessive FDG uptake has consequently been demonstrated in most cancers *in vivo*, making whole-body FDG-PET a sensitive indicator of metastatic CMM compared with conventional diagnostic imaging modalities (Blessing et al., 1995; Boni et al., 1995; Damian et al., 1996; Gritters et al., 1993; Macfarlane et al., 1998; Rinne et al., 1998; Steinert et al., 1995; Wagner et al., 1997). The improved sensitivity and potential cost-effectiveness of FDG-PET are rational arguments for PET staging of patients with recurrent CMM (Yao et al., 1994). The sensitivity of PET depends on the location and size of the tumor. A resolution of 4-6 mm is usual, which suggests that PET may lack the sensitivity to detect small nodular CMM metastasis that are usually 1-2 mm in size (Belhocine et al., 2006).

As PET alone does not provide sufficient resolution to detect small CMM metastasis, it is usually used in combination with CT (Akcali et al., 2007; Essner et al., 2006), allowing mapping of PET images onto CT images acquired simultaneously (Figure 4). Reinhardt et al studied 251 patients with PET/CT and showed a sensitivity of 98.7% compared to 88.8% for PET alone and 69.7% for CT alone (Reinhardt et al., 2006). Moreover, Iagaru et al recently reported a study involving 163 patients and showed a sensitivity of 89%, and recommended the use of PET/CT in the evaluation of high-risk CMM metastasis (Iagaru et al., 2006).

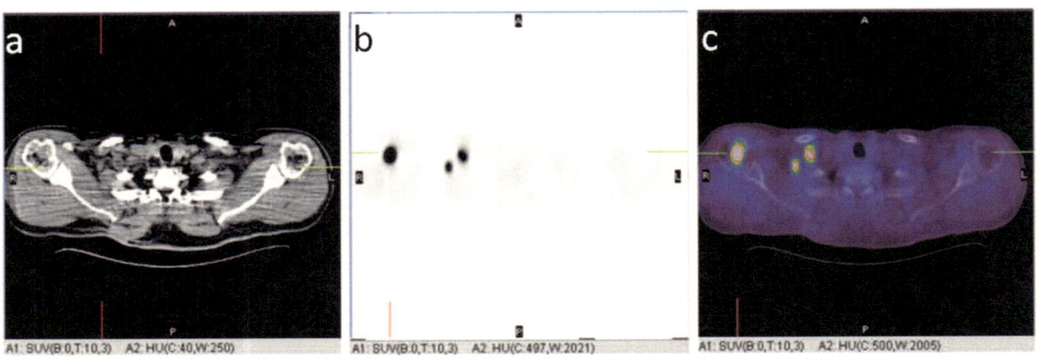

Fig. 4. ^{18}F-fluorodeoxyglucose PET/CT for restaging of a 56-year-old patient with a superficial spreading melanoma of 4.3 mm depth at the right shoulder after resection of a lymph-node metastasis at the right neck. (a) CT, (b) PET and (c) fused PET/CT images showed two lymph-node metastasis infraclavicular, and PET showed an additional metastasis that was found to be localized in the right humerus head after image fusion. Image adopted from Reinhardt et al., 2006.

2.3 High-frequency Ultrasound (HFUS)

Ultrasound (US) uses a transducer to transmit sound pulses and to receive backscattered echo signals. Because the interfaces between tissues have different acoustic impedances and, therefore, different reflectivities, the received US signal contains boundary information of tissue with different elastic properties (T. Wang et al., 2011). US frequencies of 7.5-15 MHz are routinely used to visualize subcutaneous structures deeper than 1.5 cm including muscles, tendons, vessels and internal organs to identify pathologies or lesions (Aaslid et al., 2010; Shia et al., 2007; Tuzcu et al., 2010). The traditional US equipment used in the clinical environment does not allow precise measurement of tissues due to insufficient spatial resolution (Ulrich et al., 1999). High-frequency ultrasound (HFUS), however, is capable of visualization of dermis (20 MHz) and even epidermis (50-100 MHz). The resolution of the image and depth of tissue penetration is largely dependent on the frequency of the US transducer. High-frequency scanners offer finer resolution (e.g., axial resolution of 50 µm and lateral resolution of 300 µm for a 20 MHz transducer) but poorer tissue penetration. HFUS at 20 MHz have been used with success to distinguish between benign skin lesions and CMM. Harland et al showed 100% sensitivity in distinguishing between 29 basal cell carcinomas and 25 CMMs (Harland et al., 2000). Bessoud et al in a study involving 111 patients, identified 65 of 70 CMMs (81%). There was a 100% sensitivity and specificity for melanoma and 32% specificity for non-melanoma lesions (Bessoud et al., 2003). HFUS at 20 MHz has also been shown to allow preoperative assessment of CMM thickness that correlated well with histological measurement (Dummer et al., 1995; Hoffmann et al., 1992; Lassau et al., 1999; Serrone et al., 2002; Tacke et al., 1995). A prospective study and systematic review of literature from 1987 to 2007 on CMM thickness measurement using 20 MHz HFUS reported that measurement of CMM thickness was possible except for thin CMMs (<0.4 mm) in areas with marked photoaging, and in the case of very thick CMMs exceeding the explored depth (7.6 mm) (Figure 5a) (Machet et al., 2009). This study also demonstrated a linear correlation between ultrasound and histology in CMM thickness measurements (Figure 5b). Another study using 75 MHz HFUS, involving 112 patients with suspicious CMMs, showed that 45 of 52 CMMs had clear hypoechogenic boundaries with tumor thicknesses ranging from 0 to 2.8 mm and correlation between HFUS measurement and histology was high (r=0.908) (Guitera et al., 2008).

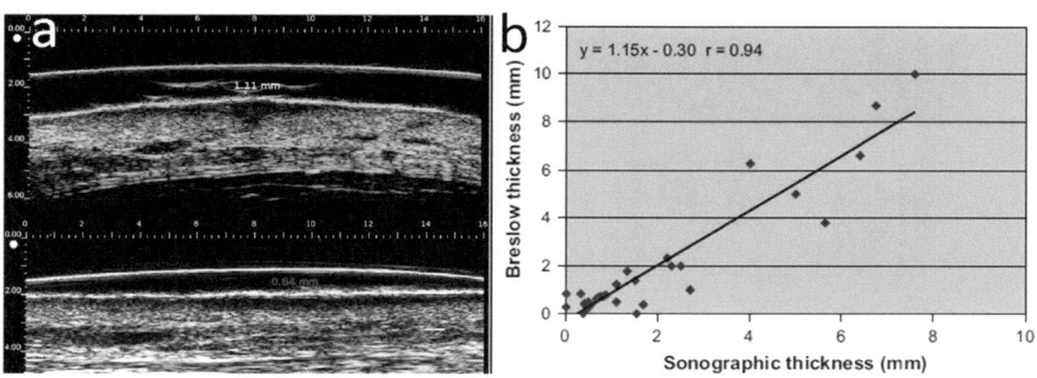

Fig. 5. (a) HFUS imaging of two CMM lesions. Lesions were generally hypoechoic and well demarcated from the dermis. (b) Linear relationship of CMM thickness between HFUS and histological measurements. Image adopted from Machet et al., 2009.

2.4 Optical Coherence Tomography (OCT)

OCT is an emerging diagnostic optical imaging technique that provides *in vivo* structure and function of tissues by measuring backscattered or backreflected light. OCT is based on the principle of Michelson interferometry. The light sources used for OCT imaging of skin are broad-band superluminescent diodes or tunable laser sources operating at a wavelength of about 1300 nm (Huang et al., 1991). The broad-band source leads to a small coherence length and achieves an axial and lateral resolution of approximately 15 µm and a penetration depth of

500 to 1000 μm (Olmedo et al., 2006; Welzel et al., 2003). OCT is a well established tool in ophthalmology (Welzel, 2003) and currently being advanced in dermatology (Fujimoto et al., 1995; Gambichler et al., 2005; Welzel, 2001), particularly for the diagnosis of CMM (Marghoob et al., 2003). A study of CMM characterization by OCT examined a panel of CMMs and benign nevi and demonstrated that CMMs showed increased architectural disarray, less defined dermal-epidermal borders, and vertically oriented icicle-shaped structures not seen in nevi (Figure 6b,c) (Gambichler et al., 2007). A recent review of OCT investigation in dermatology also showed that the intact border between epidermis and dermis disappears in infiltrative growing CMM compared with healthy skin (Figure 6a) (Smith & MacNeil, 2011).

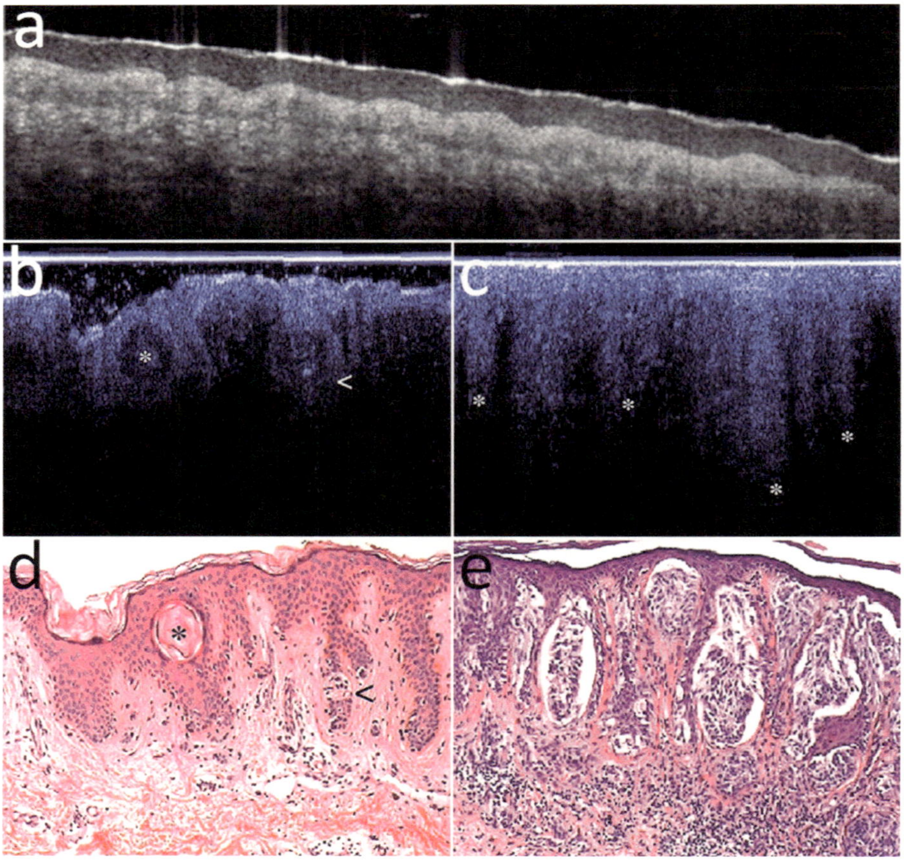

Fig. 6. (a) OCT image of health human finger tip skin. Image adopted from Smith & MacNeil, 2011. (b,d) OCT image of a compound nevi and corresponding histology, respectively. OCT displays finger-shaped elongated and broadened rete ridges including dense cell clusters (<) (b). Dermoepidermal junction zone is relatively clearly demarcated from more or less dark-appearing papillary dermis (b). Besides, epidermal horn cyst is demonstrated both on histology and OCT (*) (b and d). (c,e) OCT image of a superficial spreading CMM (0.91 mm) and corresponding histology, respectively. OCT (c) clearly displays marked architectural disarray including large vertically arranged icicle-shaped structures (*). Image adopted from Gambichler et al., 2007.

The utility of OCT for early-stage CMM thickness measurement (Figure 7) has not been fully established because correlation studies for CMM thickness determination by OCT and histology have not been reported. Furthermore, an important limitation of OCT is penetration depth. The maximum penetration depth of OCT is currently between 1-2 mm, dependent on the tissue type. Although the use of longer light wavelengths (e.g., 1750 nm) may improve penetration depth, no data is available to suggest that penetration depth greater than 4 mm is possible in the near future (Brezinski & Fujimoto, 1999). Therefore, OCT is currently not an established candidate for CMM thickness measurement.

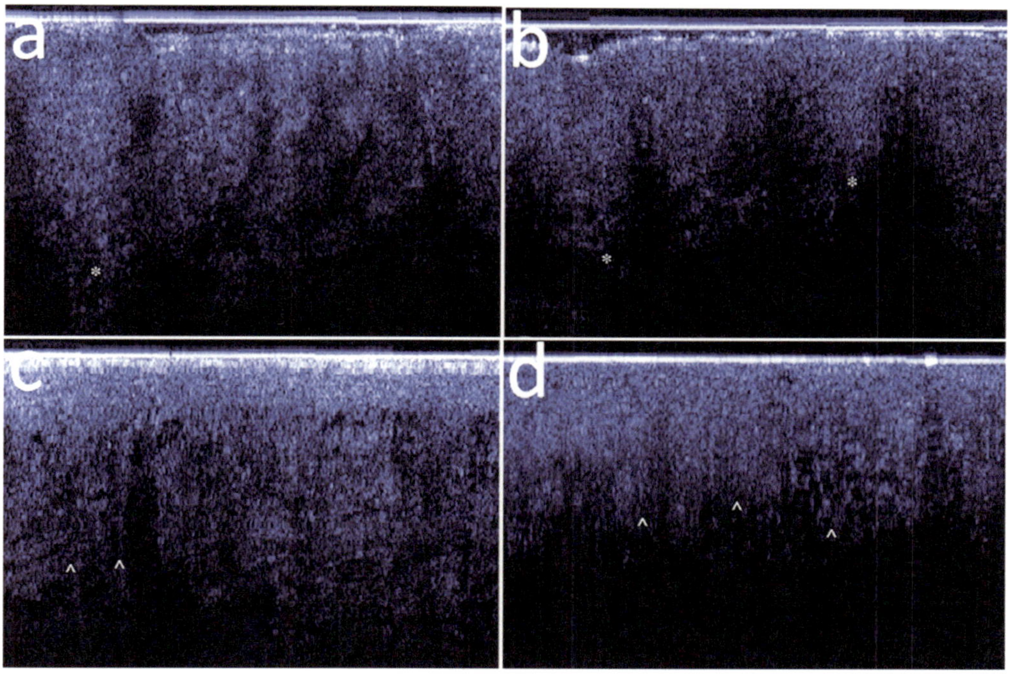

Fig. 7. OCT of 4 superficial spreading CMMs with Breslow thickness of (a) 0.45 mm, (b) 0.5 mm, (c) 0.7 mm, and (d) 1.6 mm measured by histology. CMM thickness determination is hardly possible. Despite large icicle-shaped structures (*) (a and b) and a patchy or cloudy bright dermis was observed (^) (c and d). Image adopted from Gambichler et al., 2007.

2.5 Photoacoustic Imaging (PAI)

PAI is an emerging hybrid technique that detects absorbed photons ultrasonically through the photoacoustic effect (Sun & Diebold, 1992). When a short-pulsed radiant source (e.g., laser) irradiates biological tissues, wideband ultrasonic waves (referred to as photoacoustic waves) are induced as a result of transient thermoelastic expansion. Magnitude of the photoacoustic waves is proportional to the local optical energy deposition and, hence, the waves divulge physiologically specific optical absorption contrast. As energy deposition is related to optical absorption coefficient of chromophores, concentration of multiple chromophores can be quantified by varying the laser excitation wavelength. Tissues such as blood vessels and CMM, can be imaged by PAI with the spatial resolution of ultrasound, which is not limited by the strong light scattering in biological tissues (X. Wang et al., 2003).

Images of microvasculature as deep as 3 mm were demonstrated with high-resolution PAI (Maslov et al., 2005). Recently, Oh et al used high-resolution and high-contrast PAI *in vivo* with a near-infrared (NIR) (764 nm) and a visible (584 nm) pulsed laser source, respectively, to image the 3-D CMM distribution inside nude mouse skin and the vascular system surrounding the CMM including tumor-feeding vessels (Oh et al., 2006). Maximum CMM thickness (0.5 mm) was measured with a lateral resolution of 45 µm and an axial resolution of 15 µm (Figure 8). Detection of melanoma cells in circulation was also reported (Holan & Viator, 2008; Weight et al., 2006; Zharov et al., 2006). More recently, in a pilot study Song et al proposed that non-invasive *in vivo* spectroscopic PAI can map sentinel lymph node using gold nanorods as lymph node tracers in a rodent model (Song et al., 2009).

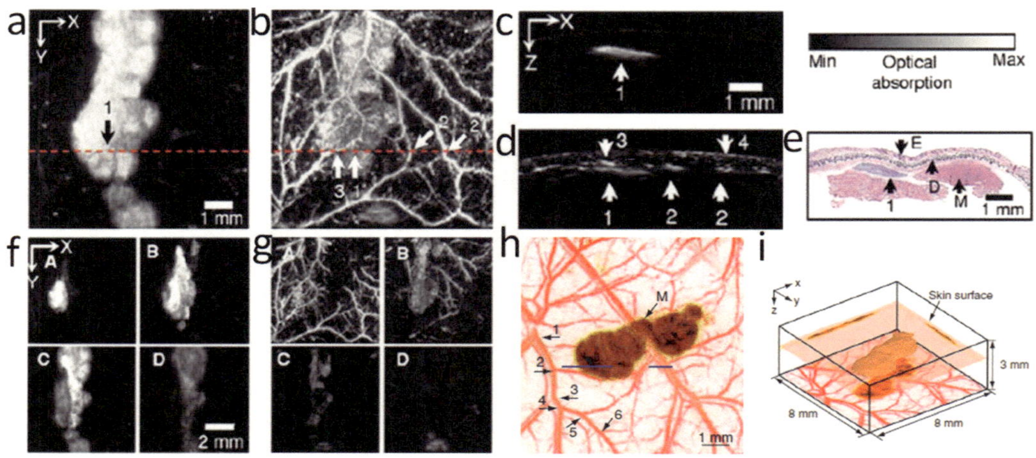

Fig. 8. *In vivo* non-invasive photoacoustic images of CMM and vascular distribution in nude mouse skin. (a,b) Enface photoacoustic images for the NIR light source (764 nm) and visible light source (584 nm), respectively: 1, CMM; 2, vessels perpendicular to image plane; 3, vessels horizontal to image plane; 4, skin. (c,d) Photoacoustic B-scan images from the NIR and visible light sources, respectively, for the dot lines in (a) and (b). (e) A cross-sectional histology image (H&E staining): E, epidermis; D, dermis; M, muscle. (f,g) Depthwise enface photoacoustic images from the NIR and visible light sources, respectively: A, 0.15-0.30 mm; B, 0.30-0.45 mm; C, 0.45-0.60 mm; D, 0.60-0.75 mm from the skin surface. Image adopted from Oh et al., 2006. (h) A composite of the two maximum amplitude projection (MAP) images projected along the z axis of a CMM region, where an MAP image is formed by projecting the maximum photoacoustic amplitudes along a direction to its orthogonal plane. Here, blood vessels are pseudocolored red in the 584 nm image and the CMM is pseudo-colored brown in the 764 nm image. As many as six orders of vessel branching can be observed in the image as indicated by numbers 1-6. (i) 3-D rendering of the CMM from the data acquired at 764 nm. Two MAP images at this wavelength projected along the x and y axes are shown on the two side walls, respectively. Image adopted from Zhang et al., 2006.

2.6 Pulsed Photothermal Radiometry (PPTR)

PPTR is a non-invasive technique that utilizes an infrared detector to measure radiometric temperature changes induced in a test material exposed to pulsed radiation. Heat generated as a result of light absorption by subsurface chromophores in the test material diffuses to the surface and results in increased infrared emission levels. By collecting emitted radiation onto an infrared detector, a PPTR signal is obtained that represents the time evolution of temperature near the test-material surface. Useful information regarding the test material may be deduced from analysis of the PPTR signal. PPTR has been applied to depth profiling of strongly absorbing tissues and tissue phantoms (Milanič et al., 2007; Milner et al., 1996), including blood vessels in port wine stain (PWS) birthmarks in human skin (Li et al., 2004). Because different chromophore thicknesses can provide different laser induced initial temperature profiles and eventually produce different radiometric temperatures (T. Wang et al., 2009), the authors proposed that relationship between CMM thickness and detected radiometric temperature increase can be determined using PPTR in tissue phantoms mimicking CMM thicknesses from 120 μm to 2.8 mm (Figure 9) with a penetration depth of 1.7 mm and axial resolution of 75 μm (T. Wang et al., 2011). However, further studies are needed to investigate the capability of PPTR in CMM thickness measurement in skin *in vivo*.

2.7 Scanning Confocal Microscopy (SCM)

SCM is a non-invasive imaging technique that permits *in vivo* examination of the epidermis and papillary dermis. The basic premise of SCM is the selective collection of light from a specific plane in tissue through a pinhole-sized aperture which allows for light collection from the single in-focus plane and the rejection of light from all out-of-focus planes (Nehal et al., 2008). SCM has been recently employed in CMM diagnosis (Gerger et al., 2005; Marghoob & Halpern, 2005), preoperative and intraoperative margin assessment (Busam et al., 2001), and followup for response to medical treatment (Ahmed & Berth-Jones, 2000; Cornejo et al., 2000; Langley et al., 2006; Tannous et al., 2000, 2002). Commercial SCM instruments have been developed that image with lateral resolution of 0.5 to 1.0 μm and an optical sectioning thickness of 1.0 to 5.0 μm, to a depth of 200 to 300 μm in human skin (depth of papillary dermis). The spatial resolution of SCM is determined by the pinhole size while imaging depth is limited by the laser wavelength (with a 488 nm laser imaging 50-100 μm into skin (Gareau et al., 2007) and longer wavelengths lasers able to image at depths of up to 300 μm (Gonzalez & Gilaberte-Calzada, 2008; Marghoob et al., 2003; Nehal et al., 2008), providing images of the basement membrane down into the papillary dermis. SCM with an 830 nm light source is ideal for detecting CMM because melanin serves as an endogenous contrast agent. Melanin presence in melanocytic nevi and CMM provides strong contrast, thereby permitting the clear visualization of the architecture and outlines of cells (Gareau et al., 2008; Rajadhyaksha et al., 1995). SCM can be used in either fluorescence or reflectance modes (Meyer et al., 2006). While dermatological research tends to use fluorescence, clinical practice uses reflectance microscopy as this does not require fluorescent labeling of cells and tissues and, therefore, is more suitable for *in vivo* imaging. SCM criteria have been established to distinguish between CMMs and benign nevi (Gerger et al., 2005; Pellacani et al., 2007). Pellacani et al proposed a diagnostic algorithm that uses 2 major (i.e., nonedged dermal papillae and cytologic atypia at the basal layer) and 4 minor criteria (i.e., roundish pagetoid cells, widespread pagetoid infiltration in the epidermis, nucleated cells within dermal papillae, and cerebriform cell clusters in the dermis) (Figure 10) (Pellacani et al., 2005). The presence of at least 2 features, 1 major and 1 minor criterion, are required for a positive CMM diagnosis.

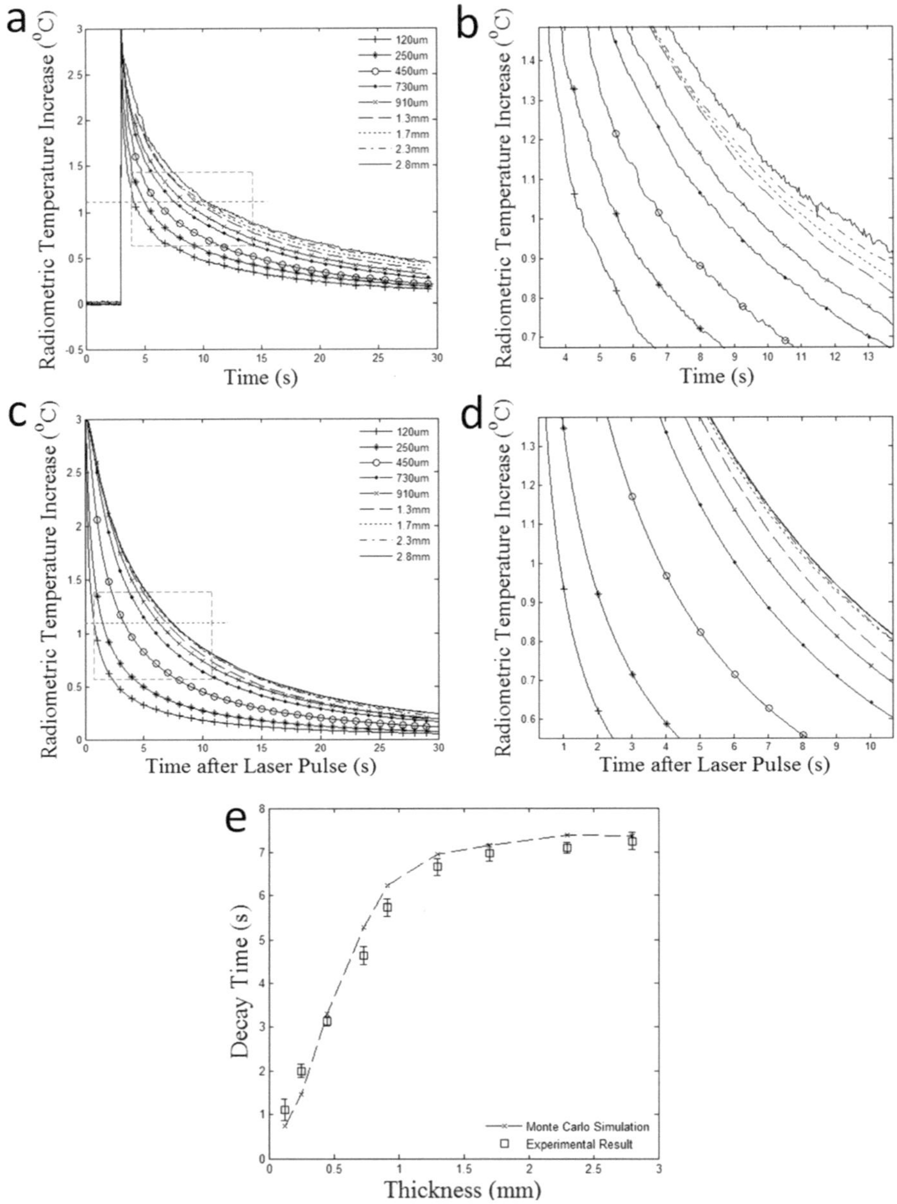

Fig. 9. (a) Measured radiometric temperature increase from PDMS tissue phantoms (top-layer is 120 μm-2.8 mm thick respectively - mimicking different CMM thicknesses). (b) Measured radiometric temperature increase in the window indicated in (a). (c) Simulated radiometric temperature increase. (d) Simulated radiometric temperature increase in the window indicated in (c). The dashed lines in (a,c) indicate when peak radiometric temperature increase decays to 37% of the maximum. (e) Decay time of the PDMS tissue phantoms with different top-layer thicknesses from experiment (square box) and simulation (dashed line). Image adopted from T. Wang et al., 2011.

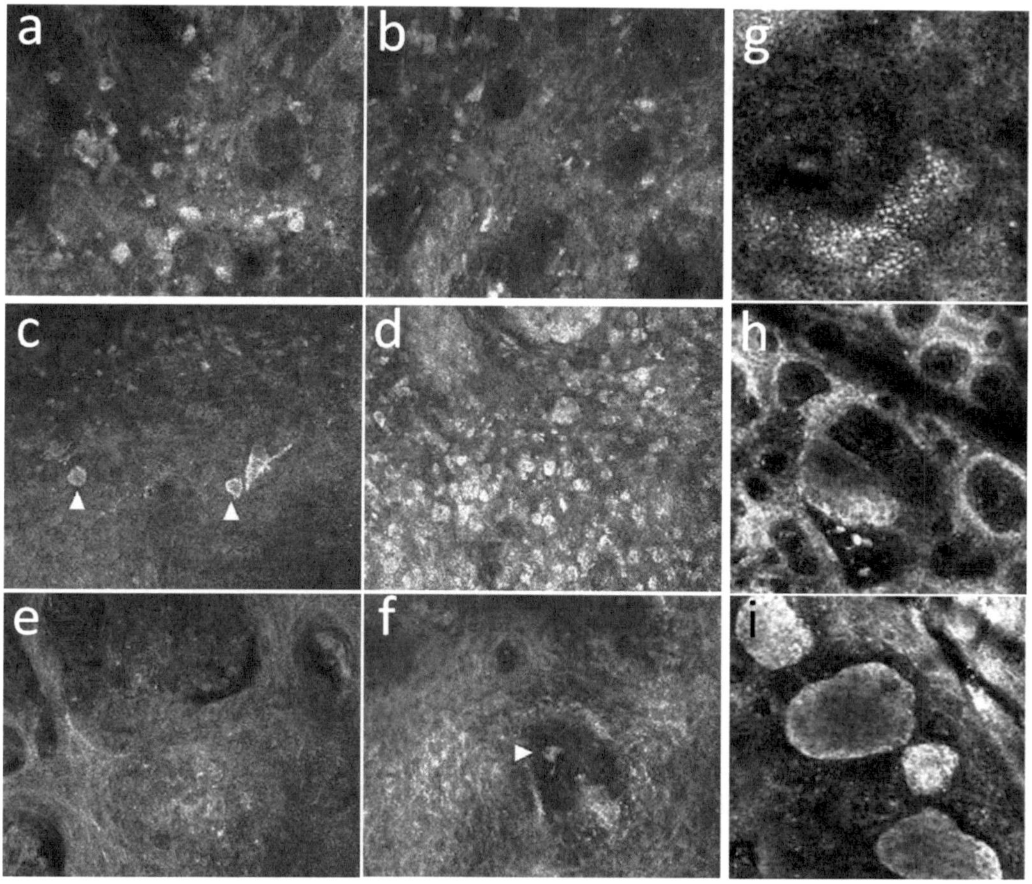

Fig. 10. *In vivo* reflectance-mode SCM images of characteristic CMM (corresponding to major (a,b) and minor (c,d,e,f) criteria) and benign nevi features (g,h,i): (a) Marked cytologic atypia at basal cell layers. (b) Nonedged papillae at dermoepidermal junction. (c) Roundish cells in superficial layers spreading upward in pagetoid fashion (arrowheads). (d) Pagetoid cells widespread throughout lesion. (e) Cerebriform clusters in papillary dermis. (f) Nucleated cells within dermal papilla (arrowhead). Image adopted from Pellacani et al., 2005. (g) Regular honeycombed and cobblestone pattern. (h) Regular junctional nests of cells (junctional cluster and junctional thickening); (i) Regular dense nests in the dermis. Image adopted from Pellacani et al., 2007.

SCM is capable to identify the lateral margins of CMM when determining the precise margins by clinical Wood's lamp or dermoscopic examination is virtually impossible. Chen et al reported a case of a patient with a recurrent CMM on the scalp that developed in a background of photodamage with diffuse melanocytic atypia and lentigines (Chen et al., 2005). SCM was able to distinguish the adjacent normal skin from CMM and the lateral tumor margin was preoperatively determined by SCM and the tumor was excised accordingly (Figure 11). Another study by Curiel-Lewandrowski also demonstrated the feasibility of using SCM in preoperative and intraoperative surgical margin assessment of indistinct CMM lesions (Curiel-Lewandrowski et al., 2004). However, SCM detection of tumor depth margins is still difficult due to insufficient penetration depth. The high cost and sophisticated design of current SCM devices are considered to be major barriers. Efforts, such as miniaturizing the device and lowering the cost of production can facilitate wider adoption.

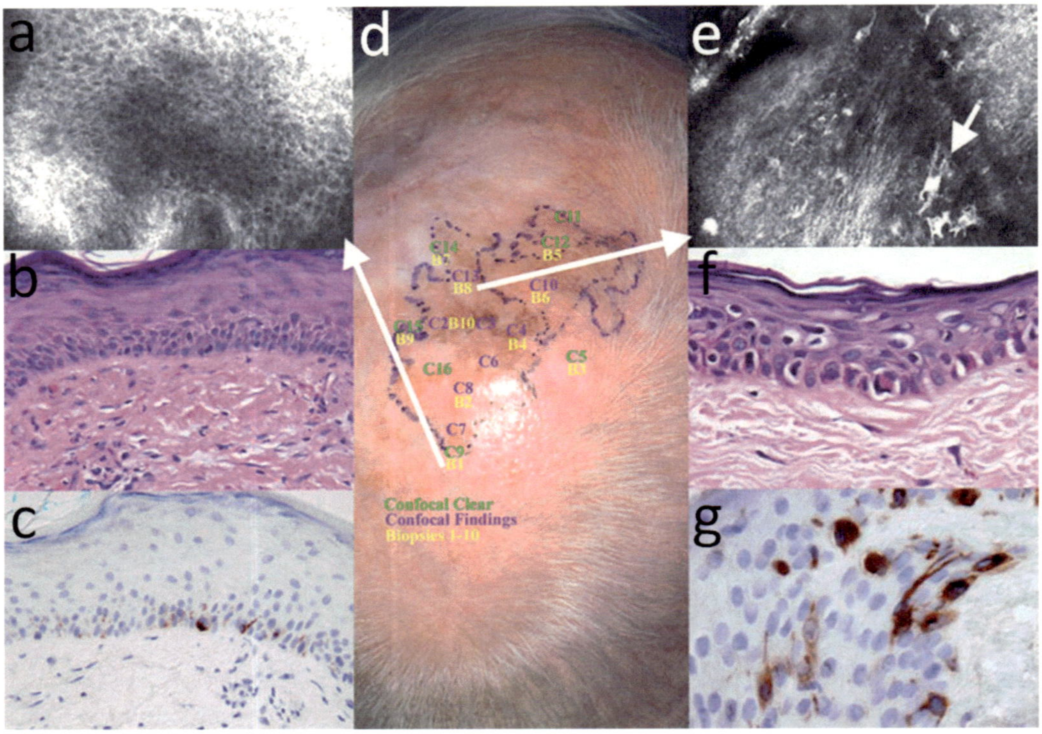

Fig. 11. (d) shows the refined border of the lentigo malignant melanoma (LMM) as determined by SCM. The SCM-examined foci are numbered 1-16 and are color-coded to indicate areas that were negative (green) and positive (purple) for LMM on SCM images. Five pairs (marked in yellow) of these foci on either side of the border were biopsied for histological confirmation. (a), (b) and (c) are the confocal, histology and Melan-A immunostained sections of one representative area of normal skin (long arrow in (d)). (a) shows the epidermal layer and demonstrates the honeycomb pattern of keratinocytes and well-defined cell to cell demarcations which is the characteristic architecture of normal skin. (b,c) The haematoxylin and eosin (H&E)-stained and Melan-A-stained histological sections of normal skin, respectively. (e,f,g) Confocal, histology and Melan-A immunostained sections of one representative area of skin with LMM (long arrow in (d)). (e) shows the spinous layer and demonstrates pagetoid spread of atypical, dendritic melanocytes (short arrow), loss of the normal architecture and a grainy background-all features consistent with LMM. (f,g) H&E-stained and Melan-A-stained histological sections of LMM, respectively. The Melan-A staining (g) shows the dendrites of the melanoma cell and correlates with the dendritic malignant melanocyte (arrow) seen in (e). Image adopted from Chen et al., 2005.

2.8 Multi-photon Luminescence Microscopy (MPLM) and Second Harmonic Generation (SHG)

MPLM is a rapidly developing imaging technique in the field of optical sectioning, which has been applied to tissue imaging with intrinsic fluorescence (Zipfel et al., 2003a, 2003b). Endogenous fluorophores such as melanin, elastin and collagen are sources of tissue fluorescence. MPLM of animal and human skin has been reported by So et al, Masters et al, Hendriks et al, König et al and Peuckert et al (Hendriks & Lucassen, 1999; König, 2000a, 2000b, 2002; Masters et al., 1998; Peuckert et al., 2000; So & Kim, 1998). Teuchner et al reported MPLM detection of melanin fluorescence (Teuchner et al., 1999). MPLM excites fluorophores by a non-linear multiphoton (e.g., two-photon) process, as opposed to the single photon excitation used in conventional microscopy. Two-photon excitation occurs when two photons of approximately half the one photon energy are absorbed nearly simultaneously by the fluorescent molecule. MPLM allows non-invasive tissue screening with subcellular spatial resolution. Wang et al demonstrated that lateral and axial resolution of MPLM can reach about 0.3 and 1 μm, respectively (H. Wang et al., 2005). Masters et al detected the autofluorescence of human skin in depths down to 200 μm (Masters et al., 1997). Figure 12 illustrates the effectiveness of MPLM in obtaining subcellular resolution images of CMM and normal skin (Dimitrow et al., 2009).

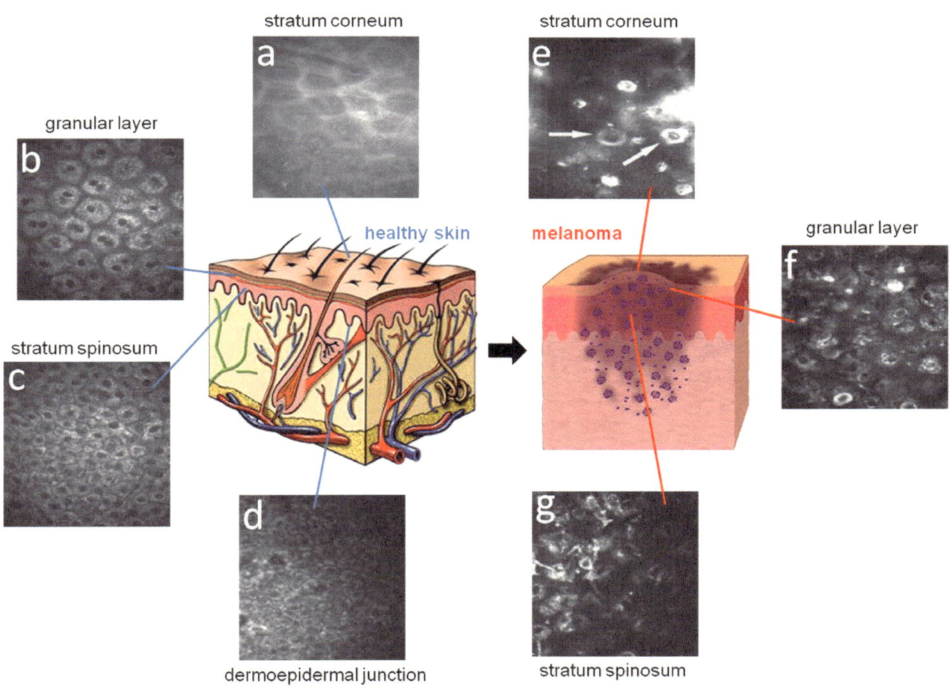

Fig. 12. MPLM of healthy human skin (a,b,c,d) and melanoma (e,f,g) with subcellular resolution. Optical sections of healthy skin were captured at the same skin site, but at different tissue depths showing: (a) the stratum corneum, (b) the granular layer, (c) the stratum spinosum and (d) the dermoepidermal junction; Optical sections of melanoma: (e) The stratum corneum characterized by highly fluorescent melanocytes marked by white arrows. (f) The granular layer characterized by large intercellular distance. (g) The spinous layer characterized by poorly defined keratinocyte cell borders. Image modified from Dimitrow et al., 2009.

Similar to SCM, MPLM has the potential to precisely measure the lateral margins of CMM, however, limited penetration depth prevents use for tumor depth margin delineation.
SHG (also called frequency doubling) is also a nonlinear optical process, in which photons interacting with a nonlinear material are effectively combined to form new photons with twice the energy and, therefore, twice the frequency and half the wavelength of the incident photons (Fine & Hansen, 1971; Roth & Freund, 1979; Theodossiou et al., 2006). Because SHG excitation wavelength is off the resonance wavelength of chromophores in tissue, less energy is absorbed, and hence, negligible thermal or photodamage is observed (Lohela & Werb, 2010). Recently, SHG imaging has been employed to detect noncentrosymmetric crystalline structures (e.g., collagen) in tissues (Campagnola et al., 2001; Cox et al., 2003; Lim et al., 2010; H. Wang et al., 2009). Thrasivoulou et al demonstrated that SHG imaging showed detailed collagen distribution in healthy skin, with total absence of SHG signal (fibrillar collagen) within the melanoma-invaded tissue (Figure 13) (Thrasivoulou et al., 2011). The presence or absence of SHG signal changed dramatically at the borders of CMM, allowing accurate demarcation of CMM margins that strongly correlated with H&E and Melan-A defined margins ($p<0.002$).

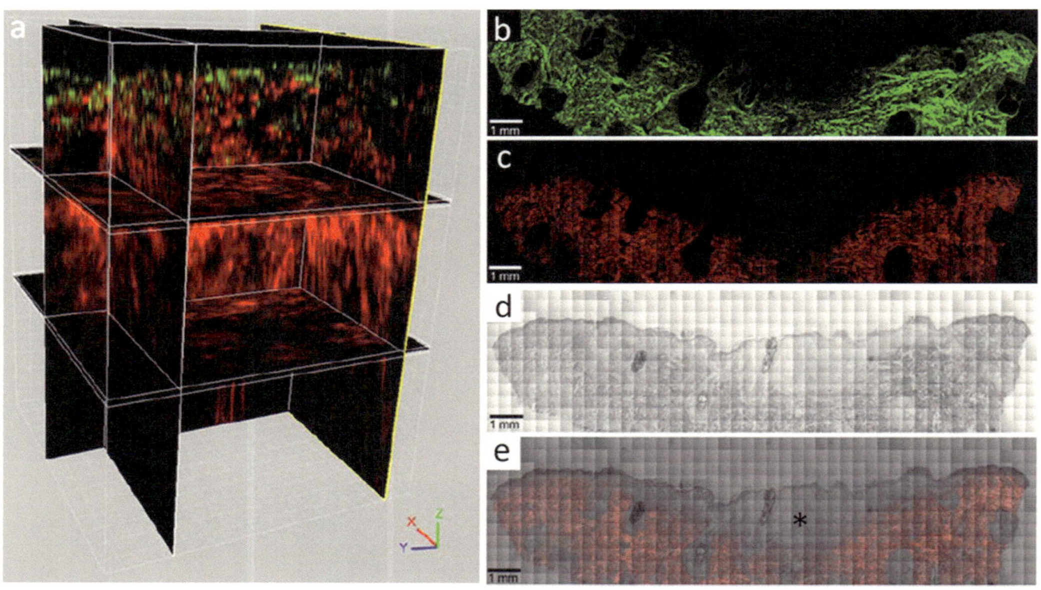

Fig. 13. (a) SHG imaging of healthy, *ex vivo*, human skin sample showing collagen morphology throughout the entire thickness when imaged from the epidermis, in the transmission (red) and backscattered (green) geometry. The whole thickness of epidermis and dermis to depths of approximately 300 μm in the backscattered geometry and over 1000 μm in the transmission geometry were imaged, respectively. Montage of SHG images of CMM in (b) transmission, (c) backscattered geometry, and (d) bright-field image. (e) Superimposed image of bright-field and SHG images indicates collagen distribution within each section. (*) indicates the CMM location in (e). Image modified from Thrasivoulou et al., 2011.

2.9 Dermoscopy

Dermoscopy (also called dermatoscopy, skin surface microscopy, epiluminescence microscopy) is a non-invasive technique for the early recognition of CMM. Dermoscopy was first introduced to evaluate pigmented lesions in 1971 (MacKie, 1971), studied rigorously in Europe and Australia during the 1980s and 1990s (Argenziano et al., 1998), and adopted slowly in the United States in recent years (Tripp et al., 2002). To date, dermoscopic and histologic correlations and algorithms for dermoscopic diagnosis of CMM have been established (Argenziano et al., 2003; Henning et al., 2007). Two types of dermoscopes are currently available: (1) nonpolarized dermoscope (NPD) and (2) polarized dermoscope (PD). NPD uses liquid (e.g., oil, water, or alcohol gel) to cover the lesion, which decreases light reflection, refraction, and diffraction, makes the epidermis essentially translucent and allows for visualization of subsurface anatomic structures of the epidermis and papillary dermis (Figure 14). PD uses a polarizer that preferentially captures backscattered light from below the surface of the skin. The liquid or direct contact with the skin is not needed. However, some subset of CMMs (e.g., amelanotic/hypomelanotic CMMs that lack pigmentations and dermoscopic structures) are difficult to diagnose with dermoscopy and, thus, impossible to determine lateral margins by dermoscopy. Although a dermoscopic image can show subsurface structures of CMM, this approach is a 2-D imaging technique that cannot obtain a depth profile of the lesion. Therefore, depth margins of melanoma are not provided by dermoscopy.

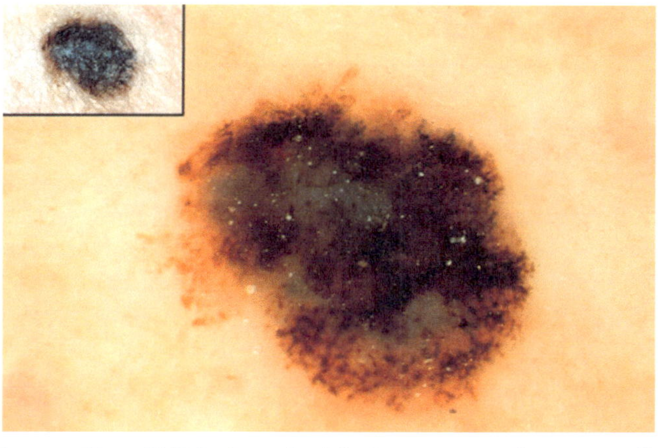

Fig. 14. Superficial spreading CMM viewed with dermoscopy (large panel) and with the unaided eye (inset panel). Compared with the unaided eye, dermoscopy reveals several additional structural features, which are typical of CMM, including irregular dots and irregular extensions (pseudopods) in the periphery and a blue-whitish veil. Image adopted from Kittler et al., 2002.

2.10 Multispectral Imaging (MSI), Diffuse Reflectance Spectroscopy (DRS) and Raman Spectroscopy (RS)

MSI has been widely used in the fields of astronomy and remote sensing (Colarusso et al., 1998; Curran, 1994) and, recently, is being applied to the field of biology and medicine (Johnson et al., 2007; Mansfield et al., 2005; Weber et al., 2011). An essential part of an MSI microscope is a spectral dispersion element that separates incident light into its spectral components (i.e., 400-1000 nm) (Bearman & Levenson, 2003). MSI of skin acquires spectrally resolved information at each pixel of a multispectral image, providing information on the distributions of collagen, melanin content and blood vessels within skin lesions (Marchesini, 1991, 1992). Carrara et al developed an algorithm for the automatic segmentation of multispectral images of 1856 cutaneous pigmented lesions including 264 CMMs, which successfully detected lateral margins of the lesions with a contour accuracy of 97.1% (Carrara et al., 2005). Marchesini et al reported that MSI and an artificial neural network could be used in the preoperative evaluation of CMM thickness with sensitivity (i.e., CMM≥0.75 mm thick correctly classified) and specificity (i.e., CMM<0.75 mm thick correctly classified) ranging from 76 to 90% and from 91 to 74%, respectively (Marchesini et al., 2007).

DRS (also called elastic scattering spectroscopy) measures the spectral modification of remitted light (i.e., light that has propagated some distance into the skin, been scattered, and recollected at skin surface). DRS was first introduced as a single-point measurement technique by Marchesini et al in 1992 to study CMM and nevus with a 5 mm probe (Marchesini et al., 1992). Wallace et al later reported that DRS in the wavelength range 320-1100 nm had the potential for improving the differential diagnosis of CMM from benign pigmented skin lesions (Wallace, 2000a, 2000b). However, further prospective study of DRS is needed to investigate its capability to detect tumor margins.

RS is a non-invasive imaging technique that has been widely used for the past 70 years for nondestructive chemical analysis. RS is based on the principle of Raman scattering, the inelastic scattering of electromagnetic radiation. The Raman scattering effect is caused by molecular vibrations in the irradiated sample and thus gives information about the structure of the molecules. Earlier studies have shown that samples of various benign skin lesions and nonmelanoma skin cancer have characteristic Raman spectra (Gniadecka et al., 1997a, 1997b, 1998). Recent studies on basal cell carcinoma by RS demonstrated its feasibility to distinguish malignant tissue from healthy surrounding tissue (Nijssen et al., 2002). More recently, Gniadecka et al developed a neural network system for the automated classification of Raman spectra, allowing CMM differentiation from other clinically similar skin tumors (Gniadecka et al., 2004). Therefore, RS is potentially capable of demarcating lateral margins of CMM.

In contrast to other imaging techniques (e.g., dermoscopy), MSI, DRS and RS are more objective and not observer dependent. However, similar to demoscopy, MSI, DRS and RS are also 2-D imaging techniques that cannot image the depth profile of CMM directly. Therefore, detection of depth margins of CMM by MSI, DRS or RS is hardly possible.

3. Conclusion

Early detection and surgical resection can reduce CMM mortality. To this end, several non-invasive imaging techniques have been developed to realize CMM screening, early diagnosis, preoperative tumor staging, surgical margin definition and *in vivo* tumor monitoring over multiple time points. Currently available instruments include MRI, CT, PET, HFUS, OCT, PAI, PPTR, SCM, MPLM, SHG, dermoscopy, MSI, DRS and RS. Dermoscopy, MSI, DRS and RS are useful in the evaluation of superficial CMMs, but they are not depth resolved. PET/CT do not have the resolution to detect early stage CMMs (e.g., <1 mm). They can, however, be used to detect tumor metastasis. MRI has comparable or higher resolution than CT and, hence, is suited to imaging advanced tumor invasion (e.g., >1 mm). SCM, MPLM and SHG provide physicians with an unprecedented capability to visualize a CMM lesion at a detail comparable to histology, but their imaging depths are limited to several hundred micrometers from skin surface, preventing them from detection of CMM depth margins beyond penetration depth. HFUS, OCT, PAI and PPTR have spatial resolutions and penetration depths between MRI/CT/PET and SCM/MPLM/SHG, therefore, they are potentially capable of detecting both lateral and depth margins of CMMs. A comparison of spatial resolution, penetration depth, sensitivity/specificity, correlation with histology and temporal monitoring (possibility to monitor CMM changes at multiple time points) of the imaging techniques discussed are summarized in Table 2 below.

From a clinical perspective, sensitivity and specificity studies of CMM diagnosis by MRI/CT/PET, HFUS, SCM/MPLM and dermoscopy/MSI/DRS/RS having been performed. Although sensitivity and specificity of OCT, PAI, PPTR and SHG on human CMM diagnosis are not yet established, they are promising imaging techniques that need further investigation on not only CMM diagnosis but also tumor lateral and depth margin delineation. To date, surgical resection is the major treatment for primary CMMs, which significantly increases the five-year survival rate. Surgical margins are currently determined by CMM thickness measured from biopsy with histology - the gold standard. The imaging techniques discussed, however, have the potential to non-invasively measure CMM thickness and detect tumor margins, and even guide CMM surgical resection in real time, which will reduce unnecessary biopsies and, eventually replace this invasive approach.

Because each of these imaging techniques has advantages and shortcomings, the best performing imaging tool for CMM evaluation is a combination of different imaging techniques - although at increased cost. A multimodal imaging tool will significantly improve the accuracy of CMM identification as well as the precision of surgical margin definition, which would achieve the five-year survival rate currently determined by biopsy-based surgical resection.

Imaging Techniques	Spatial Resolution (Lateral/Axial)	Penetration Depth	Sensitivity/Specificity in CMM Diagnosis	Correlation (R) with Histology	Temporal Monitoring
MRI	0.04-0.5 mm/ 0.3-0.5 mm†	Whole body	79.8%/76.4%①	NA	Yes
CT	0.1-0.29 mm/ 0.1-1 mm$	Whole body	77.1%/69.9%①	NA	Yes
PET	1-4 mm/ 1-4 mm*	Whole body	70.4%/83.7%①	NA	Yes
HFUS	20-300 μm/ 20-50 μm§	4-7.6 mm§	100%/32%②	>0.96②	Yes
OCT	10 μm/ 10-20 μm¶	1-2 mm	NA	NA	Yes
PAI	45 μm/15 μm	3 mm	NA	NA	Possible
PPTR	50 μm/75 μm	1.7 mm	NA	NA	Possible
SCM	0.5-1 μm/ 1-5 μm	200-300 μm	91%/99%③	NA	Possible
MPLM	0.3 μm/1 μm	200 μm	84%/76%④	NA	Possible

Imaging Techniques	Spatial Resolution (Lateral/Axial)	Penetration Depth	Sensitivity/Specificity in CMM Diagnosis	Correlation (R) with Histology	Temporal Monitoring
SHG	0.5 μm/ 1-1.9 μm[δ]	550 μm[ζ]	NA	0.9924⑤	Possible
Dermoscopy	20 μm/NA[ζ]	NA	96.3%/70.4%⑥	NA	Yes
MSI	30 μm/NA[η]	NA	76-90%/91-74%⑦	0.33⑦	Possible
DRS	200 μm/NA[κ]	NA	100%/84.4%⑧	NA	Possible
RS	100 μm/NA[μ]	NA	85%/99%⑨	NA	Possible

† Lateral resolution varies from 0.04 (9.4 T) to 0.7 mm (3 T), axial resolution varies from 0.3 (9.4 T) to 0.5 mm (3 T) (Gammal et al., 1996; Schick, 2005).
$ Lateral resolution varies from 0.1 (micro-CT) to 0.29 mm (conventional CT), axial resolution varies from 0.1 (micro-CT) to 1 mm (conventional CT) (Badea et al., 2004; Schroeder et al., 2001).
* Both lateral and axial resolution vary from nearly 1 mm FWHM (2 mm FWTM) for a 10-20 cm diameter system typical for animal studies with ^{18}F to roughly 4 mm FWHM (7 mm FWTM) for an 80 cm diameter system typical for human imaging using ^{15}O (Levin & Hoffman, 1999).
§ Lateral resolution varies from 20 (100 MHz) to 300 μm (20 MHz), axial resolution varies from 20 (100 MHz) to 50 μm (20 MHz), penetration depth varies from 4 (100 MHz) to 7.6 mm (20 MHz) (Harland et al., 1993; Passmann & Ermert, 1999; Pavlin et al., 1990).
¶ Lateral resolution can be 10 μm or better, axial resolution varies from 10 to 20 μm (Ding et al., 2002; Schenk & Brezinski, 2002).
δ Axial resolution varies from 1 to 1.9 μm (Campagnola et al., 2002; Moreaux et al., 2000).
ζ Lateral resolution is 20 μm with no axial resolution (Kopf et al., 1997).
η Lateral resolution is 30 μm with no axial resolution (Marchesini et al., 2007).
κ Lateral resolution is limited by the fiber size, no axial resolution is available (Häggblad et al., 2010).
μ Lateral resolution is limited by the laser spot size, no axial resolution is available (Gniadecka et al., 2004).
① 420 stage III/IV melanoma lesions from 64 patients were examined by MRI, CT and PET respectively (Pfannenberg et al., 2007).
② 114 pigmented skin lesions including 65 CMMs were examined by 20 MHz HFUS, ultrasound and histological measurement of melanoma thickness strongly correlated (Bessoud et al., 2003).
③ 162 skin lesions including 27 CMMs were examined by SCM (Gerger et al., 2006).
④ 100 melanocytic skin lesions including 26 CMMs from 83 patients were examined by MPLM (Dimitrow et al., 2009).
⑤ Correlation of collagen fiber density was examined from mid-point of CMM lesion to deep area of non-lesion skin (Thrasivoulou et al., 2011).
⑥ 128 pigmented skin lesions including 33 CMMs were examined by dermoscopy and ABCD diagnosis rule (Argenziano et al., 2003).
⑦ 1939 pigmented skin lesions including 250 CMMs were examined by MSI, the correlation coefficient value between tumor thickness and area is not so great to fully assess that lesion dimension increases with thickness (Marchesini et al., 2007).
⑧ 15 CMMs and 32 compound naevi were examined by DRS (Wallace, 2000a).
⑨ 134 pigmented skin lesions including 22 CMMs were examined by RS and neural network analysis (Gniadecka et al., 2004).

Table 2. Comparison of non-invasive imaging techniques for CMM diagnosis and tumor margin detection in terms of spatial resolution, penetration depth, sensitivity/specificity, correlation with histology and temporal monitoring (possibility to monitor CMM changes at multiple time points)

4. Acknowledgement

We thank Jingjing Sun for her technical assistance with the preparation of references for this book chapter.

5. References

Aaslid, R.; Huber, P. & Nornes, H. (1984). Evaluation of Cerebrovascular Spasm with Transcranial Doppler Ultrasound. *Journal of Neurosurgery*, Vol.60, No.1, (January 1984), pp. 37-41

Ahmed, I. & Berth-Jones, J. (2000). Imiquimod: a Novel Treatment for Lentigo Maligna. *British Journal of Dermatology*, Vol.143, No.4, (October 2000), pp. 843–845

Akcali, C.; Zincirkeser, S.; Erbagcy, Z.; Akcali, A.; Halac, M.; Durak, G.; Sager, S. & Sahin, E. (2007). Detection of Metastases in Patients with Cutaneous Melanoma Using FDG-PET/CT. *Journal of International Medical Research*, Vol.35, No.4, (July 2007), pp. 547-553

American Cancer Society, (Last medical review: March 5, 2010), 06.01.2011, Available from http://www.cancer.org/Cancer/SkinCancerMelanoma/DetailedGuide/melanoma-skin-cancer-key-statistics

Argenziano, G.; Fabbrocini, G.; Carli, P.; Giorgi, V. D.; Sammarco, E. & Delfino, M. (1998). Epiluminescence Microscopy for the Diagnosis of Doubtful Melanocytic Skin Lesions. Comparison of the ABCD Rule of Dermatoscopy and a New 7-Point Checklist Based on Pattern Analysis. *Archives of Dermatology*, Vol.134, (December 1998), pp. 1563-1570

Argenziano, G.; Soyer, H. P.; Chimenti, S.; Talamini, R.; Corona, R.; Sera, F.; Binder, M.; Cerroni, L.; Rosa, G. D. & Ferrara, G. (2003). Dermoscopy of Pigmented Skin Lesions: Results of a Consensus Meeting via the Internet. *Journal of the American Academy of Dermatology*, Vol.48, No.5, (May 2003), pp. 679-693

Armstrong, P. & Wastie, M. L. (Eds.). (2001). *A Concise Textbook of Radiology*, Arnold, pp. 536-594, ISBN 0340759380-9780340759387, London, UK

Baddeley, H. (1984). *Radiological Investigation. A Guide to the Use of Medical Imaging in Clinical Practice*, Wiley Medical Publications, Ann Arbor, MI, USA

Badea, C.; Hedlund, L. W. & Johnson, G. A. (2004). Micro-CT with Respiratory and Cardiac Gating. *Medical Physics*, Vol.31, No.12, (November 2004), pp. 3324-3329

Balch, C. M. & Ross, M. I. (1999). Sentinel Lymphadenectomy for Melanoma-Is It a Substitute for Elective Lymphadenectomy?. *Annals of Surgical Oncology*, Vol.6, No.5, (May 1999), pp. 416-417

Balch, C. M.; Buzaid, A.C.; Soong, S.J.; Atkins, M. B.; Cascinelli, N.; Coit, D. G.; Fleming, I. D.; Gershenwald, J. E.; Houghton, A.; Kirkwood, Jr J. M.; McMasters, K. M.; Mihm, M. F.; Morton, D. L.; Reintgen, D. S.; Ross, M. I.; Sober, A.; Thompson, J. A. & Thompson, J. F. (2001). Final Version of the American Joint Committee on Cancer (AJCC) Staging System for Cutaneous Melanoma. *Journal of Clinical Oncology*, Vol.19, No.16, (August 2001), pp. 3635–3648

Bearman, G. & Levenson, R. (2003). Biological Imaging Spectroscopy, In: *Biomedical Photonics Handbook*, Vo-Dinh, T. (Ed.), CRC Press, pp. 8.1–8.26, ISBN 0849311160, Boca Raton, FL, USA

Belhocine, T. Z.; Scott, A. M.; Even-Sapir, E.; Urbain, J. L. & Essner, R. (2006). Role of Nuclear Medicine in the Management of Cutaneous Malignant Melanoma. *Journal of Nuclear Medicine*, Vol.47, No.6, (June 2006), pp. 957–967

Bessoud, B.; Lassau, N.; Koscielny, S.; Longvert, C.; Avril, M.; Duvillard, P.; Rouffiac, V.; Leclère, J. & Roche, A. (2003). High-frequency Sonography and Color Doppler in the Management of Pigmented Skin Lesions. *Ultrasound in Medicine and Biology*, Vol.29, No.6, (June 2003), pp. 875-879

Bittoun, J.; Saint-Jalmes, H.; Querleux, B. G.; Darrasse, L.; Jolivet, O.; Idy-Peretti, I.; Wartski, M.; Richard, S. B. & Leveque, J. L. (1990). In Vivo High-Resolution MR Imaging of the Skin in a Whole-Body System at 1,5 T. *Radiology*, Vol.176, (August 1990), pp. 457–460

Blessing, C.; Feine, U.; Geiger, L.; Carl, M.; Rassner, G. & Fierlbeck, G. (1995). Positron Emission Tomography and Ultrasonography: a Comparative Retrospective Study Assessing the Diagnostic Validity in Lymph Node Metastases of Malignant Melanoma. *Archives of Dermatology*, Vol.131, No.12, (1995), pp. 1394-1398, ISSN 0003-987X

Boni, R.; Böni, R.; Steinert, H.; Burg, G.; Buck, A.; Marincek, B.; Berthold, T.; Dummer, R.; Voellmy, D.; Ballmer, B. & Von Schulthess, G. (1995). Staging of Metastatic Melanoma by Whole-Body Positron Emission Tomography Using 2-fluorine-18-fluoro-2-deoxy-D-glucose. *British Journal of Dermatology*, Vol.132, No.4, (April 1995), pp. 556–562

Breslow, A. (1970). Thickness, Cross Sectional Areas and Depth of Invasion in the Prognosis of Cutaneous Melanoma. *Annals of Surgery*, Vol.172, (November 1970), pp. 902-908

Brezinski, M. E. & Fujimoto, J. G. (1999). Optical Coherence Tomography: High-Resolution Imaging in Nontransparent Tissue, *IEEE Journal of Selected Topics in Quantum Electronics*, Vol.5, No.4, (July-August 1999), pp. 1185-1192

Busam, K. J.; Hester, K.; Charles, C.; Sachs, D. L.; Antonescu, C. R.; Gonzalez, S. & Halpern, A. C. (2001). Detection of Clinically Amelanotic Malignant Melanoma and Assessment of Its Margins by In Vivo Confocal Scanning Laser Microscopy. *Archives of Dermatology*, Vol.137, (July 2001), pp. 923-929

Campagnola, P. J.; Clark,H. A.; Mohler, W. A.; Lewis, A. & Loew, L. M. (2001). Second-Harmonic Imaging Microscopy of Living Cells. *Journal of Biomedical Optics*, Vol.6, No.3, (July 2001), pp. 277–286

Campagnola, P. J.; Millard, A. C.; Terasaki, M.; Hoppe, P. E.; Malone, C.J. & Mohler, W.A. (2002). Three-Dimensional High-Resolution Second-Harmonic Generation Imaging of Endogenous Structural Proteins in Biological Tissues. *Biophysical Journal*, Vol.82, No.1, (January 2002), pp. 493-508

Cancer Facts and Figures 2010. (2010). *American Cancer Society*, 06.06.2011, Available from http://www.cancer.org/acs/groups/content/@epidemiologysurveilance/documents/document/acspc026238.pdf

Carrara, M.; Tomatis, S.; Bono, A.; Bartoli, C.; Moglia, D.; Lualdi, M.; Colombo, A.; Santinami M. & Marchesini, R. (2005). Automated Segmentation of Pigmented Skin Lesions in Multispectral Imaging. *Physics in Medicine and Biology*, Vol.50, No.22, (November 2005), pp. N345-N357

Chen, C. S.; Elias, M.; Busam, K.; Rajadhyaksha, M. & Marghoob, A. (2005). Multimodal In Vivo Optical Imaging, Including Confocal Microscopy, Facilitates Presurgical Margin Mapping for Clinically Complex Lentigo Maligna Melanoma. *British Journal of Dermatology*, Vol.153, No.5, (November 2005), pp. 1031–1036

Colarusso, P.; Kidder L. H.; Levin, I. W.; Fraser, J. C.; Arens, J. F. & Lewis, E. N. (1998). Infrared Spectroscopic Imaging: from Planetary to Cellular Systems. *Applied Spectroscopy*, Vol.52, No.3, (March 1998), pp. 106A-120A

Cornejo, P.; Vanaclocha, F.; Polimon, I. & Del Rio, R. (2000). Intralesional Interferon Treatment of Lentigo Maligna. *Archives of Dermatology*, Vol.136, No.3, (March 2000), pp. 428-430

Cox, G.; Kable, E.; Jones, A.; Fraser, I.; Manconi, F. & Gorrell, M. D. (2003). 3-dimensional Imaging of Collagen Using Second Harmonic Generation. *Journal of Structural Biology*, Vol.141, No.1, (January 2003), pp. 53-62

Curiel-Lewandrowski, C.; Williams, C. M.; Swindells, K. J.; Tahan, S. R.; Astner, S.; Frankenthaler, R. A. & Gonzalez, S. (2004). Use of In Vivo Confocal Microscopy in Malignant Melanoma: an Aid in Diagnosis and Assessment of Surgical and Nonsurgical Therapeutic Approaches. *Archives of Dermatology*, Vol.140, No.9, (2004), pp. 1127-1132, ISSN 0003-987X

Curran, P. J. (1994). Imaging Spectrometry. *Progress in Physical Geography*, Vol.18, No.2, (June 1994), pp. 247-266

Damian, D. L.; Fulham, M. J.; Thompson, E. & Thompson, J. F. (1996). Positron Emission Tomography in the Detection and Management of Metastatic Melanoma. *Melanoma Research*, Vol.6, No.4, (August 1996), pp. 325-329

Dimitrow, E.; Ziemer, M.; Koehler, M. J.; Norgauer, J.; König, K.; Elsner, P. & Kaatz, M. (2009). Sensitivity and Specificity of Multiphoton Laser Tomography for In Vivo and Ex Vivo Diagnosis of Malignant Melanoma. *Journal of Investigative Dermatology*, Vol.129, (January 2009), pp. 1752-1758

Ding, Z; Ren, H; Zhao, Y.; Nelson, J. S. & Chen, Z. (2002). High-resolution Optical Coherence Tomography over a Large Depth Range with an Axicon Lens. *Optics Letters*, Vol.27, No.4, (February 2002), pp. 243-245

Dummer, W.; Blaheta, H. J.; Bastian, B. C.; Schenk, T.; Brocker, E. V. & Remy, W. (1995). Preoperative Characterization of Pigmented Skin Lesions by Epiluminescence Microscopy and High-frequency Ultrasound. *Archives of Dermatology*, Vol.131, No.3, (1995), pp. 279–285

Edge, S. B.; Byrd, D. R.; Compton, C. C.; Fritz, A. G.; Greene, F. L. & Trotti, A. (October 2010). *AJCC Cancer Staging Manual (7th ed)*, Springer, ISBN 978-0-387-88440-0, New York, NY, USA

el Gammal, S.; Hartwig R.; Aygen S.; Bauermann,T.; Gammal, C. el & Altmeyer, P. (1996). Improved Resolution of Magnetic Resonance Microscopy in Examination of Skin Tumors. *Journal of Investigative Dermatology*, Vol.106, (February 1996), pp. 1287–1292

Essner, R.; Belhocine, T.; Scott, A. M. & Even-Sapir, E. (2006). Novel Imaging Techniques in Melanoma. Surgical Oncology Clinics of North America, Vol.15, No.2, (April 2006), pp. 253–283

Fine, S. & Hansen, W. P. (1971). Optical Second Harmonic Generation in Biological Systems. *Applied Optics*, Vol.10, No.10, (October 1971), pp. 2350–2353

Foster, P. J.; Dunn, E. A.; Karl, K. E.; Snir, J. A.; Nycz, C. M.; Harvey, A. J. & Pettis, R. J. (2008). Cellular Magnetic Resonance Imaging: In Vivo Imaging of Melanoma Cells in Lymph Nodes of Mice. *Neoplasia*, Vol.10, No.3, (March 2008), pp. 207–216

Fujimoto, J. G.; Brezinski, M. E.; Tearney, G. J.; Boppart, S. A.; Bourna, B.; Hee, M. R.; Sourthern, J. F. & Swanson, E. A. (1995). Optical Biopsy and Imaging Using Optical Coherence Tomography. *Nature Medicine*, Vol.1, No.9, (September 1995), pp. 970–972

Gambichler, T.; Moussa, G.; Sand, M.; Sand, D.; Altmeyer, P. & Hoffmann, K. (2005). Applications of Optical Coherence Tomography in Dermatology. *Journal of Dermatological Science*, Vol.40, No.2, (November 2005), pp. 85-94

Gambichler, T.; Matip, R.; Moussa, G.; Altmeyer, P. & Hoffmann, K. (2006). In Vivo Data of Epidermal Thickness Evaluated by Optical Coherence Tomography: Effects of Age, Gender, Skin Type, and Anatomic Site. *Journal of Dermatological Science*, Vol.44, No.3, (December 2006), pp. 145–152

Gambichler, T.; Regeniter, P.; Bechara, F. G.; Orlikov, A.; Vasa, R.; Moussa, G.; Stücker, M.; Altmeyer, P. & Hoffmann, K. (2007). Characterization of Benign and Malignant Melanocytic Skin Lesions Using Optical Coherence Tomography In Vivo. *Journal of the American Academy of Dermatology*, Vol.57, No.4, (October 2007), pp. 629-637

Gareau, D. S.; Merlino, G.; Corless, C.; Kulesz-Martin, M. & Jacques, S. L. (2007). Noninvasive Imaging of Melanoma with Reflectance Mode Confocal Scanning Laser Microscopy in a Murine Model. *Journal of Investigative Dermatology*, Vol.127, (April 2007), pp. 2184–2190

Gareau, D. S.; Patel, Y. G. & Rajadhyaksha, M. (2008). Basic Principles of Reflectance Confocal Microscopy, In: *Reflectance Confocal Microscopy of Cutaneous Tumors*, Gonzalez, S., Gill, M., Halpern, A. C. (Eds.), pp. 1-3, Informa Healthcare, ISBN 0415451043, London, UK

Gerger, A.; Koller, S.; Kern, T.; Massone, C.; Steiger, K.; Richtig, E.; Kerl, H. & Smolle, J. (2005). Diagnostic Applicability of In Vivo Confocal Laser Scanning Microscopy in Melanocytic Skin Tumors. *Journal of Investigative Dermatology*, Vol.124, (March 2005), pp. 493–498

Gerger, A.; Koller, S.; Weger, W.; Richtig, E.; Kerl, H.; Samonigg, H.; Krippl, P. & Smolle, J. (2006). Sensitivity and Specificity of Confocal Laser-Scanning Microscopy for In Vivo Diagnosis of Malignant Skin Tumors. *Cancer*, Vol.107, No.1, (July 2006), pp. 193–200

Gniadecka, M.; Wulf, H. C.; Mortensen, N. N.; Nielsen, O. F. & Christensen, D. H. (1997). Diagnosis of Basal Cell Carcinoma by Raman Spectroscopy. *Journal of Raman Spectroscopy*, Vol.28, (February 1997), pp.125–129

Gniadecka, M.; Wulf, H. C.; Nielsen, O. F.; Christensen, D. H.; Hercogova, J. (1997). Distinctive Molecular Abnormalities in Benign and Malignant Skin Lesions: Studies by Raman Spectroscopy. *Photochem and Photobiol*, Vol.66, No.4, (June 1997), pp. 418–423

Gniadecka, M.; Wulf, H. C.; Nielsen, O. F.; Christensen, D. H.; Hercogova, J. & Rossen, K. (1998). Potential of Raman Spectroscopy for In Vitro and In Vivo Diagnosis of Malignant Melanoma, In: *Proceedings of the XVI International Conference on Raman Spectroscopy*. Heyns, E. M. (Ed.), pp. 764–765, John Wiley and Sons, ISBN 0471983616, Chichester, UK

Gniadecka, M.; Philipsen, P. A.; Sigurdsson, S.; Wessel, S.; Nielsen, O. F.; Christensen, D. H.; Hercogova, J.; Rossen, K.; Thomsen, H. K.; Gniadecki, R.; Hansen, L. K. & Wulf, H. C. (2004). Melanoma Diagnosis by Raman Spectroscopy and Neural Networks: Structure Alterations in Proteins and Lipids in Intact Cancer Tissue. *Journal of Investigative Dermatology*, Vol.122, No.2 (February 2004), pp. 443–449

Gonzalez, S. & Gilaberte-Calzada, Y. (2008). In Vivo Reflectance-Mode Confocal Microscopy in Clinical Dermatology and Cosmetology. *International Journal of Cosmetic Science*, Vol.30, No.1, (February 2008), pp. 1–17

Gritters, L. S.; Francis, I. R.; Zasadny, K. R. & Wahl, R. L. (1993). Initial Assessment of Positron Emission Tomography Using 2-Fluorine- 18-Fluoro-2- Deoxy-D-Glucose in the Imaging of Malignant Melanoma. *Journal of Nuclear Medicine*, Vol. 34, No. 9, (September 1993), pp. 1420-1427

Guitera, P.; Li, L.; Crotty, K.; FitzGerald, P.; Mellenbergh, R.; Pellacani, G. & Menzies, S. (2008). Melanoma Histological Breslow Thickness Predicted by 75-Mhz Ultrasonography. *British Journal of Dermatology*, Vol.159, No.2, (August 2008), pp. 364–369

Häggblad, E.; Petersson, H.; Ilias, M. A.; Anderson, C. D. & Salerud, E. G. (2010). A Diffuse Reflectance Spectroscopic Study of UV-induced Erythematous Reaction across Well-defined Borders in Human Skin. *Skin Research and Technology*, Vol.16, No.3, (August 2010), pp. 283–290

Halton, K. P. (1992). Radiological Considerations in Diagnosis of Metastatic Melanoma: Modern Management of Malignant Melanoma. *The Mount Sinai Journal of Medicine*, Vol.59, No.3, (1992), pp. 211-216, ISSN 0027-2507

Harland, C. C.; Bamber, J. C.; Gusterson, B. A. & Mortimer, P. S. (1993). High Frequency, High Resolution B-Scan Ultrasound in the Assessment of Skin Tumours. *British Journal of Dermatology*, Vol.128, No.5, (May 1993), pp. 525–532

Harland, C. C.; Kale, S.; Jackson, P.; Mortimer, P. S. & Bamber, J. C. (2000), Differentiation of Common Benign Pigmented Skin Lesions from Melanoma by High-Resolution Ultrasound. *British Journal of Dermatology*, Vol.143, No.2, (August 2000), pp. 281–289

Heaston, D. K.; Putman, C. E.; Rodan, B. A.; Nicholson, E.; Ravin, C. E.; Korobkin, M.; Chen, J. T. & Seigler, H. F. (1983). Solitary Pulmonary Metastasis in High Risk Melanoma Patients: a Prospective Comparison of Conventional and Computed Tomography. *American Journal of Roentgenology*, Vol.141, No.1, (1983), pp. 169-174

Hendriks, R. F. M. & Lucassen, G. W. (2000). Two Photon Fluorescence Microscopy of In Vivo Human Skin, *Proceedings of SPIE 2000 Conference on Laser Microscopy*, Vol.4164, pp. 116-121, Amsterdam, Netherlands, July 2000

Henning JS, Dusza SW, Wang SQ, Marghoob, A. A.; Rabinovitz, H. S.; Polsky, D. & Kopf, A. W. (2007). The CASH (Color, Architecture, Symmetry, and Homogeneity) Algorithm for Dermoscopy. *Journal of the American Academy of Dermatology*, Vol.56, No.1, (January 2007), pp. 45-52

Hoffmann, K.; Jung, J.; el Gammal, S. & Altmeyer, P. (1992). Malignant Melanoma in 20-Mhz B Scan Sonography. *Dermatology*, Vol.185, No.1, (1992), pp. 49–55

Holan, S. H. & Viator, J. A. (2008). Automated Wavelet Denoising of Photoacoustic Signals for Circulating Melanoma Cell Detection and Burn Image Reconstruction. *Physics in Medicine and Biology*, Vol.53, No.12, (June 2008), pp. N227–N236

Huang, D.; Swanson, E. A.; Lin, C. P.; Schuman, J. S.; Stinson, W. G.; Chang, W.; Hee, M. R.; Flotte, T.; Gregory, K.; Puliafito, C. A. & Fujimoto, J. G. (1991). Optical Coherence Tomography. *Science*, Vol.254, No.5035, (November 1991), pp. 1178-1181

Hyde, J. S.; Jesmanowicz, A. & Kneeland, J. B. (1987). Surface Coil for MR Imaging of the Skin. *Magnetic Resonance in Medicine*, Vol.5, No.5, (November 1987), pp. 456–461

Iagaru, A.; Quon, A.; Johnson, D.; Gambhir, S. S. & McDougall, I. R. (2006). 2-Deoxy-2-[F-18]fluoro-Dglucose Positron Emission Tomography/Computed Tomography in the Management of Melanoma. *Molecular Imaging and Biology*, Vol.8, No.1, (October 2006), pp. 309-14

Jerant, A. F.; Johnson, J. T.; Sheridan, C. D. & Caffrey T. J. (2000). Early Detection and Treatment of Skin Cancer. *American Family Physician*, Vol.62, No.2, (July 2000), pp. 357-368

Johnson, W. R.; Wilson, D.W.; Fink, W.; Humayun, M. & Bearman, G. (2007). Snapshot Hyperspectral Imaging in Ophthalmology. *Journal of Biomedical Optics*, Vol.12, No.1, (January-February 2007), pp. 0140361-0140367

Kanzler, M. H. & Mraz-Gernhard, S. (2001). Treatment of Primary Cutaneous Melanoma. *Journal of American Medical Association*, Vol.285, No.14, (April 2001), pp. 1819-1821

King, D.M. (2004). Imaging of Metastatic Melanoma. Journal of Hong Kong College of Radiologists, Vol.7, No.2, (2004), pp. 66-69

Kittler, H.; Pehamberger, H.; Wolff, K. & Binder, M. (2002). Diagnostic Accuracy of Dermoscopy. *The LANCET Oncology*, Vol.3, (March 2002), pp. 159-165

König, K. (2000). Laser Tweezers and Multiphoton Microscopes in Life Sciences. *Histochemistry and Cell Biology*, Vol.114, No.2, (July 2000), pp. 79–92

König, K. (2000). Multiphoton Microscopy in Life Sciences. *Journal of Microscopy*, Vol.200, No.2, (November 2000), pp. 83–104

König, K.; Wollina, U.; Riemann, I.; Peuckert, C.; Halbhuber, K. J.; Konrad, H.; Fischer, P.; Fünfstück, V.; Fischer, T. W. & Elsner, P. (2002). Optical Tomography of Human Skin with Subcellular Spatial and Picosecond Time Resolution Using Near Infrared Femtosecond Laser Pulses, *Proceedings of SPIE 2002 Conference on Multiphoton Microscopy in the Biomedical Sciences II*, Vol.4620, pp. 190–201, June 2002

Kopf, A. W.; Elbaum, M. & Provost, N. (1997). The Use of Dermoscopy and Digital Imaging in the Diagnosis of Cutaneous Malignant Melanoma. *Skin Research and Technology*, Vol.3, No.11, (February 1997), pp. 1–7

Langley, R. G.; Burton, E.; Walsh, N.; Propperova, I. & Murray, S. J. (2006). In Vivo Confocal Scanning Laser Microscopy of Benign Lentigines: Comparison to Conventional Histology and In Vivo Characteristics of Lentigo Maligna. *Journal of American Academy of Dermatology*, Vol.55, No.1, (July 2006), pp. 88-97

Lassau, N.; Mercier, S.; Koscielny, S.; Avril, M. F.; Margulis, A.; Mamelle, G.; Duvillard, P. & Leclere, J. (1999). Prognostic Value of High-frequency Sonography and Color Doppler Sonography for the Preoperative Assessment of Melanomas. *American Journal of Roentgenology*, Vol.172, (February 1999), pp. 457–461

Levin, C. S. & Hoffman E. J. (1999). Calculation of Positron Range and Its Effect on the Fundamental Limit of Positron Emission Tomography System Spatial Resolution. *Physics in Medicine and Biology*, Vol.44, No.3, (March 1999), pp. 781-799

Li, B.; Majaron, B.; Viator, J. A.; Milner, T. E.; Chen, Z.; Zhao, Y.; Ren, H. & Nelson, J. S. (2004). Accurate Measurement of Blood Vessel Depth in Port Wine Stained Human Skin In Vivo Using Pulsed Photothermal Radiometry. *Journal of Biomedical Optics*, Vol.9, No.5, (September-October 2004), pp. 961-966

Lim, R. S.; Kratzer, A.; Barry, N. P.; Miyazaki-Anzai, S.; Miyazaki, M.; Mantulin, W. W.; Levi, M.; Potma, E. O. & Tromberg, B. J. (2010). Multimodal CARS Microscopy Determination of the Impact of Diet on Macrophage Infiltration and Lipid Accumulation on Plaque Formation in ApoE-deficient Mice. *Journal of Lipid Research*, Vol.51, No.7, (July 2010), pp. 1729-37

Link, T. M.; Vieth V.; Stehling, C.; Lotter, A.; Beer, A.; Newitt, D. & Majumdar, S. (2002). High-Resolution MRI vs Multislice Spiral CT: Which Technique Depicts the Trabecular Bone Structure Best?. *European Radiology*, Vol.13, No.4, (September 2002), pp. 663-671

Lohela, M. & Werb, Z. (2010). Intravital Imaging of Stromal Cell Dynamics in Tumors. *Current Opinion in Genetics and Development*, Vol.20, No.1, (February 2010), pp. 72-78

Macfarlane, D. J.; Sondak, V.; Johnson, T. & Wahl, R. L. (1998). Prospective Evaluation of 2-(18F)-2-deoxyglucose Positron Emission Tomography in Staging of Regional Lymph Nodes in Patients with Cutaneous Malignant Melanoma. *Journal of Clinical Oncology*, Vol.16, No.5, (May 1998), pp. 1770-1776

Machet, L.; Belot, V.; Naouri, M.; Boka, M.; Mourtada, Y.; Giraudeau, B.; Laure, B.; Perrinaud, A.; Machet, M. & Vaillant, L. (2009). Preoperative Measurement of Thickness of Cutaneous Melanoma Using High-Resolution 20 MHz Ultrasound Imaging: A Monocenter Prospective Study and Systematic Review of the Literature, *Ultrasound in Medicine and Biology*, Vol.35, No.9, (September 2009), pp. 1411-1420

MacKie, R. M. (1971). An Aid to the Preoperative Assessment of Pigmented Lesions of the Skin. *British Journal of Dermatology*, Vol.85, No.3, (September 1971), pp. 232-238

Mansfield, J. R.; Hoyt, C. C.; Miller, P. J. & Levenson, R. M. (2005). Distinguished Photons: Increased Contrast with Multispectral In Vivo Fluorescence Imaging. *Biotechniques*, Vol.39, (December 2005), pp. S33–S37

Marchesini, R.; Brambilla, M.; Clemente, C.; Maniezzo, M.; Sichirollo, A. E.; Testori, A.; Venturoli, D. R. & Cascinelli, N. (1991). In Vivo Spectrophotometric Evaluation of Neoplastic and Non-Neoplastic Skin Pigmented Lesions–I. Reflectance Measurements. *Photochemistry and Photobiology*, Vol.53, No.1, (January 1991), pp. 77–84

Marchesini, R.; Cascinelli, N.; Brambilla, M.; Clemente, C.; Mascheroni, L.; Pignoli, E.; Testori, A. & Venturoli, D. R. (1992). In Vivo Spectrophotometric Evaluation of Neoplastic and Non-Neoplastic Skin Pigmented Lesions. II: Discriminant Analysis between Nevus and Melanoma. *Photochemistry and Photobiology*, Vol.55, No.4, (April 1992), pp. 515–522

Marchesini, R.; Bono, A.; Tomatis, S.; Bartoli, C.; Colombo, A.; Lualdi, M. & Carrara, M. (2007). In Vivo Evaluation of Melanoma Thickness by Multispectral Imaging and an Artificial Neural Network. A Retrospective Study on 250 Cases of Cutaneous Melanoma. *Tumori*, Vol.93, No.2, (March-April 2007), pp. 170-177

Marghoob, A. A.; Swindle, L. D.; Moricz, C. Z. M. S.; Sanchez-Negron, F. A.; Slueb, B.; Halpern, A. C. & Kopf, A. W. (2003). Instruments and New Technologies for the In Vivo Diagnosis of Melanoma. *Journal of the American Academy of Dermatology*, Vol.49, No.5, (November 2003), pp. 777-797

Marghoob, A. A. & Halpern, A. C. (2005). Confocal Scanning Laser Reflectance Microscopy: Why Bother?. *Archives of Dermatology*, Vol.141, No.2, (February 2005), pp. 212-215

Maslov, K.; Stoica, G. & Wang, L. V. (2005). In Vivo Dark-Field Reflectionmode Photoacoustic Microscopy. *Optics Letters*, Vol.30, No.6, (March 2005), pp. 625-627

Masters, B. R.; So, P. T. C. & Gratton, E. (1997). Multiphoton Excitation Fluorescence Microscopy and Spectroscopy of In Vivo Human Skin. *Biophysical Journal*, Vol.2, No.6, (June 1997), pp. 2405-2412

Masters, B. R.; So, P. T. C. & Gratton, E. (1998). Multiphoton Excitation Microscopy of In Vivo Human Skin, In: *Advances in Optical Biopsy and Optical Mammography*, Alfano, R. R. (Ed.), Vol.838, pp. 58–67, New York Academy of Sciences, New York, NY, USA

Meyer, L. E.; Otberg, N.; Sterry, W. & Lademann, J. (2006). In Vivo Confocal Scanning Laser Microscopy: Comparison of the Reflectance and Fluorescence Mode by Imaging Human Skin. *Journal of Biomedical Optics*, Vol.11, No.4, (August 2006), pp. 11–17

Mihm, M. C.; Murphy, G. F. & Kaufman, N. (1988). *Pathobiology and Recognition of Malignant Melanoma*, United States and Canadian Academy of Pathology, New York, NY, USA

Milanič, M.; Majaron B. & Nelson, J. S. (2007). Pulsed Photothermal Temperature Profiling of Agar Tissue Phantoms, *Lasers in Medical Science*, Vol.22, No.4, (May 2007), pp. 279-284

Milner, T. E.; Smithies, D. J.; Goodman, D. M.; Lau, A. & Nelson, J. S. (1996). Depth Determination of Chromophores in Human Skin by Pulsed Photothermal Radiometry. *Applied Optics*, Vol.35, No.19, (June 1996), pp. 3379-3385

Moreaux, L.; Sandre, O. & Mertz, J. (2000). Membrane Imaging by Second-harmonic Generation Microscopy. *Journal of the Optical Society of America B: Optical Physics*, Vol.17, No.10, (October 2000), pp. 1685-1694

Nehal, K. S.; Gareau, D. & Rajadhyaksha, M. (2008). Skin Imaging with Reflectance Confocal Microscopy. *Seminars in Cutaneous Medicine and Surgery*, Vol.27, No.1, (March 2008), pp. 37-43

Nijssen, A., Bakker Schut, T. C.; Heule, F.; Caspers, P. J.; Hayes, D. P.; Neumann, M. H. A. & Puppels, G. J. (2002). Discriminating Basal Cell Carcinoma from Its Surrounding Tissue by Raman Spectroscopy. *Journal* of *Investigative Dermatology*, Vol.119, No.1, (July 2002), pp. 64–69

Oh, J.; Li, M.; Zhang, H. F.; Maslov, K. & Wang, L. V. (2006). Three-dimensional Imaging of Skin Melanoma In Vivo by Dual-Wavelength Photoacoustic Microscopy. *Journal of Biomedical Optics*, Vol.11, No.3, (June 2006), pp. 0340321-0340324

Olmedo, J. M.; Warschaw, K. E.; Schmitt, J. M. & Swanson, D. L. (2006). Optical Coherence Tomography for the Characterization of Basal Cell Carcinoma In Vivo: a Pilot Study. *Journal of the American Academy of Dermatology*, Vol.55, No.3, (September 2006), pp. 408-412

Ono, I. & Kaneko, F. (1995), Magnetic Resonance Imaging for Diagnosing Skin Tumors. *Clinics in Dermatology*, Vol.13, No.4, (July-August 1995), pp. 393-399

Passmann, C. & Ermert, H. (1999). A 100-MHz Ultrasound Imaging System for Dermatologic and Ophthalmologic Diagnostics. *IEEE Transactions on Ultrasonics, Ferroelectrics, and Frequency Control*, Vol.43, No.4, (July 1999), pp. 545-552

Pavlin, C. J.; Sherar, M. D. & Foster, F. S. (1990). Subsurface Ultrasound Microscopic Imaging of the Intact Eye. *Ophthalmology*, Vol.97, No.2, (February 1990), pp. 244-250

Pellacani, G.; Cesinaro, A. M. & Seidenari, S. (2005). Reflectance-mode Confocal Microscopy of Pigmented Skin Lesions-Improvement in Melanoma Diagnostic Specificity. *Journal of the American Academy of Dermatology*, Vol.53, No.6, (December 2005), pp. 979-985

Pellacani, G.; Guitera, P.; Longo, C.; Avramidis, M.; Seidenari, S. & Menzies, S. (2007). The Impact of In Vivo Reflectance Confocal Microscopy for the Diagnostic Accuracy of Melanoma and Equivocal Melanocytic Lesions. *Journal of Investigative Dermatology*, Vol.127, (July 2007), pp. 2759-2765

Peuckert, C.; Riemann, I. & König, K. (2000). Two Photon Induced Autofluorescence of In Vivo Human Skin with Femtosecond Laser Pulses-a Novel Imaging Tool of High Spatial, Spectral and Temporal Resolution. *Cellular and Molecular Biology*, Vol.46, (2000), abstract 179

Pfannenberg, C.; Aschoff, P.; Schanz, S.; Eschmann, S. M.; Plathow, C.; Eigentler, T. K.; Garbe, C.; Brechtel, K.; Vonthein, R.; Bares, R.; Claussen C. D. & Schlemmer, H. P. (2007). Prospective Comparison of ^{18}F-fluorodeoxyglucose Positron Emission

Tomography/Computed Tomography and Whole-body Magnetic Resonance Imaging in Staging of Advanced Malignant Melanoma. *European Journal of Cancer*, Vol.43, No.3, (February 2007), pp. 557-564

Querleux, B. (1995). Nuclear Magnetic Resonance (NMR) Examination of the Epidermis In Vivo, In: *Handbook of Non-Invasive Methods and the Skin*, Serup, J. & Jemec, G. B. E. (Eds.), pp. 133–139, CRC, ISBN 0849314372, Boca Raton, FL, USA

Querleux, B.; Yassine, M. M.; Darrasse, L.; Saint-Jalmes, H.; Sauzade, M. & Leveque, J. L. (1988). Magnetic Resonance Imaging of the Skin. A Comparison with the Ultrasonic Technique. *Bioengineering and the Skin*, Vol.4, No.1, (1988), pp. 1–14, ISSN 0266-3082

Rajadhyaksha, M.; Grossman, M.; Esterowitz, D.; Webb, R. H. & Anderson, R. R. (1995). In Vivo Confocal Scanning Laser Microscopy of Human Skin: Melanin Provides Strong Contrast. *Journal of Investigative Dermatology*, Vol.104, No.6, (June 1995), pp. 946–952

Rajeswari, M. R.; Jain, A; Sharma, A.; Singh, D.; Jagannathan, N. R.; Sharma, U. & Degaonkar, M. N. (2003). Evaluation of Skin Tumors by Magnetic Resonance Imaging. *Laboratory Investigation*, Vol.83, (May 2003), pp. 1279–1283

Reinhardt, M. J.; Joe, A. Y.; Jaeger, U.; Huber, A.; Matthies, A.; Bucerius, J.; Roedel, R.; Strunk, H.; Bieber, T.; Biersack, H. & Tüting T. Diagnostic Performance of Whole Body Dual Modality 18F-FDG PET/CT Imaging for N- and M-Staging of Malignant Melanoma: Experience with 250 Consecutive Patients. *Journal of Clinical Oncology*, Vol.24, No.7, (March 2006), pp. 1178-1187

Richard, S.; Querleux, B.; Bittoun, J.; Idy-Peretti, I.; Jolivet, O.; Cermakowa, E. & Leveque, J. L. (1991). In Vivo Proton Relaxation Times Analysis of Skin Layers by Magnetic Resonance Imaging. *Journal of Investigative Dermatology*, Vol.97, (February 1991), pp. 120–125

Ries, L.; Eisner, M.; Kosary, C.; Hankey, B.; Miller, B. & Clegg, L. (2003). SEER Cancer Statistics Review, 1975-2000. *National Cancer Institute*, (2003), Tables XV1-9

Rinne, D.; Baum, R.P.; Hor, G. & Kaufmann, R. (1998). Primary Staging and Followup of High Risk Melanoma Patients with Whole Body 18 F-fluorodeoxyglucose Positron Emission Tomography: Results of a Prospective Study of 100 Patients. *Cancer*, Vol.82, No.9, (1998), pp. 1664-1671, ISSN 0008-543X

Roth, S. & Freund, I. (1979). Second Harmonic-Generation in Collagen. *Journal of Chemical Physics*, Vol.70, No.4, (February 1979), pp. 1637–1643

Rubin, K. M. (2010). Melanoma Staging: A Review of the Revised American Joint Committee on Cancer Guidelines. Journal of the Dermatology Nurses' Association, Vol.2, No.6, (November-December 2010), pp. 254-259

Schenk, J. O. & Brezinski, M. E. (2002). Ultrasound Induced Improvement in Optical Coherence Tomography (OCT) Resolution. *Proceedings of the National Academy of Sciences of the United States of America*, Vol.99, No.15, (July 2002), pp. 9761-9764

Schick, F. (2005). Whole-Body MRI at High Field: Technical Limits and Clinical Potential. *European Radiology*, Vol.31, No.5, (May 2005), pp. 946–959

Schroeder, S.; Kopp, A. F.; Baumbach, A.; Meisner, C.; Kuettner, A.; Georg, C.; Ohnesorge, B.; Herdeg, C.; Claussen, C. D. & Karsch, K. R. (2001). Noninvasive Detection and Evaluation of Atherosclerotic Coronary Plaques with Multislice Computed Tomography. *Journal of the American College of Cardiology*, Vol.37, No.5, (April 2001), pp. 1430-1435

Serrone, L.; Solivetti, F. M.; Thorel, M. F.; Eibenschutz, L.; Donati, P. & Catricala, C. (2002). High Frequency Ultrasound in the Preoperative Staging of Primary Melanoma: a Statistical Analysis. *Melanoma Research*, Vol.12, No.3, (June 2002), pp. 287–290

Shi, J.; Zheng,Y. P.; Chen, X. & Huang, Q. H. (2007). Assessment of Muscle Fatigue Using Sonomyography: Muscle Thickness Change Detected from Ultrasound Images. *Medical Engineering and Physics*, Vol.29, No.4, (May 2007), pp. 472-479

Sladden, M. J.; Balch, C.; Barzilai, D. A.; Berg, D.; Freiman, A.; Handiside, T.; Hollis, S.; Lens, M. B. & Thompson, J. F. (2009). Surgical Excision Margins for Primary Cutaneous Melanoma. *Cochrane Database of Systematic Reviews*, No.4, (October 2009), pp. 1-34

Smith, L. & MacNeil, S. (2011), State of the Art in Non-Invasive Imaging of Cutaneous Melanoma. *Skin Research and Technology*, Vol.17, (February 2011), doi: 10.1111/j.1600-0846.2011.00503.x

So, P. T. C. & Kim, H. (1998). Two-photon Deep Tissue Ex Vivo Imaging of Mouse Dermal and Subcutaneous Structures. *Optics Express*, Vol.3, No.9, (October 1998), pp. 339–350

Song, K. H.; Kim, C.; Maslov, K. & Wang, L. V. (2009). Noninvasive In Vivo Spectroscopic Nanorod-Contrast Photoacoustic Mapping of Sentinel Lymph Nodes. *European Journal of Radiology*, Vol.70, No.2, (May 2009), pp. 227-231

Steinert, H. C.; Huch Böni, R. A.; Buck, A.; Böni, R.; Berthold, T.; Marincek, B.; Burg, G. & von Schulthess, G. K. (1995). Malignant Melanoma: Staging with Whole Body Positron Emission Tomography and 2-(F-18)-fluoro-2-deoxy-D-glucose. *Radiology*, Vol.195, (June 1995), pp. 705-709

Strobel, K.; Dummer, R.; Husarik, D. B.; Lago, M. P.; Hany, T. F. & Steinert, H. C. (2007). High-Risk Melanoma: Accuracy of FDG PET/CT with Added CT Morphologic Information for Detection of Metastases. *Radiology*, Vol.244, No.2, (August 2007), pp. 566-574

Sun, T. & Diebold, G. J. (1992). Generation of Ultrasonic Waves from a Layered Photoacoustic Source. *Nature*, Vol.355, (February 1992), pp. 806–808

Tacke, J.; Haagen, G.; Hornstein, O. P.; Huettinger, G.; Kiesewetter, F.; Schell, H. & Diepgen, T. L. (1995). Clinical Relevance of Sonometry-derived Tumour Thickness in Malignant Melanoma: a Statistical Analysis. *British Journal of Dermatology*, Vol.132, No.2, (February 1995), pp. 209–214

Tannous, Z. S.; Lerner, L. H.; Duncan, L. M.; Mihm Jr, M. C. & Flotte, T. J. (2000). Progression to Invasive Melanoma from Malignant Melanoma In Situ, Lentigo Maligna Type. *Human Pathology*, Vol.31, No.6, (June 2000), pp. 705-708

Tannous, Z. S.; Mihm, M. C.; Flotte, T. J. & Gonzalez, S. (2002). In Vivo Examination of Lentigo Maligna and Malignant Melanoma In Situ, Lentigo Maligna Type by Near-Infrared Reflectance Confocal Microscopy: Comparison of In Vivo Confocal Images with Histologic Sections. *Journal of American Academy of Dermatology*, Vol.46, No.2, (February 2002), pp. 260-263

Teuchner, K.; Freyer, W.; Leupold, D.; Volkmer, A.; Birch, D. J. S.; Altmeyer, P.; Stucker, M. & Hoffmann, K. (1999). Femtosecond Two-photon Excited Fluorescence of Melanin. *Photochemistry and Photobiology*, Vol.70, No.2, (August 1999), pp. 146–151

Theodossiou, T. A.; Thrasivoulou, C.; Ekwobi, C. & Becker, D. L. (2006). Second Harmonic Generation Confocal Microscopy of Collagen Type I from Rat Tendon Cryosections. *Biophysical Journal*, Vol.91, No.12, (December 2006), pp. 4665-4677

Thrasivoulou, C.; Virich, G.; Krenacs, T.; Korom, I. & Becker, D. L. (2011). Optical Delineation of Human Malignant Melanoma Using Second Harmonic Imaging of Collagen. *Biomedical Optics Express*, Vol.2, No.5, (May 2011), pp. 1282-1295

Totty, W. G.; Murphy, W. A. & Lee, J. K. T. (1986). Soft-tissue Tumors: MR Imaging. *Radiology*, Vol.160, (July 1986), 135-141.

Tripp, J. M.; Kopf, A. W.; Marghoob, A. A. & Bart, R. S. (2002). Management of Dysplastic Nevi: a Survey of Fellows of the American Academy of Dermatology. *Journal of the American Academy of Dermatology*, Vol.46, No.5, (May 2002), pp. 674-682

Tuzcu, E. M.; Bayturan, O. & Kapadia, S. (2010). Coronary Intravascular Ultrasound: a Closer View. *Heart*, Vol.96, No.16, (2010), pp. 1318-1324

Ulrich, J.; Petereit, S. & Gollnick, H. (1999). The Preoperative Diagnostics of Malignant Melanoma - Comparison of 7.5-MHz- and 20-MHz-Sonography. *Ultraschall in Medicine*, Vol.20, No.5, (1999), pp. 197-200

Wagner, J. D.; Schauwecker, D.; Hutchins, G. & Coleman, J. J. (1997). Initial Assessment of Positron Emission Tomography for Detection of Nonpalpable Regional Lymphatic Metastases in Melanoma. *Journal of Surgical Oncology*, Vol.64, No.3, (March 1997), pp. 181–189

Wagner, J. D.; Schauwecker, D.; Davidson, D.; Coleman III, J. J.; Saxman, S.; Hutchins, G.; Love, C. & Hayes, J. T. (1999). Prospective Study of Fluorodeoxyglucose–Positron Emission Tomography Imaging of Lymph Node Basins in Melanoma Patients Undergoing Sentinel Node Biopsy. *Journal of Clinical Oncology*, Vol. 17, No. 5, (May 1999), 1508-1515

Wallace, V. P.; Crawford, D. C.; Mortimer, P. S.; Ott, R. J. & Bamber, J. C. (2000). Spectrophotometric Assessment of Pigmented Skin Lesions: Methods and Feature Selection for Evaluation of Diagnostic Performance. *Physics in Medicine and Biology*, Vol.45, No.3, (January 2000), pp. 735–751

Wallace, V. P.; Bamber, J. C.; Crawford, D. C.; Ott, R. J. & Mortimer P. S. (2000). Classification of Reflectance Spectra from Pigmented Skin Lesions, a Comparison of Multivariate Discriminant Analysis and Artificial Neural Networks. *Physics in Medicine and Biology*, Vol.45, No.10, (March 2000), pp. 2859-2871.

Wang, H.; Huff, T. B.; Zweifel, D. A.; He, W.; Low, P. S.; Wei, A. & Cheng, J. (2005). In Vitro and In Vivo Two-photon Luminescence Imaging of Single Gold Nanorods. *Proceedings of the National Academy of Sciences of the United States of America*, Vol.102, No.44, (November 2005), pp. 15752-15756

Wang, H.; Langohr, I. M.; Sturek M. & Cheng, J. (2009). Imaging and Quantitative Analysis of Atherosclerotic Lesions by CARS-Based Multimodal Nonlinear Optical Microscopy. *Arteriosclerosis, Thrombosis, and Vascular Biology*, Vol.29, (June 2009), pp. 1342-1348

Wang, T.; Qiu, J.; Paranjape, A. S. & Milner, T. E. (2009). Melanoma Thickness Measurement in Two-layer Tissue Phantoms Using Pulsed Photothermal Radiometry (PPTR), *Proceedings of SPIE 2009 Conference on Optical Interactions with Tissue and Cells XX*, Vol.7175, pp. 71750L1-71750L9, San Jose, CA, USA, January 2009

Wang, T.; Mallidi, S.; Qiu, J.; Ma, L. L.; Paranjape, A. S.; Sun, J.; Kuranov, R. V.; Johnston, K. P. & Milner, T. E. (2011). Comparison of Pulsed Photothermal Radiometry, Optical Coherence Tomography and Ultrasound for Melanoma Thickness Measurement in PDMS Tissue Phantoms. *Journal of Biophotonics*, Vol.4, No.5, (May 2011), pp. 335–344

Wang, X.; Pang, Y.; Ku, G.; Xie, X.; Stoica, G. & Wang, L. V. (2003). Noninvasive Laser-Induced Photoacoustic Tomography for Structural and Functional In Vivo Imaging of the Brain. *Nature Biotechnology*, Vol.21, (June 2003), pp. 803-806

Weber, J. R.; Cuccia, D. J.; Johnson, W. R.; Bearman, G. H.; Durkin, A. J.; Hsu, M.; Lin, A.; Binder, D. K.; Wilson D. & Tromberg, B. J. (2011). Multispectral Imaging of Tissue Absorption and Scattering Using Spatial Frequency Domain Imaging and a Computed-Tomography Imaging Spectrometer. *Journal of Biomedical Optics*, Vol.16, No.1, (January 2011), pp. 0110151-0110157

Weeks, R. G.; Berquist, T. H.; McLeod, R. A. & Zimmer, W. D. (1985). Magnetic Resonance Imaging of Soft-Tissue Tumors: Comparison with Computed Tomography. *Magnetic Resonance Imaging*, Vol.3, No.4, (September 1985), pp. 345-352

Weight, R. M.; Viator, J. A.; Dale, P. S.; Caldwell, C. W. & Lisle, A. E. (2006). Photoacoustic Detection of Metastatic Melanoma Cells in the Human Circulatory System. *Optics Letters*, Vol.31, No.20, (October 2006), pp. 2998–3000

Welzel, J. (2001). Optical Coherence Tomography in Dermatology: a Review. *Skin Research and Technology*, Vol.7, No.1, (February 2001), pp. 1–9

Welzel, J.; Bruhns, M. & Wolff, H. H. (2003). Optical Coherence Tomography in Contact Dermatitis and Psoriasis. *Archives of Dermatological Research*, Vol.295, No.2, (April 2003), pp. 50-55

Yao, W. J.; Hoh, C.K. & Glaspy, F. (1994). Whole Body FDG-PET Imaging for Staging Of Malignant Melanoma: Is It Cost Effective?. *Journal of Nuclear Medicine*, Vol.35, (May 1994), pp. 8P, ISSN 0161-5505

Zemtsov, A.; Lorig, R.; Bergfield, W. F.; Bailin, P. L. & Ng, T. C. (1989). Magnetic Resonance Imaging of Cutaneous Melanocytic Lesions. *Journal of Dermatologic Surgery and Oncology*, Vol.15, No.8, (August 1989), pp. 854-858

Zhang, H. F.; Maslov, K.; Stoica, G. & Wang, L. V. (2006). Functional Photoacoustic Microscopy for High-Resolution and Noninvasive In Vivo Imaging. *Nature Biotechnology*, Vol.24, (June 2006), pp. 848 - 851

Zharov, V. P.; Galanzha, E. I.; Shashkov, E. V.; Khlebtsov, N. G. & Tuchin, V. V. (2006). In Vivo Photoacoustic Flow Cytometry for Monitoring of Circulating Single Cancer Cells and Contrast Agents. *Optics Letters*, Vol.31, No.24, (December 2006), pp. 3623–3625

Zipfel, W. R.; Williams, R. M.; Christie, R.; Nikitin, A. Y.; Hyman, B. T. & Webb, W. W. (2003). Live Tissue Intrinsic Emission Microscopy Using Multiphotonexcited Native Fluorescence and Second Harmonic Generation. *Proceedings of the National Academy of Sciences of the United States of America*, Vol.100, No.12, (June 2003), pp. 7075–7080

Zipfel, W. R.; Williams, R. M. & Webb, W. W. (2003). Nonlinear Magic: Multiphoton Microscopy in the Biosciences. *Nature Biotechnology*, Vol.21, No.11, (November 2003), pp. 1369 –1377

6

Differential Scanning Calorimetry, as a New Method to Monitor Human Plasma in Melanoma Patients with Regional Lymph Node or Distal Metastases

Andrea Ferencz, Tamás Fekecs and Dénes Lőrinczy
University of Pécs, Medical School, Department of the Surgical Research and Techniques, Department of Dermatology, Venereology and Oncodermatology, Department of Biophysics
Hungary

1. Introduction

Cutaneus malignant melanoma (MM) is a highly malignant tumour of the skin and is responsible for more deaths than any other skin cancer (Imko-Walczuk et al., 2009). Melanocytes originate from the neural crest and in contrast to Langerhans' cells are located amongst the basal layer of the epidermis, hair bulb, eyes, ears, and meninges (Bandarchi et al., 2010; Fitzpatrick, 1971; Nordlund & Boissy, 2001). The pigmentary system of the skin is a complex set of reactions with many potential sites for dysfunction (Grichnik, 1998). Melanin pigment is produced by melanocytes in their specific cytoplasmic organelles called melanosomes. MM arises from the malignant transformation of melanocytes at the dermal-epidermal junction or from the nevomelanocytes of melanocytic nevi that become invasive and may metastasise.

The incidence of MM has been increasing in white populations. Although MM comprises less than 5% of malignant skin tumours; however, it is responsible for almost 60% of lethal skin neoplasia. With increased life expectancy of the elderly population, melanoma will be a public health challenge (Riker et al., 2010). Increased incidence of melanoma is partly due to early detection (thin melanomas) and partly due to true increase of incidence. Despite the increase in the incidence of melanoma, the prognosis has been improving due to earlier diagnosis of thin melanomas and hence in a curable stage (MacKie, 2000). The incidence of melanoma is equal in men and women and uncommon in children although there are reports that the incidence may be higher in women. A typical patient is usually a Caucasian adult in the 4th decade of life with lesion on the back and leg in male and female, respectively. One typical study revealed that the most common sites in decreasing order are the trunk (43.5%), extremities (33.9%), acral sites (11.9%), and head and neck (10.7%) (Bandarchi et al., 2010).

There is a complex interaction of environmental (exogenous) and endogenous factors. Up to 65% of MM is sun-related (Whiteman & Green, 1999). It is now widely accepted that the major environmental risk factor for the development of primary cutaneous melanoma is Ultraviolent (UV) radiation, which can be subdivided into UVA, UVB, and UVC. UV radiation in sunlight is cytotoxic and, in over dosages, clearly detrimental cells die in apoptosis („sunburn cells") and strong inflammation occurs (Imko-Walczuk et al., 2009). The list of risk factors in developing MM includes pale skin, blond or red hair, numerous freckles and tendency to burn and tan poorly, presence of more than 50 acquired nevi, more than five dysplastic (atypical, Clark's) nevi, large congenital nevi, nevi larger than 6 mm, PUVA therapy, tendency to sunburn and tan poorly, use of tanning salons, Xeroderma pigmentosum, immunosuppression, chemical exposures, scars, Marjolin's ulcer, and genetic factors (Bandarchi et al., 2010; Halpern et al., 1991).

2. Diagnosis of melanoma malignum

2.1 Routine diagnostic methods and prognostic factors

During the past 30 years, there has been significant evolution in the diagnosis of early melanoma. Several factors have contributed to a marked improvement in detection of cutaneous melanomas at an early, curable stage (Rigel & Carucci, 2000). Early detection of MM remains the key factor in lowering mortality from this cancer. Recognizing the importance of this issue 25 years ago, Rigel's group at New York University published the mnemonic "ABCD" to facilitate the early diagnosis of melanoma (Rigel et al., 2010). The ABCD rule of typical MM means: asymmetry, border irregularity, colour variegation, diameter more than 6 mm. However, many exceptions may occur as they may do in other medical disciplines. Studies have demonstrated the usefulness of this paradigm in enhancing early melanoma diagnosis as a part of clinical examinations, mass screenings, and public education programs. Even though dermascopy, even in the hands of a relatively inexpert practitioner, may show high diagnostic accuracy and boost the clinical suspicion in diagnosing MM; however, the definitive diagnosis is confirmed done by biopsy.

The clinicopathological stage of the melanoma patients can determine by pathological evaluation of the primary lesion and of the dissected lymph nodes, as well as by routine examinations (lactate dehydrogenase test, chest X-ray, ultrasound of the abdominal cavity, and computed tomography (CT) or positron emission tomography combined with CT) (Neila & Soyer, 2011).

There are three classes of adverse prognostic factors in melanoma: pathological, clinical, and other factors including genetic alteration (Bataille, 2000). Among others the first group includes increasing the Breslow thickness and Clark level. In 1969, Clark et al. proposed staging criteria for lesions on the basis of skin invasion levels (Clark et al., 1969). Subsequently, Breslow evidenced the importance of the primary melanoma thickness in millimetres, and this index became one of the most important prognostic indicators, in association with data on ulceration, mitosis, regression, microscopic satellites, histopathologic subtype, and presence of vertical growth phase (Breslow & Macht, 1977; Byers & Bhawan 1998; Clemente et al., 1996). Proliferation of the primary melanoma as defined by the mitotic rate was identified as a powerful and independent predictor of survival. As a result, primary tumour mitotic rate is now a required element for the seventh edition melanoma staging system. Multiple thresholds of mitotic rate were examined statistically, and the most significant correlation with survival was identified at a threshold of at least $1/mm^2$. Data from the American Joint Committee on Cancer Melanoma Staging Database demonstrated a highly significant correlation between increasing mitotic rate and declining survival rates. In a multifactorial analysis of 10,233 patients with clinically localized melanoma, mitotic rate was the second most powerful predictor of survival, after tumour thickness (Balch, et al., 2009). Clinical adverse factors include increasing age, male, location of the lesion, and metastasis. Moreover, regional lymph node (Sentinel) status has emerged as an accurate method for evaluating the draining lymph node basin, allowing for the generation of valuable prognostic information (Mraz-Gernhard et al., 1998). Sentinel lymph node biopsy became a compulsory phase for patients with tumour thickness > 1 mm (Patnana, et al., 2011; Petrescu, et al., 2010). Beside routine clinical follow-up with the unaided eye additional techniques are being used to follow these high risk patients sequentially. Recently, there is a need for more studies to diagnose and monitor MM patients in any different clinical stages (as far as possible) with non-invasive methods.

2.2 New diagnostic method: A DSC technique

Differential Scanning Calorimetry (DSC) is a thermoanalytical technique which monitors small heat changes between a sample and reference. The technique was developed by Watson and O'Neill in 1960 (Watson & O'Neill, 1966). For biological samples, a dilute aqueous solution of a biomolecule is loaded into a sample chamber and a matched reference buffer loaded into a reference chamber. Both chambers are heated, and as the temperature increases, thermally-induced processes occurring in the sample cell result in heat either being absorbed or released. This creates a thermal imbalance between the sample and reference chambers which is compensated for by electrically-powered feedback heaters. This electrical power output is directly proportional to the apparent heat capacity of the sample and reference solutions and is the raw data recorded during a DSC experiment (Biltonen & Freire, 1978; Brandts & Lin, 1990).

The DSC thermogram, is an unique signature for bio-molecules reflecting the normal or pathomorphological changes under given solution conditions. Therefore, DSC technique allows demonstrating the thermal consequences of conformation changes in different bio-molecules (Zielenkiewicz, 2011). Moreover, DSC is useful method to evaluate local and global conformation changes in the structure of different tissue elements not only in the animal experiences, but in the orthopaedic and traumatologic, surgical, oncological and dermatological clinical studies (Ferencz, et al., 2011; Szántó & Lőrinczy, 2011; Wiegand, et al., 2011).

Depending on the structural nature of the protein, denaturation might reflect the independent melting of individual domains within the tertiary structure of the protein resulting in a complex thermogram with multiple transitions. A primary DSC thermogram is an extensive property of a protein solution and is therefore directly proportional to the mass of protein in solution. For plasma, assuming there are no significant interactions between the plasma proteins, the DSC thermogram will reflect the melting of a complex mixture of proteins with the observed thermogram representing the sum of the individual protein thermograms weighted according to their mass in solution (Garbett, et al., 2009). The high sensitivity of DSC towards binding interactions means that dramatic shifts in DSC thermograms can result from binding interactions. This represents an intrinsic advantage of the DSC method over other methods applied to the study of the plasma protein, such as electrophoresis and mass spectrometry.

The result of a DSC experiment is a curve of heat flux versus temperature or versus time. As the temperature increases the sample eventually reaches its melting temperature (T_m). The melting process results in an endothermic peak in the DSC curve. A biomolecule in solution is in equilibrium between the native (folded) conformation and its denatured (unfolded) state. The higher the thermal transition midpoint, when 50% of the biomolecules are unfolded, the more stable the molecule. The ability to determine T_m temperatures (T_1, T_2) and enthalpies makes DSC a valuable tool in producing phase diagrams for various chemical systems. $T_{1/2}$ indicates the cooperatively of thermal domens. The calorimetric enthalpy (ΔH) is an absolute measurement of the heat energy uptake, given by the area under the transition peak. It depends on the total amount of (active) protein in the calorimeter cell (Fig. 1.).

Recently, numerous articles confirmed that DSC is widely used as a new diagnostic method for detection of diseases' seriousness, and as an applicable technique during monitoring of patients. Garbett and co-workers demonstrated in these calorimetric studies average thermograms for individuals diagnosed with various diseases (Lyme disease, rheumatoid arthritis) and cancers (endometrial, ovarian, lung), among others in 5 patients with MM.

These data suggest that each type of cancer or disease may have a characteristic signature in their thermogram (Garbett, et al., 2007, 2009; Michnik, 2011). This method is based on the biophysical technique of DSC, which monitors heat changes in a sample as a function of temperature. Analysis of plasma proteins using DSC is therefore based on an entirely different physical property than those of size, charge and chemical interactions that are utilized by the techniques of electrophoresis, mass spectrometry and immunochemistry, which have been mainstays of plasma protein analysis to-date.

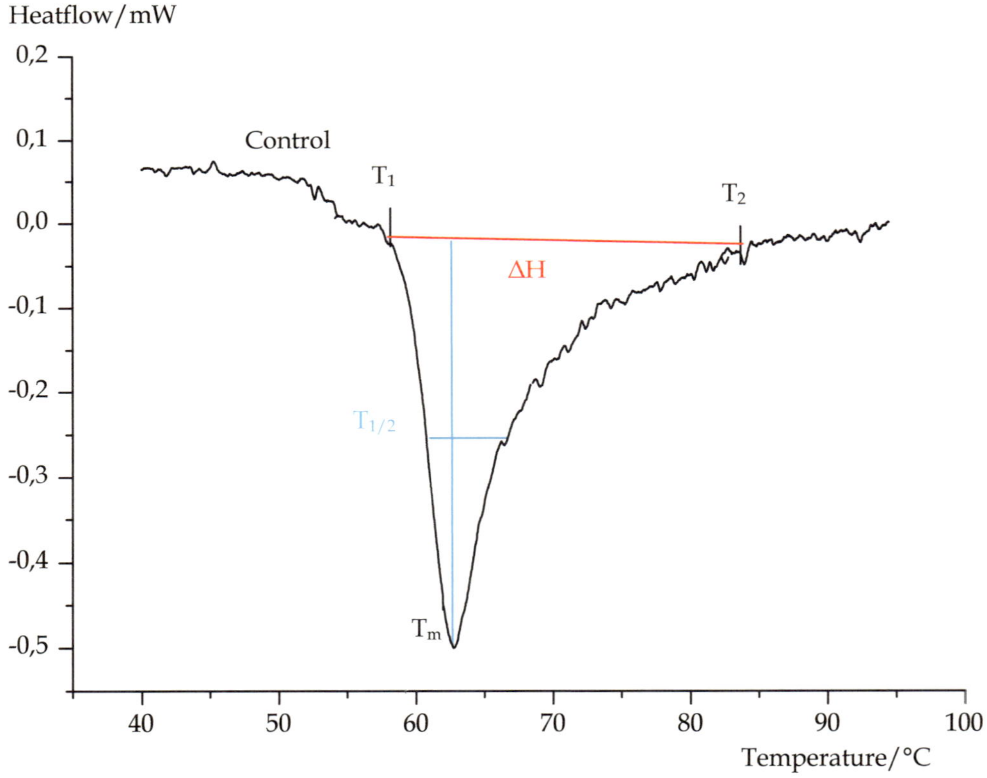

Fig. 1. DSC curve of human healthy control blood plasma
Transition temperatures: T_1: beginning of denaturation, T_2: end of denaturation;
Melting temperature: T_m; Calorimetric enthalpy: ΔH

This chapter will discuss the application of a DSC approach as a new diagnostic method for MM diagnosis and monitoring of patients with different clinical stages.

2.2.1 DSC examination of blood plasma of MM patients

In this study the primary melanoma and the sentinel lymph nodes painted with patent blue and labelled with ^{99m}Tc radiotracer were removed from 36 white adult patients (26 men and 10 women; median age, 61.3 years), who had histopathologically diagnosed operable MM. Surgery and follow-up were made in the Department of Dermatology, Venereology and Oncodermatology of the University Pecs, Hungary. MM was located on the head and neck (11%), on trunk (39%), on the upper limbs (27%), and on the lower limbs (23%). Regional lymph nodes were positive in 12 patients, while distant metastases (lung, brain) were diagnosed in 5 cases. From histopathological parameters tumour thickness were evaluated according to Breslow's, which is a prognostic factor of MM. This parameter changed from 0.5 mm to 8.3 mm in our patients. Clark's level is a related staging system, used in conjunction with Breslow's depth, which describes the level of anatomical invasion of the melanoma in the skin. Clark's level has prognostic significance only in patients with very thin (Breslow's depth <1 mm) melanomas. Invasion value was between Clark level II and IV in this study. The protocol was approved by regional ethical committee of Pecs University (27.06.2008/3220).

Peripheral blood samples of healthy controls (n=10) and preoperatively from MM patients (n=35) were collected and plasma components were analyzed by DSC technique. The thermal unfolding of the human plasma components were monitored by SETARAM Micro DSC II calorimeter. All experiments were conducted between 0 and 100 °C. The heating rate was 0.3 K/min in all cases. Conventional Hastelloy batch vessels were used during the denaturation experiments with 850μL sample volume in average. Reference sample was contained normal saline (0.9% NaCl). The sample and reference samples were equilibrated with a precision of ±0.1 mg. There was no need to do any correction from the point of view of heat capacity between sample and reference samples. The repeated scan of denatured sample was used as baseline reference, which was subtracted from the original DSC curve. Calorimetric enthalpy was calculated from the area under the heat absorption curve by using two-point setting SETARAM peak integration.

Comparison of DSC scans of healthy controls to the curves of cases with regional metastases, the DSC measurements showed 2 different thermal domains during the denaturation (Fig. 1., Fig. 2.). DSC measurements showed at least two marked different thermal domains during the denaturation. The first T_ms were only slightly influenced by the Breslow's depth and the Clark level (see Table 1 and 2), but it can be seen a difference in the melting enthalpies (Fig. 2.). The second T_ms and the calorimetric enthalpy changes demonstrated a significant difference of the melanoma depth dependence in 0.95-8 mm range and in Clark levels of II-IV (Fig. 2. as well as Table 1. and 2). These thermal parameters have been changed significantly in comparing with the control samples which were: T_ms 56 °C and 63 °C, ΔH~1.5 J/g. In the pathologic samples and in the progress of the decease one can separate a third thermal component between the first and second T_m (Fig. 2.). It is at around 62 °C, and it is shifted to higher temperature in case of regional metastasis. In cases of MM with distal metastases plasma denaturation exhibited an increase in second T_m, but a decrease in the calorimetric enthalpy (Fig. 2.).

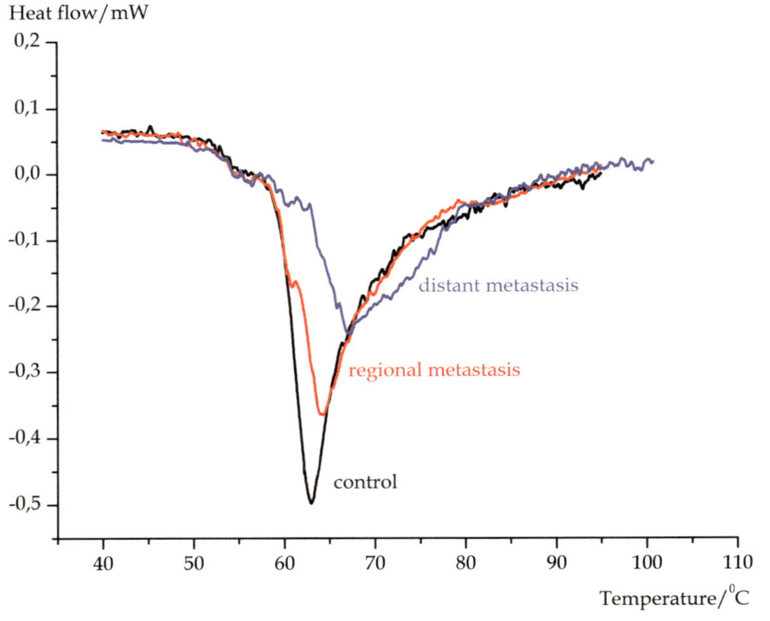

Fig. 2. DSC scans of human plasma in healthy controls, in MM patients with regional or distant metastases. Downward deflection represents endotherm process. (Black line: control, red line: MM with regional metastasis, blue line: MM with distant metastasis)

	T_{m1}/°C (mean±se)	T_{m2}/°C (mean±se)	ΔH(J/g) (mean±se)
Control (n=10)	56 ± 0.2	63.3 ± 0.3	1.53 ± 0.02
Breslow's depth (mm)			
0.5-1.0 (n=7)	55.8 ± 0.2	64.1 ± 0.3	1.13 ± 0.02
1.1-1.5 (n=2)	56.3 ± 0.3	63.5 ± 0.02	1.61 ± 0.01
1.6-2.0 (n=2)	55.75 ± 0.3	67.15 ± 0.4	1.3 ± 0.02
2.1-3.0 (n=5)	56.16 ± 0.2	62.18 ± 0.02	1.45 ± 0.03
3.1-4.0 (n=3)	55.8 ± 0.04	63.2 ± 0.2	1.37 ± 0.02
4.1-6.0 (n=2)	55.7 ± 0.2	63.9 ± 0.4	1.25 ± 0.01
6.1-8.5 (n=3)	55.8 ± 0.01	64.5 ± 0.1	1.23 ± 0.04

Table 1. DSC data according to Breslow's depth of melanoma

Clark level	T_{m1}/°C (mean±se)	T_{m2}/°C (mean±se)	ΔH(J/g) (mean±se)
I. (n=2)	55.2 ± 0.3	64.6 ± 0.1	1.14 ± 0.02
II. (n=1)	55.8 ± 0.03	63 ± 0.01	1.45 ± 0.04
III. (n=10)	55.7 ± 0.4	64.63 ± 0.2	1.286 ± 0.03
IV. (n=12)	56.05 ± 0.2	60.4 ± 0.02	1.43 ± 0.03

Table 2. DSC data according to Clark level of melanoma

3. Conclusion

Malignant melanoma is one of the most aggressive malignancies in human and is responsible for almost 60% of lethal skin tumours. Its incidence has been increasing in white population in the past two decades. Moreover, metastatic MM is an incurable disease with high mortality rate. Patients with metastatic disease have an average survival of <1 year. This high mortality rate is largely the result of the resistance to chemotherapy and radiotherapy (Palmieri, et al., 2009; Uong & Zon, 2010).

Although for most tumours, diameter is a powerful prognostic attribute, this is not so for melanomas, which can be very broad and yet have a good prognosis. This is because most melanomas have an extensive in situ or superficially invasive component that does not contribute to metastatic potential. It is therefore misleading and not recommended to report the breadth of a melanoma in a pathology diagnosis (Elder, 2011). The extent of penetration of melanoma cells into the skin was recognized as a better predictor of survival than breadth in a few early studies and was first codified into a powerful model in 1967 by Clark and co-workers. The disease was classified into intraepidermal (Clark level I), invades papillary dermis (Clark level II), fills papillary dermis (Clark level III), invades reticular dermis (Clark level IV), and invades subcutaneus fat (Clark level V) (Clark et al., 1969). Clark's level is a related staging system, used in conjunction with Breslow's depth, which describes the level of anatomical invasion of the melanoma in the skin. In 1970, Breslow described a simple system for measuring the thickness of melanomas. The Breslow thickness is determined by measuring from the top of the granular layer of the overlying skin, or from the base of an overlying ulcer, to the deepest invasive melanoma cell. Clark's level has prognostic significance only in patients with very thin (Breslow's depth <1 mm) melanomas.

Adequate resection of the specimens and sentinel lymph node biopsies are important factors in management of MM. But, there is no definite proof that longevity of patients is affected by routine laboratory tests (Bandarchi et al., 2010). New diagnostic methods in development and progression of MM could be helpful to identify the molecular profiles underlying aggressiveness, clinical behaviour, and response to therapy as well as to better classify the subsets of melanoma patients with different prognosis and/or clinical outcome. The human plasma proteome holds great promise as a convenient specimen for disease diagnosis and therapeutic monitoring. Moreover, blood samples may be easily obtained from patients by minimally invasive, safe procedure. The novel calorimetric assays are described that provides a new window through which to view the properties of the human plasma proteome (Anderson, N.L. & Anderson, N.G., 2002; Bruylants, et al., 2005; Ebert, et al., 2006).

This study investigated the thermal changes of human blood plasma components in melanoma patients with or without regional lymph node metastases by DSC. Overview 36 patients' thermograms, we observed their individual characteristics compare to healthy controls. Similar observations have been described by Garbett et al. in their important calorimetric studies, where demonstrated average thermograms for individuals diagnosed with various diseases (Lyme disease, rheumatoid arthritis) and cancers (endometrial, ovarian, lung), among others in 5 patients with MM. These data suggest that each type of cancer or disease may have a characteristic signature in their thermogram (Garbett, et al., 2009).

In the present study, DSC scan of healthy controls and the curves of MM cases showed 2 different thermal domains during the denaturation. Moreover, patients' thermograms are shifted towards higher denaturation temperatures. These changes were confirmed in the literature, where the average thermogram was obtained from duplicate DSC runs on samples from 100 healthy individuals and from 5 MM patients' sample also. Moreover, the disease thermograms are apparently localized in a higher temperature range. These unique appearances present a key utility of this technology as a diagnostic method (Garbett, et al., 2008).

Examination of DSC data in different clinical stages of MM patients should observed closed correlation with melanoma thickness and the extent of regional invasion. The first T_m was slightly influenced by the Breslow's depth and the Clark level (I. and III.). But, the second T_m and the calorimetric enthalpy changes demonstrated the melanoma depth dependence in 0.95-8 mm range and in Clark levels of II-IV. The surprising jump out of all thermal data in 1.1-2.0 mm Breslow's depth range as well as the opposite change in the tendency of T_{m2} and ΔH need further investigation with increased number of patients and with finer filtering. The same could be the conclusion in case of Clark level II. and IV.

These facts are important for many reasons: DSC measurement is suitable not only to clear skin cancer diagnosis, but to separate the different stages of MM patients and to monitor the actual stage of individual's disease. However, there are no data in the literature indicating the possible diagnostic and staging method of human blood plasma by DSC in MM patients. Similar findings have been described in another report, where applied the DSC method to investigate its utility for disease staging. Gynaecologic oncology samples analyzed by the method yielded progressively shifted thermograms charting the advance of cervical cancer from pre-invasive cervical lesions through each stage of invasive carcinoma. The distinction between normal and high-grade squamous intraepithelial lesions is significant and indicates the utility of the DSC method for the rapid screening of cervical cancer (Garbett, et al., 2009). The exact explanations of these results are not yet known. However, DSC analysis of plasma from diseased individuals revealed significant changes in the thermogram which are suggested to result not from changes in the concentration of the major plasma proteins but from interactions of small molecules or peptides with these proteins.

From clinical perspective, MM is generally considered to be a highly aggressive cancer, although a small subset of patients with metastatic melanoma has a relatively indolent disease course (Tsao, et al., 2004). Histologically, mitoses are frequently apparent in sections of melanoma tumours and staining for proliferative markers such as Ki67 is usually positive (Ohsie, et al., 2008). In the earliest descriptions of melanoma, the disease was regarded as a tumour mass that developed in the skin and was often surrounded by satellites at the time of presentation. A few studies recognized that more superficial melanomas have a better prognosis.

DSC thermograms of MM cases with distant metastases are shifted more towards higher denaturation temperatures. No other DSC data in the literature in MM patient with metastatic phase. But, there was a progressive shift of the thermogram to higher denaturation temperatures in cases of invasive cervical cancer compare to high-grade squamous intraepithelial lesions. The thermograms appear to be distinct from all the other diseases and unique for high-grade squamous intraepithelial lesions and invasive cervical cancer. The distinction between normal and high-grade squamous intraepithelial lesions is significant and indicates the utility of the DSC method for the rapid screening of cervical

cancer. A more detailed analysis of the data has revealed a progressively shifted thermogram for each stage of the disease (Garbett, et al., 2009).
In summary, this is the first report examined thermal changes by DSC on human blood plasma in MM patients with different clinical stages. Blood collection is a simple procedure and convenient to perform, and the DSC thermogram confirmed unique signature for human plasma components reflecting the normal, the pathomorphological changes and staging differences in melanoma patients. Further studies are needed to elucidate these relationships, but this preliminary study indicates great potential for the application of DSC as a clinical diagnostic tool, for example during disease grading and staging processes.

4. Acknowledgment

This work was supported by grants OTKA C272 (for D. L.), OTKA PD77474 and PTE AOK Research Grant 114-603/2009(for A. F.).

5. References

Anderson, N.L. & Anderson, N.G. (2002). The human plasma proteome: history, character, and diagnostic prospects, *Molecular and Cellular Proteomics*, Vol.1, No.11, pp. 845-867

Balch, C.M. Gershenwald, J.E. Soong, S. Thompson, J.F. Atkins, M.B. Byrd, D.R. Buzaid, A.C. Cochran, A.J. Coit, D.G. Ding, S. Eggermont, A.M. Flaherty, K.T. Gimotty, P.A. Kirkwood, J.M. McMasters, K.M. Mihm, M.C. Morton, D.L. Ross, M.I. Sober, A.J. & Sondak, V.K. (2009). Final version of 2009 AJCC melanoma staging and classification, *Journal of Clinical Oncology*, Vol.20, No.36, pp. 6199-6206

Bandarchi, B. Ma, M. Navab, R. Seth, A. & Rasty G. (2010). From melanocyte to metastatic malignant melanoma, In: *Hindawi Publishing Corporation Dermatology Research and Practice*, 15.07.2010, ID 583748, 8 pages, doi:10.1155/2010/583748

Bataille, V. (2000). Genetics of familial and sporadic melanoma, *Clinical and Experimental Dermatology, Vol.*25, No.6, pp. 464–470

Biltonen, R.L. & Freire, E. (1978). Thermodynamic characterization of conformational states of biological macromolecules using differential scanning calorimetry, *CRC Critical Reviews in Biochemistry*, Vol.5, No.2, pp. 85–124

Brandts, J.F. & Lin, L-N. (1990). Study of strong to ultratight protein interactions using differential scanning calorimetry, *Biochemistry*, Vol.29, No.29, pp. 6927–6940

Breslow, A. & Macht, S.D. (1977). Optimal size of resection margin for thin cutaneous melanoma, *Surgery, Gynecology and Obstetrics*, Vol.145, No.5, pp. 691-692.

Bruylants, G. Wouters, J. & Michaux, C. (2005). Differential scanning calorimetry in life science: thermodynamics, stability, molecular recognition and application in drug design, *Current Medical Chemistry*, Vol.12, No.17, pp. 2011-2020

Byers, H.R. & Bhawan, J. (1998). Pathologic parameters in the diagnosis and prognosis of primary cutaneous melanoma, *Hematology/Oncology Clinics of North America*, Vol.12, No.4, pp. 717–735

Clark, W.H. From, L. Bernardino, E.A. & Mihm, M.C. (1969). The histogenesis and biologic behaviour of primary human malignant melanomas of the skin, *Cancer Research,* Vol.29, pp. 705-727

Clemente, C.G. Mihm, M.C. Bufalino, R. Zurrida, S. Collini, P. & Cascinelli, N. (1996). Prognostic value of tumour infiltrating lymphocytes in the vertical growth phase of primary cutaneous melanoma, *Cancer, Vol.77, No.7, pp.* 1303–1310

Dolianitis, C. Kelly, J. Wolfe, R. & Simpson, P. (2005). Comparative performance of 4 dermoscopic algorithms by nonexperts for the diagnosis of melanocytic lesions, *Archives of Dermatology,* Vol.141, No.8, pp. 1008–1014

Ebert, M.P. Korc, M. Malfertheiner, P. & Röcken, C. (2006). Advances, challenges, and limitations in serum-proteome-based cancer diagnosis, *Journal of Proteome Research,* Vol.5, No.1, pp. 19–25

Elder, D.E. (2011). Thin melanoma, Archives of Pathology & Laboratory Medicine, Vol.135, No.3, pp. 342-346

Ferencz, A. Nedvig, K. & Lőrinczy, D. (2011). DSC examination of the intestinal tissue following ischemic injuries, In: *Thermal Analysis in Medical Application,* D. Lőrinczy, (Ed.), 255-269, Akadémiai Kiadó, ISBN 978-963-05-8992-5, Budapest, Hungary

Fitzpatrick, T.B. (1971). The biology of pigmentation, *Birth Defects Original Article Series,* Vol.7, No.8, pp. 5–12

Garbett, N.C. Miller, J.J. Jenson, A.B. & Chaires, J.B. (2007). Calorimetric analysis of the plasma proteome, *Seminars in Nephrology,* Vol.27, No.6, pp. 621-626

Garbett, N.C. Miller, J.J. Jenson, A.B. & Chaires, J.B. (2008). Calorimetry outside the box: a new window into the plasma proteome, *Biohysical Journal,* Vol.94, No.4, pp. 1377-1383

Garbett, N.C. Mekmaysy, C.S. Helm, C.W. Jenson, A.B. & Chaires, J.B. (2009). Differential scanning calorimetry of blood plasma for clinical diagnosis and monitoring, *Experimental and Molecular Pathology,* Vol.86, No.3, pp. 186-191

Grichnik, J.M. Burch, J.A. Burchette, J. & Shea, C.R. (1998). The SCF/KIT pathway plays a critical role in the control of normal human melanocyte homeostasis, *Journal of Investigative Dermatology,* Vol.111, No.2, pp. 233–238

Halpern, A.C. Guerry, D. Elder, D.E. Clark, W.H. Synnestvedt, M. Norman, S. & Ayerle, R. (1991). Dysplastic nevi as risk markers of sporadic (nonfamilial) melanoma. A case-control study, *Archives of Dermatology,* Vol.127, No.7, pp. 995-999

Imko-Waczuk, B. Turner, R. & Wojnarowska, F. (2009). Malignant melanoma, In: *Skin cancer after transplantation,* S.T. Rosen, (Ed.), pp. 311-328, Springer, ISBN 978-0-387-78573-8, Berlin, Germany

MacKie, R.M. (2000). Melanoma and the dermatologist in the third millennium, *Archives of Dermatology,* Vol.136, No.1, pp. 71–73

Michnik, A. (2011). Blood plasma, serum andserum proteins microcalorimetric studies aimed at diagnosis support, In: *Thermal Analysis in Medical Application,* D. Lőrinczy, (Ed.), 171-190, Akadémiai Kiadó, ISBN 978-963-05-8992-5, Budapest, Hungary

Mraz-Gernhard, S. Sagebiel, R.W. Kashani-Sabet, M. Miller, J.R.III & Leong, S.P.L. (1998). Prediction of sentinel lymph node micrometastasis by histological features in primary cutaneous malignant melanoma, *Archives of Dermatology, Vol.134, No.8, pp.* 983–987

Neila, J. & Soyer, H.P. (2011). Key points in dermoscopy for diagnosis of melanomas, including difficult to diagnose melanomas, on the trunk and extremities, *The Journal of Dermatology*, Vol.38, No1, pp. 3-9

Nordlund, J.J. & Boissy, R.E. (2001). The biology of melanocytes, In: *The biology of the skin*, R.K. Frenkel & D.T. Woodley, (Eds.), pp. 113–131, Parthenon Publishing, New York, USA

Ohsie, S.J. Sarantopoulos, G.P. Cochran, A.J. & Binder, S.W. (2008). Immunohistochemical characteristics of melanoma, *Journal of Cutaneus Pathology*, Vol.35, No.5, pp. 433–444

Palmieri, G. Capone, M. Ascierto, M.L. Gentilcore, G. Stroncek, D.F. Casula, M. Sini, M.C. Palla, M. Mozzillo, N. & Ascierto, P.A. (2009). Main roads to melanoma, *Journal of Translational Medicine*, Vol.7, No.86, pp. 1-17

Patnana, M. Bronstein, Y. Szklaruk, J. Bedi. D.G. Hwu, W.J. Gershenwald, J.E. Prieto, V.G. & Ng, C.S. (2011). Multimethod imaging, staging, and spectrum of manifestations of metastatic melanoma, *Clinical Radiology*, Vol.66, No.3, pp. 224-236

Petrescu, I. Condrea, C. Alexandru, A. Dumitrescu, D. Simion, G. Severin, E. Albu, C. & Albu, D. (2010). Diagnosis and treatment protocols of cutaneous melanoma: latest approach 2010, *Chirurgia (Bucharest, Romania: 1990)*, Vol.105, No.5, pp. 637-643

Riker, A.I. Zea, N. & Trinh, T. (2010). The epidemiology, prevention, and detection of melanoma, *Ochsner Journal*, Vol.10, No.2, pp. 56–65

Rigel, D.S. & Carucci J.A. (2000). Malignant melanoma: prevention, early detection, and treatment in the 21st century, *A Cancer Journal for Clinicians*, Vol.50, No:4, pp. 215-236

Rigel, D.S. Russak, J. & Friedman, R. (2010). The evolution of melanoma diagnosis: 25 years beyond the ABCDs, *A Cancer Journal for Clinicians*, Vol.60, No5, pp. 301-316

Szántó, Z. & Lőrinczy, D. (2011). Differential calorimetric examination of the tracheal cartilage following primary reconstruction, In: *Thermal Analysis in Medical Application*, D. Lőrinczy, (Ed.), 111-125, Akadémiai Kiadó, ISBN 978-963-05-8992-5, Budapest, Hungary

Tsao, H. Atkins, M.B. Sober, A.J. (2004). Management of cutaneous melanoma, *The New England Journal of Medicine*, Vol.351, No.10, pp. 998-1012

Uong, A. & Zon, L.I. (2010). Melanocytes in development and cancer, *Journal of Cellular Physiology, Vol.*222, No.1, pp. 38–41

Watson, E.S. & O'Neill, M.J. (1966). Differential microcalorimeter, United States Patient Office, Vol.185, No.499, 1-9

Whiteman, D.C. & Green, A.C. (1999). Melanoma and sun exposure: where are we now?, *International Journal of Dermatology*, Vol.38, No.7, pp. 481–489

Wiegand, N. Vámhidy, L. & Lőrinczy, D. (2011). Connective tissue degenerations of the hand, In: *Thermal Analysis in Medical Application*, D. Lőrinczy, (Ed.), 75-94, Akadémiai Kiadó, ISBN 978-963-05-8992-5, Budapest, Hungary

Zielenkiewicz, W. (2011). Calorimetry and its application in medical research, In: *Thermal Analysis in Medical Application*, D. Lőrinczy, (Ed.), 9-35, Akadémiai Kiadó, ISBN 978-963-05-8992-5, Budapest, Hungary

7

New Technology in High-Dose-Rate Brachytherapy with Surface Applicators for Non-Melanoma Skin Cancer Treatment: Electronic Miniature X-Ray Brachytherapy

Yi Rong[1,2] and James S. Welsh[1]
[1]*Departments of Human Oncology, University of Wisconsin School of Medicine and Public Health, Madison, WI*
[2]*Department of Radiation Oncology, James Cancer Center, Ohio State University, Columbus, OH*
USA

1. Introduction

The number of skin cancers diagnosed in the United States is higher than all other cancers combined, and approximately one in five Americans will develop skin cancer in their life [1]. Non-melanoma skin cancer (NMSC) is estimated to affect more than 1 million persons in the United States annually[2]. Of these, the majority (75-80%) of them are basal cell carcinoma (BCC) [3]. Non-melanoma skin cancers very rarely metastasize, with a few rare exceptions such as Merkel cell carcinomas. The remainder of non-melanoma skin cancers are squamous cell carcinomas (SCC). Squamous cell skin cancers are more aggressive than BCC and have a tendency to spread into fatty tissues beneath the skin and in contrast to BCC, SCC has a small but definite risk of metastasizing to distant organs. When this happens, SCC can become a life-threatening disease, similar to metastatic squamous cell cancer from any other organ. Most NMSCs are curable with less than 1000 deaths reported annually [2]. If identified at an early stage and given appropriate treatment, excellent local control and cosmesis can be achieved for many patients. Treatment options include, but are not limited to, simple surgical excision [4], Moh's micrographic surgery [5], radiation therapy (RT) [6,7,8,9], laser surgery [10,11], topical chemotherapy [12] and cryosurgery [13]. Flexibility in the application of these modalities is important for offering patients the best method for the skin cancer treatment. Selection of the appropriate modality requires professional considerations of effective tumor control, cosmetic outcome, possible toxicities, and patient's preference. Many factors, including the cancer type, size, specific location of the cancer, primary or recurrent disease, and the extent of the invasion affect treatment options. The National Comprehensive Cancer Network (NCCN) has established guidelines and treatment algorithms for the evaluation and management of BCC and SCC [14].

NMSC is generally treated with surgical excision or Moh's micrographic surgery. Standard surgical excision is simple and effective, providing complete clearance with an appropriate margin assessment [15,16]. Moh's micrographic surgery has been shown to have superior cure rates for primary and recurrent BCCs (1% and 5.6%, respectively) and for primary and recurrent SCCs (3% and 10%, respectively) [17,18]. Treatment with RT provides a viable alternative for those patients who refuse or are medically unsuitable for surgery or when surgery might lead to unacceptable cosmesis. It is generally reserved for patients at the age of 60 years or older, given concerns of potential long-term sequelae. Clinical considerations are required from the radiation oncologist when RT is selected, such as the appropriate dose-fractionation regimen, patient setup, bolus use, field size, and the specific RT treatment modality. Several groups have reported results for NMSC treatment using different RT modalities. Treatments with superficial x-rays presented a 93-100% tumor control in one group [6] but 78% tumor control in another group [19]. Differences are mainly attributed to tumor size, dose fractionation scheme, and the total dose. Excellent tumor control was observed in treatments with fraction size between 3Gy and 5Gy, and total dose <60Gy [6]. RT treatment with orthovoltage x-rays or megavoltage electrons achieved 72-88% 5-year overall tumor control [6,7,9,20]. Sykes et al reported 100% local control with a median follow-up of 31months for T1/2 SCC on the lip using electron beams. Lesion size may explain some of the discrepancies in reported results. The continuous technology advances in the field of brachytherapy have made possible the use of precise after-loader equipment for high-dose-rate (HDR) irradiation using radioactive sources, i.e. ^{192}Ir. Isotope-based HDR brachytherapy, in conjunction with the standard surface applicators or custom-made molds, has become a highly effective treatment method of skin carcinomas in recent years. Favorable cosmetic outcomes and excellent local control with minimal complications have been reported with this method [8, 21, 22]. Post-operative RT is also considered an adjuvant therapy to surgery for multimodality treatment of NMSCs with favorable outcomes [23].

The increased demand for RT of small superficial lesions has revived the interest in HDR brachytherapy techniques using skin surface applicators or surface molds [8, 22, 23]. The available HDR afterloaders and applicators on the market include Varian GammaMedPlus™ afterloader unit with Varian surface applicators (Varian Brachytherapy, Charlottesville, VA) and Nucletron microSelectronHDR system with Leipzig and Valencia surface applicators (Nucletron, Veenendaal, The Netherlands). Both of these units utilize an HDR ^{192}Ir source, which requires experienced personnel with NRC Authorized User and Authorized Medical Physicist status, a shielded radiation treatment room, special handling of the isotopes, etc. A recently available alternative is the electronic brachytherapy (EBT) miniature tube, such as the model S700 Axxent® X-ray source (Xoft Inc., Fremont, CA), which generates an x-ray beam in the low kilovoltage (kV) energy range and provides dose-rates comparable to 7-Ci ^{192}Ir sources, with similar dose distributions [24, 25]. In contrast to a conventional radioisotope-based HDR unit, the radiation from the EBT system can be switched on and off through this water-cooled miniature x-ray tube. It has been used for accelerated partial breast irradiation (APBI) treatments [26, 27] with breast balloon applicators and endometrial treatments [28] with dedicated endometrial applicators. Dosimetric advantages have been demonstrated for normal lung and heart tissues in APBI treatment and rectum in endometrial treatments [25-29]. The advantages of the EBT device include less shielding requirements for the 50kVp x-ray source and lower exposure rate to personnel that allows staff to remain in the treatment room in close proximity to the patient [29, 30], compared to isotope based brachytherapy (HDR ^{192}Ir source has a mean energy 380keV). The dosimetric properties and energy spectrum of the 50kVp miniature x-ray source have been well studied [25, 26, 31]. System commissioning procedures have been well described in several publications [30, 31] for breast intracavitary treatment using breast applicators. The new surface applicators for skin cancer treatments were approved by the FDA in March 2009 and first used for patient treatments at our facility (University of Wisconsin Riverview Cancer Center, Wisconsin Rapids, WI) in July 2009. In contrast to prior applications of the EBT device for APBI and endometrial treatments, the soft x-rays are delivered through surface applicators externally to the patient's skin for skin treatments. Thus, this delivery setup is quite different from most brachytherapy delivery. The output calibration and treatment planning procedures for such applications have recently been reported [30].

2. Novel technology on isotope-free brachytherapy using miniature x-ray tube

2.1 System description

2.1.1 Axxent Xoft EBT controller and miniature x-ray source

The EBT system consists of the Xoft controller, miniature x-ray source, and the treatment applicators. The Xoft controller, as shown in Figure 1, includes a touch-screen monitor, USB port, barcode reader, pullback arm, x-ray source cooling system, Standard Imaging Well Chamber, and a Standard Imaging Max-4000 Electrometer. The pullback arm, as indicated in Figure 1(a) and 1(b), has three adjustable joints and they are all adjustable for better positioning the source. There is a high voltage port on the arm for the source connection (not shown on the figure). The on-board well chamber (Figure 2a) and electrometer (Figure 2b) make the source pre-treatment calibration possible. The most essential part of this novel system is the design of the miniature x-ray source, as shown in Figure 3.

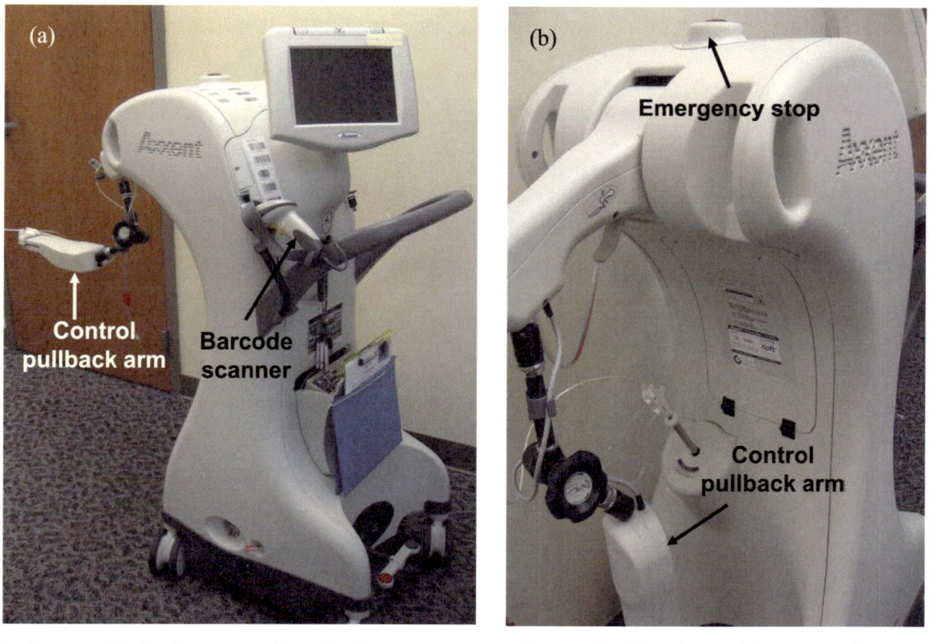

Fig. 1. Axxent Xoft electronic brachytherapy controller with (a) adjustable control pullback arm and barcode scanner; and (b) emergency stop and pullback arm pointing down

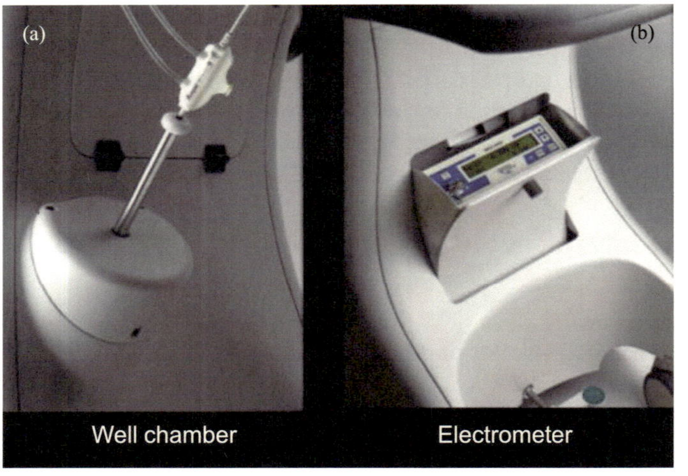

Fig. 2. (a) The well chamber and (b) electrometer are monted on the controller

Figure 3a shows the overview of the x-ray source, which consists of an x-ray tube as small as a finger tip (Figure 3b) located at the tip of a flexible cooling catheter (25 cm in length and 5.4 mm in diameter, as shown in Figure 3c), a white mounting clip with a pair of cooling connection tubes (which need to be connected with the cooling system on the Xoft controller during the treatment), and a high voltage connector. Water circulating inside the catheter cools the surface of the source, this allows maximum air kerma strength of 1400 Gy/hr at 1cm for 50kV and 300 μA beam current [25]. The miniature x-ray tube is only 2.3 mm in diameter and 1.5 cm in length and generates 50kVp bremsstrahlung x-rays with a mean energy of 26.7 kV photons.

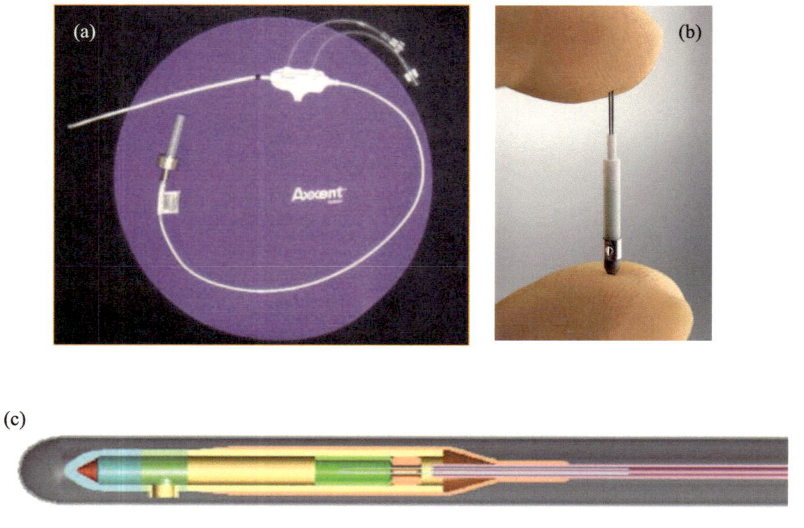

Fig. 3. (a) Axxent Xoft miniature x-ray source inserted into to a flexible cooling catheter; (b) The actual size of the miniature x-ray source; (c) The x-ray source tip detail including miniature x-ray tube and HV cable.

2.1.2 Xoft surface applicators and target collimator

For treating superficial lesions on skin, Xoft surface applicators are used, as shown in Figure 4. The cone connects to one end of the applicator source channel, whose other end connects to an adapter that is designed to lock the source in place for treatment (Figure 4a). Four applicator cone sizes are available including 10 mm, 20 mm, 35 mm, and 50 mm. A disposable end cap that is made of 0.5mm plexiglas is used to cover the cone in order to protect it from the direct contact with patient and to ensure a flat treatment area. X-ray beams are further shaped for the clinical target with the custom-made lead shields (Axxent® FlexiShield Mini) (Figure 4b), which are disposable, non-sterile, flexible devices with a circular shape (12.7 cm in diameter and 1mm in thickness). It has a lead equivalency of 0.45mm at 50kVp, which provides about a 30-fold reduction in radiation.

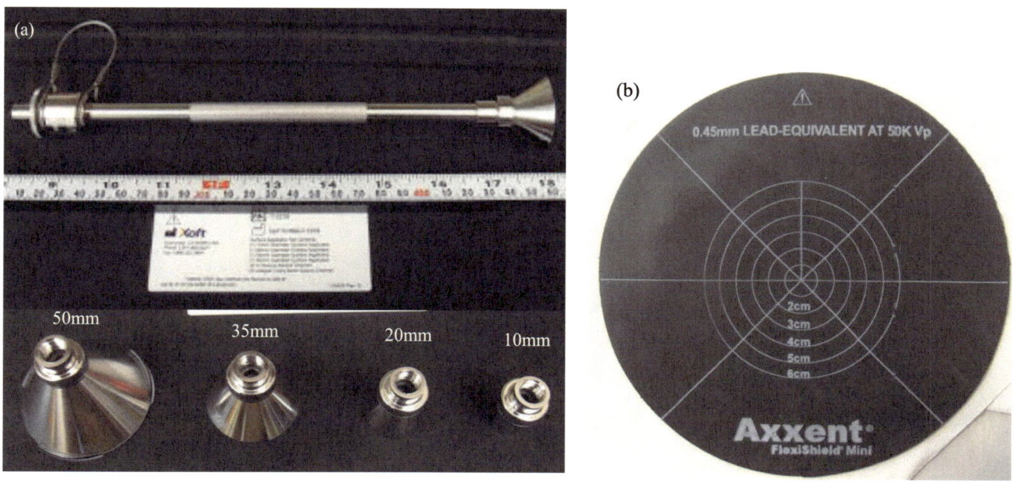

Fig. 4. (a) Applicator source channel connecting to the 35mm cone on the right end and the Touhy Burst adaptor on the left. Below are four skin applicator cones with different sizes; (b) The Axxent® FlexiShield Mini with drawn circles representing different field sizes

2.2 Physics aspects

2.2.1 Dose rate output calibration and stability

The source nominal dose rate at the skin surface with the applicator needs to be calibrated prior to treatment. It is recommended to use the protocol AAPM TG-61 in-air method[32] for the soft x-ray dose calibration, using a soft x-ray parallel plate chamber (PTW T34013) mounted to a L-shaped in-air calibration fixture (Figure 5), which is commercially available through Xoft, Inc.

Dose to water at surface can be determined by:

$$D_w = MN_k B_w P_{stem,air} [(\frac{\bar{\mu}_{en}}{\rho})^w_{air}]_{air} \tag{1}$$

Where M is the corrected ion chamber reading, $M = M_{raw} P_{TP} P_{pol} P_{ion} P_{elec}$

N_k is the air-kerma calibration factor for the given beam's quality. B_w is the backscatter factor which accounts for the effect of the phantom scatter and $P_{stem,air}$ is the stem correction factor which accounts for the change in photon scatter from the chamber stem between the calibration and measurement (mainly due to the change in field size). The mass energy-absorption coefficient ratio of water-to-air $[(\frac{\overline{\mu}_{en}}{\rho})^{w}_{air}]_{air}$ can be determined by the look-up table given in TG-61 Table IV. The dose rate to water at surface can be calculated by

$$\dot{D}_w = \frac{D_w}{t} \text{ (Gy/min)} \tag{2}$$

Finally, the nominal dose rate to skin at surface can be calculated by

$$\dot{D}_{skin,n} = C_w^{med}\dot{D}_w \frac{\text{No min al}S_k}{\text{Actual}S_k} \tag{3}$$

Where C_w^{med} is the conversion factor from dose-to-water to dose-to-medium, which can be looked-up from the table provided in TG-61 Table X. For skin treatment, C_w^{skin} has a value of 0.91. S_k is the air-kerma strength. The nominal S_k is set to be 110000U in the EBT system and the actual S_k is obtained from the well chamber measurement.

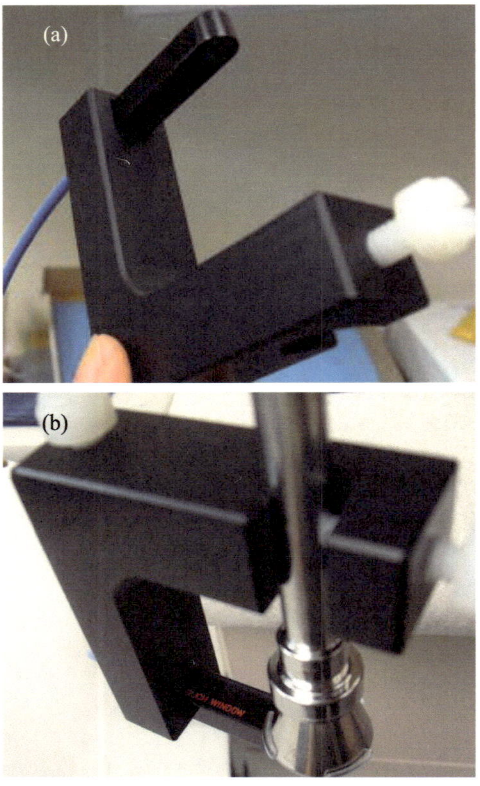

Fig. 5. L-shaped in-air calibration fixture with the PTW T34013 parallel plate chamber centrally placed under the 10mm applicator for the in-air measurement.

The nominal skin surface dose-rate of 35mm applicator cone is reported to be 1.35 Gy/min averaged over sixteen sources, with a ±5% variation [31]. For the same source, the output variation is within 2%. Due to the differences in the design of the flattening filters and cone sizes, the dose rate output varies. The average dose-rates are 1.52, 1.39, 1.35, and 0.67 Gy/min for 10, 20, 35, and 50mm applicators. Smaller cone sizes produce higher dose rates, due to the design of the flattening filter and the in-field scattering from the applicator.

2.2.2 Field flatness and symmetry

The reported beam flatness and symmetry (mean and standard deviation) for ten sources over the central 80% of the field width are well within 5% from all four sizes of the applicator cones. With a flattening filter built in the applicator cone, it is possible to obtain a uniform dose distribution on the surface of the applicator as well as at a depth beneath the skin. As shown in Figure 6(a), the radiation field was tightly conformed by the applicator cone. Film profiles (background subtracted) for five sources all normalized to the profile center at 100% are shown in Figure 6b and 6c. The dose penumbra region is smaller than 2.0 mm at surface, sharp enough to spare surrounding normal tissues.

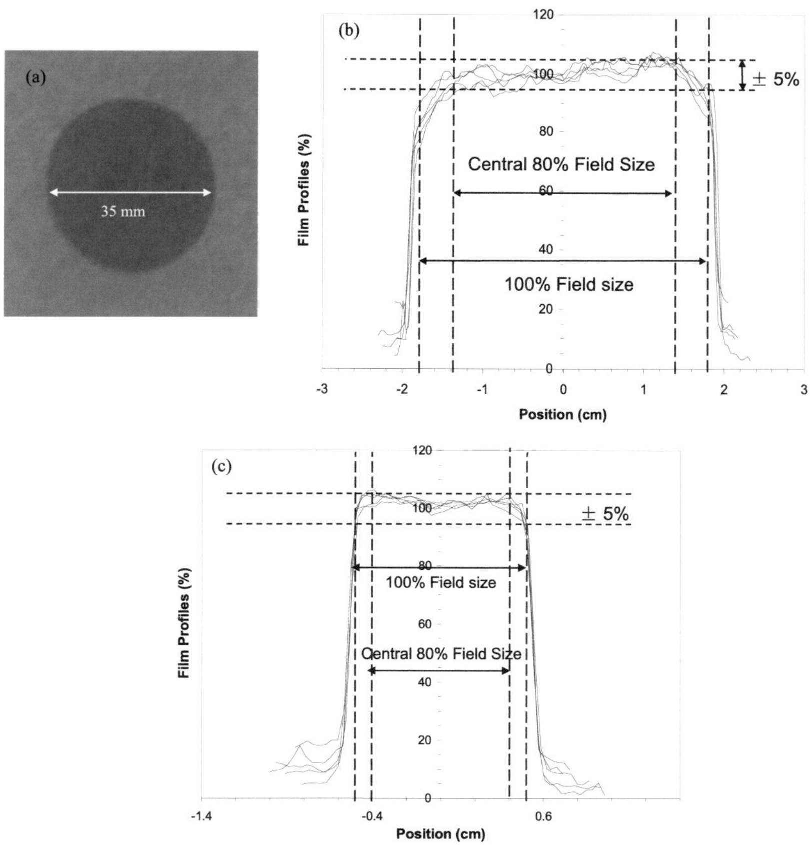

Fig. 6. (a) EBT Gafchromic film exposure at surface for a 35 mm cone. (b) Relative dose profiles for the 35mm cone from the EBT Gafchromic films exposed to five sources. (c) Relative dose profiles for the 10mm cone from the EBT Gafchromic films exposed to five sources.

2.2.3 Percentage depth dose (PDD)

The factory data is provided for clinical use based on the measurements averaging over ten sources for all four applicators. Factory PDD data was obtained using a water tank with sealed ion-chamber and applicators (Figure 7). Surface dose was obtained by extrapolation. Skin dose is about 126%-174% for a standard prescription depth of 2-5 mm. For the treatment range up to 6 mm, the dose fall-off is more rapid for smaller cone size, except for 10mm size, which resides between 20 mm and 35 mm probably due to the scattered electron contamination, which is more significant with such a small size.

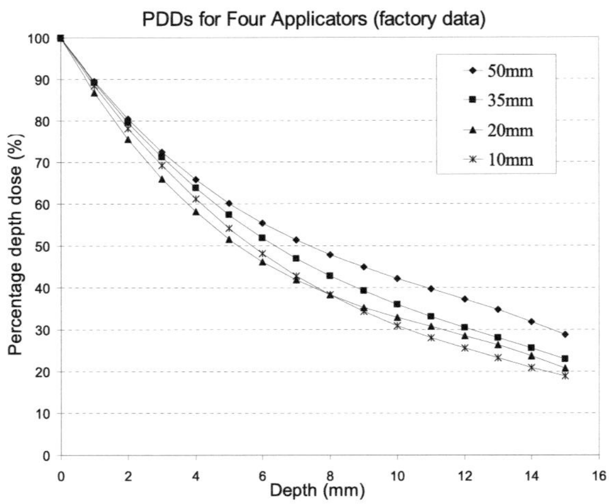

Fig. 7. Factory data of PDDs for four applicator cones: diamonds, squares, rectangles and stars represent the PDD curves for 50, 35, 20 and 10 mm cones.

2.2.4 Nominal SSD and correction factors

Low energy x-ray beam should also obey the inverse square law, $\frac{I_o}{I_g} = \left(\frac{f + d_m + g}{f + d_m}\right)^2$ where d_m is the measurement depth, g is the air gap, and f is the nominal SSD. By plotting $\sqrt{\frac{I_o}{I_g}}$ as a function of gap g, a straight line is obtained, the slope of which is $\frac{1}{f + d_m}$. Thus $f = \frac{1}{slope} - d_m$. Therefore, the nominal SSD can be verified clinically by measuring the correction factors with different air-gaps. The nominal SSD were calculated for all four applicators.

Moreover, if an air gap is inevitable in a treatment setup, the correction factor for the dose output (CF_{air}) can be calculated using the nominal SSD:

$$CF_{air} = \left(\frac{f + d}{f + g + d}\right)^2 \tag{4}$$

where d is the calculating depth.
The presence of an air-gap greatly affects the output at the skin surface. The dose fall off can be higher than 10% when there is more than 1mm air gap. The nominal SSDs are determined to be 20 mm for the 10 mm cone, 20 mm cone and 35 mm cone; and the nominal SSD is 30 mm for the 50 mm cone. Note that the nominal SSD varies with different cones due to the different filter manufacturing.
The cutouts made by the Xoft Axxent® Mini lead shield can be used to collimate the beam to accommodate the treatment area. Cutout correction factors (CF_{cone}) need to be measured prior to the treatment by qualified personnel to correct for the output change due to the use of the lead collimation. It can be calculated by:

$$CF_{cone} = M_{cone}\,(\text{uncollimated}) / M_{cone}(\text{collimated}) \tag{5}$$

Measurements of the specific cutout factors were performed using the surface applicator QA test fixture (Figure 8). The applicator QA text fixture consists of inserts for the ion chamber (left figure) and the applicator (right figure). A custom-made plastic slab with a groove can be used to accommodate the parallel-plate chamber, so that the chamber surface is flush to the phantom surface. This fixture allows measurements with additional solid water slabs placed on top of the chamber and centrally fixed applicator.

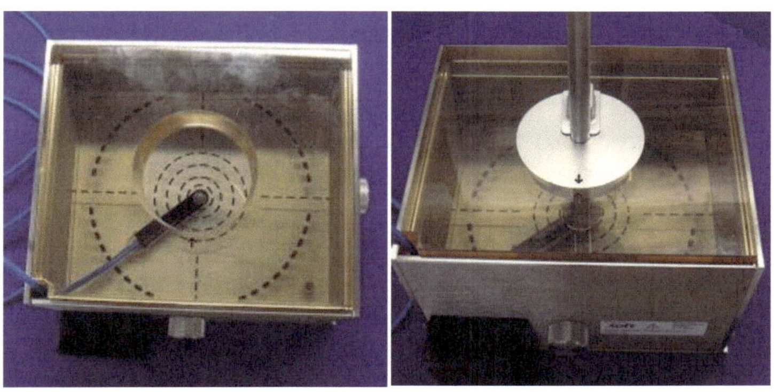

Fig. 8. Surface applicator QA test fixture with the PTW T34013 parallel plate chamber centrally inserted under the applicator for shielded measurements.

2.3 Clinical management
2.3.1 Prescription and treatment time calculation

The treatment area was determined by physician as the visible tumor (i.e. gross tumor volume or GTV) plus estimated microscopic extension (i.e. clinical target volume or CTV), with an additional margin depending on tumor size (planning target volume or PTV). A smaller margin (typical 5 mm) than typically used with electron beam or ^{192}Ir HDR brachytherapy is recommended, given the beam flatness of the Xoft 35 mm surface applicator (with a mean and SD of 3.2%±1.2% as stated in the Xoft Axxent® system manual). Physicians make the selection of applicator cone size depending on the treatment area. Common prescription doses are 3 Gy per fraction to 45~48 Gy total for larger lesions or 5 Gy per fraction to 40 Gy total for smaller lesions. The prescription depth varies from 2 to 6 mm, depending on the characteristics of the tumor. Patient with lesion thicknesses larger than 6 mm generally should not be treated with EBT treatment, due to the rapid dose fall-off with depth. Very close contact should be maintained between the applicator end-cap and skin so that the air gaps can be eliminated.

Treatment duration (in seconds) can be calculated based on the prescribed fractionated dose D_p, the nominal dose-rate $\dot{D}_{skin,n}$ (Gy/min), the percentage depth dose at depth $PDD(d)$, and the cutout factor CF_{cone} using the equation:

$$T(s) = \frac{D_p}{\dot{D}_{skin,n} \times PDD(d) \times CF_{cone}} \times 60$$

Cutout factors need to be pre-measured for each patient case since patients have very different target areas, as shown in Figure 9, using the method mentioned in section B.4. Bolus materials have multiple purposes for skin cancer treatment including immobilizing the collimation material and attenuating radiation outside the treatment field. For cases shown in Figure 9a and 9b, bolus materials are used for filling the gap between the collimator cutouts and the mask in order to ensure minimum air gap and for protecting the scalp area behind the ear.

Treatment time usually takes 4 to 6 minutes for each session. The source stays in one position inside the applicator throughout the entire session. In the early clinical application of this new technology there were no cases of interruption of treatment resulting from malfunction of the applicator or patient movements. Source arcing did occur a few times during a few treatments, leading to an interruption of the treatment and recalculation for the remaining dose. The air-kerma strength was re-measured prior to the continuation of the treatment using the on-board well chamber and electrometer. In all cases, the treatment was successfully continued and finished after replacing the source.

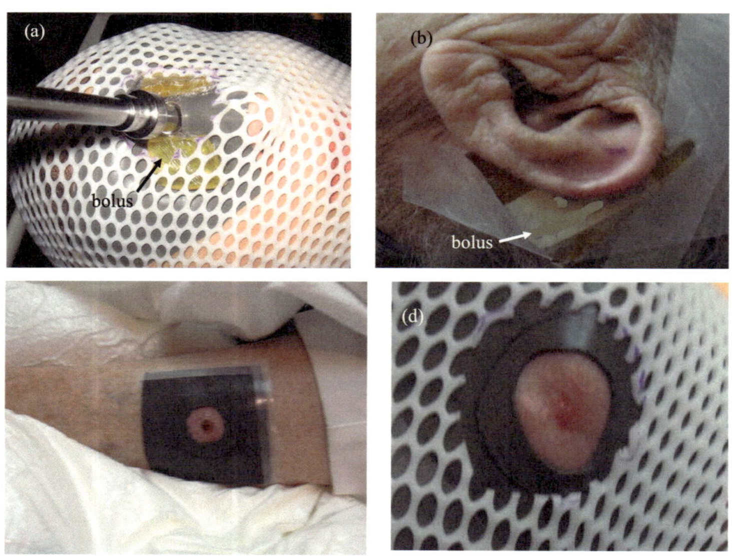

Fig. 9. Different collimations using the Flexishield lead material for targets located at (a) the bridge of the nose, (b) the left ear, (c) the left leg, and (d) the left temple.

2.3.2 Room setup and exposure to the personnel

In our clinic, patients lie on a flat "couch" (a linac table is what we use in our clinic) with clinically appropriate immobilization systems devised by the radiation therapists and physician to ensure minimal patient motion at applicator placement and during the treatment. For example, a thermoplastic facemask (WFR-Aquaplast, Avondale, PA) is normally used for lesions located on the face and other areas in the head and neck (Figure 10a). Patient positioning is not essential in this type of treatment since physicians can visually locate the treatment area and accurately place the applicator (although it is preferable to have the applicator oriented downwards rather than upwards or horizontally when possible for ease of set-up and reproducibility). A 0.5 cm lead equivalent rolling shield (2 meter tall and 1 meter wide) is used to reduce radiation exposure to the therapy personnel (Figure 10b). The therapy team can stay in the room and monitor the treatment through a small viewing window on the rolling shield. The room exposure measured with a survey meter was reported for three patients with the skin lesions located at their scalp, left ear, and left leg [31]. These three patients were scheduled on the same day for treatment using the same x-ray source. Seven positions in the treatment room were surveyed during the treatment session (Figure 11). As shown in Table 1, the highest room exposures were 70 mR/hr, 43 mR/hr, and 6.7 mR/hr at 1 m superior to the lesion for the scalp, left ear, and left leg. As expected, the further away from the source, the lower the exposure. The exposure rate was consistently at background reading (<1 mR/hr) behind the rolling shield. Therefore, the clinical personnel are safe and receive essentially no radiation behind the rolling shield.

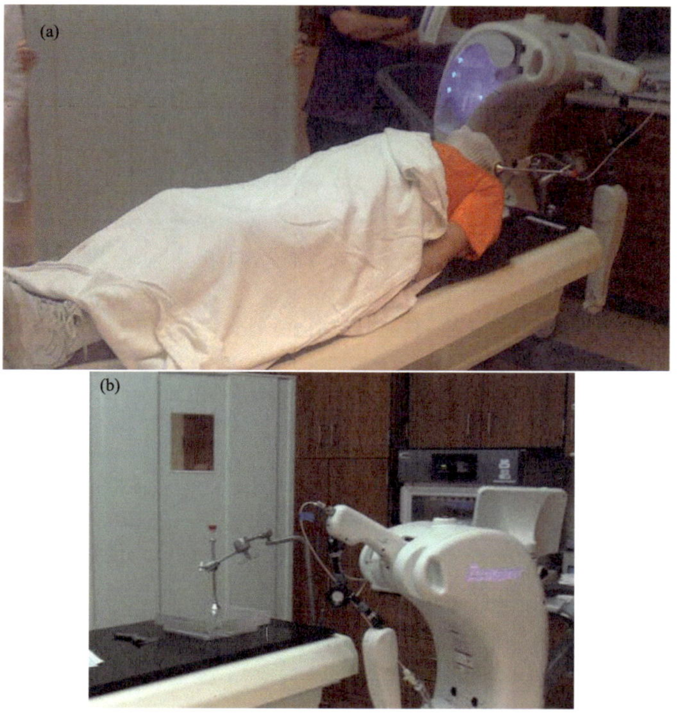

Fig. 10. (a) Patient setup with a thermoplastic facemask for skin treatment on the ear; (b) Radiation protection with the rolling shield in place.

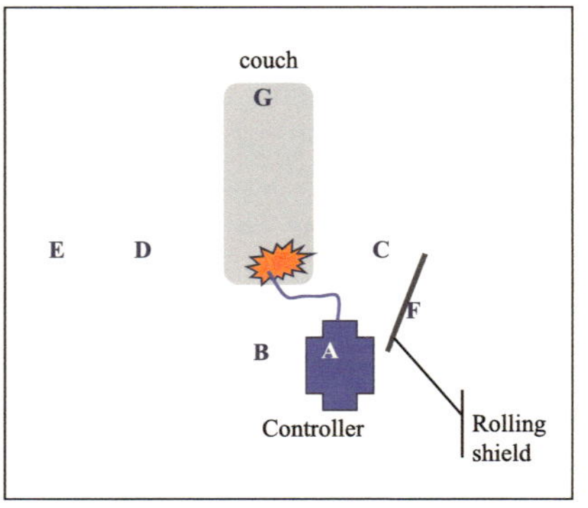

Fig. 11. Diagram of measurement points with clinical setup for ear, scalp and leg cases. Point A is right behind the controller. Point B, G, C, and D are 1 meter from the source superior, inferior, right and left. Point E is 1 meter from the source to the left. Point F is behind the rolling shield.

Table 1: Room Exposure (mR/hr)			
Measured points	Scalp	Left Ear	Left Leg
A (controller)	1.2	1.8	0.5
B (1meter Sup)	70	43	6.7
C (1meter right)	24	18	7.2
D (1meter left)	50	37	26
E (2meter left)	18	9.3	4.1
F (lead shield)	0.8	0.1	0.2
G (1meter Inf)	0.7	0.3	0.9

Table 1. Room exposure at different locations during the treatment of several patient setups

2.3.3 Initial clinical experience and patient follow-up

Similar to isotope-based HDR brachytherapy, the primary radiation oncologist and a medical physicist are currently required to be present for each treatment. After patient is comfortably lying down on the table, the radiation oncologist directly visualizes the target location and places the applicator with minimal air gap and at an appropriate angle. The physicist and therapists help the physician to secure the applicator using a clamp system. As shown in Figure 12, the surface applicator needs to be placed close to the target or pressing the collimator for various lesion locations, such as on the left ear, the left leg, and the scalp.
As in Figures 13, 14, and 15, most non-melanoma skin cancers responded fully to the treatment. During the course of treatment, most lesions demonstrated increased erythema. Many lesions became slightly ulcerated or turned into eschars in the first one to four weeks following the completion of treatment. However, by three to six months of follow up most cases showed resolution of acute radiodermatitis and no evidence of remaining malignancy.
Due to the early stage of clinical practice using the surface applicators and EBT system, there is only one publication so far to provide the initial experience for treatment of 37 patients

with 44 cutaneous malignancies in terms of tumor control, acute toxicity, and cosmesis [33]. No recurrences had been seen for a median of 4.1 months (range 1-9 months) follow-up, with acceptable acute toxicity and good to excellent early cosmesis.

Early clinical experience of EBT shows favorable tumor control as well as cosmetic outcomes. Using the hypofractionated approach, the treatment duration is short and convenient for patients. Direct visualization of the target location helps radiation oncologist to accurately place the applicator, thus accurately direct the radiation.

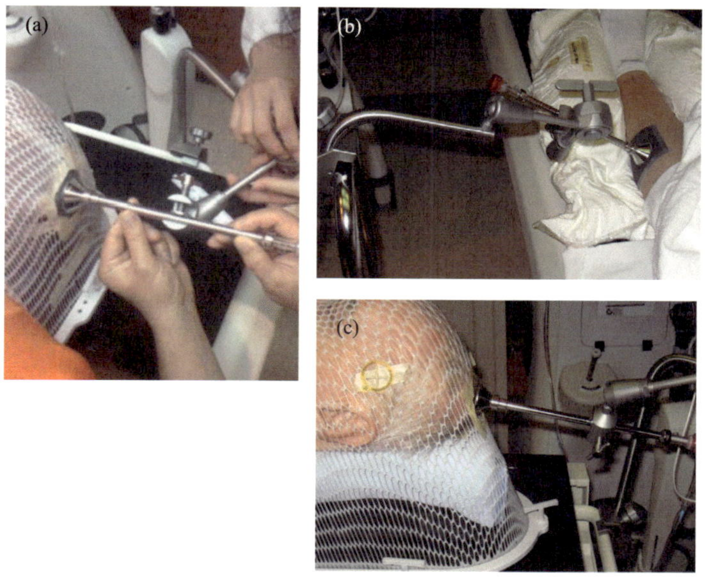

Fig. 12. The surface applicator setup immobilized with an Elmed Retract-Robot clamp system for different lesion locations, including (a) the left ear, (b) the left leg, and (c) the scalp.

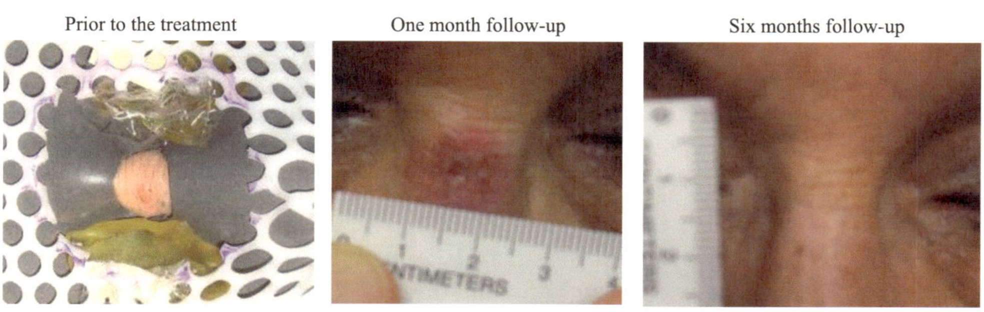

Fig. 13. Patient follow-ups for basal cell carcinoma on the nose, with pictures showing (a) prior to the treatment, (b) one month after the treatment, and (c) six months after the treatment.

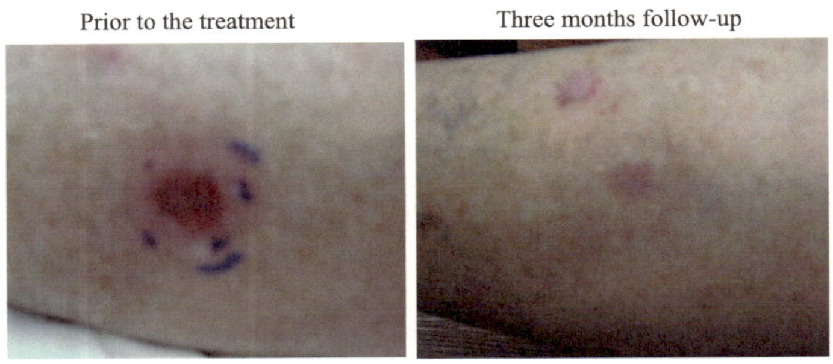

Fig. 14. Patient follow-ups for basal cell carcinoma on the left leg, with pictures showing (a) prior to the treatment and (b) three month after the treatment.

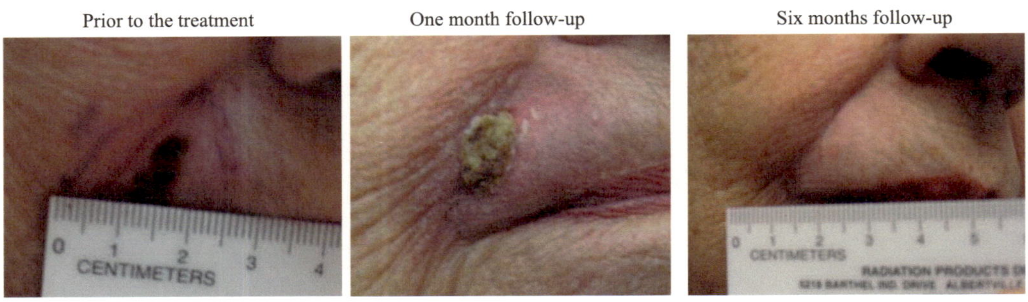

Fig. 15. Patient follow-ups for basal cell carcinoma on the face, with pictures showing (a) prior to the treatment, (b) one month after the treatment, and (c) six months after the treatment.

2.4 Technical and clinical considerations

2.4.1 Dose output uncertainty

As suggested in TG-61, the in-air method is recommended for measuring the absorbed dose to water at surface for low energy x-rays with tube potential between 40 kV and 300 kV. The Xoft source has an operating voltage of 50 kV, which falls within this region. Based on equation (1), several factors need to be pre-determined for the surface dose measurements. Similar to TG-51 for high-energy external beam, the calibration factor N_k and the electrometer correction *(P_{elec})* are provided by the Accredited Dosimetry Calibration Laboratory (ADCL) or **National Institute of Standards and Technology** (NIST). The mass energy-absorption coefficient ratio $[(\frac{\overline{\mu}_{en}}{\rho})^{w}_{air}]_{air}$ is a function of half value layer (HVL) in Al of the beam. The nominal beam quality (1st HVL in mm Al) is provided by factory measurements to be 1.39, 1.53, 1.57 and 1.56 mm Al for 10, 20, 35, and 50mm cones for the Xoft 50kVp x-ray beam. Thus, based on AAPM TG-61 Table IV, $[(\frac{\overline{\mu}_{en}}{\rho})^{w}_{air}]_{air}$ is 1.017. The backscatter factor B_w is a function of nominal SSD, field size, and HVL. Interpolated from

Table V in TG-61, the backscatters used in the calculation are 1.049, 1.081, 1.102, and 1.130 for 10, 20, 35, and 50 mm cone sizes, respectively. The stem correction factor $P_{stem,air}$ is set to 1 if the change of field size and beam quality between the calibration and actual measurements is minimal. Including all calibration parameters, the combined uncertainty at the surface in low energy x-ray beams using the in-air calibration method is 5%. Since the other part of uncertainty associated with the clinical setup and immobilization during treatment can be considered negligible due to the ease and stability of the setup using this skin applicator system, the final uncertainty in the absorbed dose should satisfy a tolerance of ±5% [34].

2.4.2 Treatment consideration

The presence and specific magnitude of electron contamination generated in air and on the inside surface of the treatment cone might contribute to an enhanced surface dose, which largely depends on the material from which the treatment cone is fabricated. A five-fold increase was reported in relative surface dose with lead lined treatment cones[35, 36]. The selection of an ionization chamber for a proper window thickness used in surface dose determination is crucial to the x-ray source calibration. The entrance window thickness should not be so thick that it absorbs low-energy photons nor so thin that it can be contaminated by photoelectrons. The surface points on the PDD curves provided by the company were determined by extrapolation. Its accuracy is questionable due to the possible effect of enhanced surface dose with the applicator cone. Further studies with Monte Carlo simulation are needed for accurately modeling the PDD in tissue with the surface applicators. It also implies that correction factors, i.e. cutout factors or air gap factors are more accurate if measured at depth.

It is recommended that close contact between skin surface and applicator end-cap be maintained to avoid underdosing due to the presence of an air-gap. The effective SSD is different for different applicators, but it can be determined for all applicators by measuring the air-gap correction factors as we described above. For treatment areas where a flat surface is hard to achieve, thin bolus material can be use to facilitate the treatment.

As to date, the largest available cone size is 50 mm in diameter for the Xoft surface applicators. This limits the application of EBT for lesions with a diameter larger than 40 mm. One possible solution is to combine multiple fields to cover the target. However, with the round shape of the field and manual positioning of the applicator, this technique might requires more practice and better design, to avoid overdosing or underdosing at the junction of two fields.

2.4.3 Room exposure to personnel

Room exposure varies with patient setups. As shown in Table 1, the scalp case represents an extreme scenario where no lead collimation was used due to a large treatment area and a very loose contact with the skin (due to patient discomfort when the applicator was pressed onto the lesion). The left ear case has an oblique skin surface but the use of bolus and lead collimation helped to reduce radiation exposure to staff. The left leg case was a small lesion and had very flat skin surface and thus close contact was achieved. This case represents the other extreme. Even for the scalp case, where the room exposure was maximal, the survey meter reading was below 1 mR/hr behind the rolling shield. The rolling shield does effectively minimize radiation exposure to personnel when properly used. Moreover, the use of Flexi-shield or bolus significantly reduces the room exposure, thus is recommended when possible.

2.4.4 Comparison with isotope-based HDR brachytherapy

Overall, it has been shown that Xoft miniature x-ray source can produce comparable dose distribution for intracavitory brachytherapy treatment compared to ^{192}Ir source [26-28]. One major concern is the relatively more rapid dose fall off with distance in tissue compared to ^{192}Ir source, which results in a higher surface dose near the MammoSite balloon applicator for APBI treatment or the Vaginal cylinder applicator for endometrial treatment. This is due to the lower energy (50keV) emitted from the miniature x-ray tube, compared to the effective energy of about 380keV for ^{192}Ir [37]. The size of the source is also a limitation. The miniature x-ray source is 2.3 mm in diameter, and it has to be housed in a cooling catheter in order to maintain a long time function. The apparent size of the source is 5.4 mm in diameter, which is too large for interstitial brachytherapy treatments. However the economics and safety favor the use of EBT over ^{192}Ir, in terms of minimal shielding required, less regulations over radioactive materials, initial cost of the unit, etc.

Favorable cosmetic outcomes and excellent local control (97~98% for primary tumors and 87% for recurrence) with minimal complications have been reported with isotope-based brachytherapy method for a follow-up study of 117 patients[8]. Clinical follow-up of a total of 85 patients have shown that the local control for the skin cancer using the isotope-based brachytherapy is 97%, with good cosmetic results (grade 1 (58%) and grade 2 (24%) acute skin toxicity)[22]. Since the electronic brachytherapy for skin cancer is still at its early stage for clinical management, patient follow-up reports are limited. Initial experience at University of Pittsburgh was published for treatment of 37 patients with 44 cutaneous malignancies using the electronic brachytherapy in terms of tumor control, acute toxicity, and cosmesis. No recurrences had been seen for a median of 4.1 months (range 1-9 months) follow-up, with acceptable acute toxicity and good to excellent early cosmesis [33]. We anticipate increased clinical applications of this technology in the near future.

3. Summary

The application of EBT for skin treatment is still relatively new and consequently is unfamiliar to many medical physicists and physicians. It is relatively simple to implement technically. With limited clinical experience and short follow-up it appears to be safe and effective for small non-melanoma skin cancers. Each source needs to be carefully calibrated with the surface applicator prior to treatment. The electronic brachytherapy is a feasible approach for treatment of non-melanoma skin cancer.

4. References

[1] Christenson LJ, Borrowman TA, Vachon CM, et al. Incidence of basal cell and squamous cell carcinomas in a population younger than 40 years. JAMA 294, 681-690 (2005)

[2] http://www.cancer.gov/cancertopics/types/skinCancer, National Cancer Institute 2009, Website last accessed January 11, 2010.

[3] http://www.cancer.org/downloads/STT/2008CAFFfinalsecured.pdf, American Cancer Society. Cancer Facts and Figures 2008.

[4] Freeman RG, Knox JM, Heaton CL. The treatment of skin cancer: A statistical study of 1341 skin tumors comparing results obtained with irradiation, surgery and curettage followed by electrodesiccation. Cancer 17, 535–538 (1964)
[5] Mohs FE. The chemosurgical method for microscopical controlled excision of cancer of the skin. NY State J. Med. 56, 3486 –3492 (1956)
[6] Lovett RD, Perez CA, Shapiro SJ, et al. External irradiation of epithelial skin cancer. Int. J. Radiat. Oncol. Biol. Phys. 19, 235–242 (1990)
[7] Silva JJ, Tsang RW, Panzarella P, et al. Results of radiotherapy for epithelial skin cancer of the pinna: the Princess Margaret Hospital experience, 1982-1993. Int. J. Radiat. Oncol. Biol. Phys. 47, 451-459 (2000)
[8] Guix B, Finestres F, Tello J, et al. Treatment of skin carcinomas of the face by high dose rate Brachytherapy and custom made surface molds. Int. J. Radiat. Oncol. Biol. Phys. 47, 95-102 (2000)
[9] Kwan W, Wilson D, Moranvan V. Radiotherapy for locally advanced basal cell and squamous cell carcinomas of the skin. Int. J. Radiat. Oncol. Biol. Phys. 60, 406-411 (2004)
[10] Klein E, Fine S, Laor Y et al., Laser irradiation of the skin. J. Invest. Dermatol. 43, 565–570 (1964)
[11] Spicer MS, Goldberg DJ, Lasers in dermatology. J. Am. Acad. Dermatol. 34, 1-25 (1996)
[12] Heidary N, Naik H, Burgin S, Chemotherapeutic agents and the skin: an update. J Am Acad Dermatol. 58, 545-570 (2008)
[13] Kuflik EG, Gage AA, The five-year cure rate achieved by cryosurgery for skin cancer. J. Am. Acad. Dermatol. 24, 1002-1004 (1991)
[14] Lee DA, Miller SJ, Nonmelanoma Skin Cancer. Facial Plast Surg Clin N Am 17, 309-324 (2009)
[15] Wolf DJ, Zitelli JA. Surgical margins for basal cell carcinoma. Arch Dermatol. 123, 340-344 (1987)
[16] Brodland DG, Zitelli JA. Surgical margins for excision of primary cutaneous squamous cell carcinoma. J Am Acad Dermatol. 27, 241-248 (1992)
[17] Greene F, Page DL, Fleming ID. AJCC cancer staging manual. 6th edition. New York: AJCC Springer-Verlag; 2001. Berlin, Heidelberg.
[18] Rowe D, Caroll RJ, Day CL Jr. Mohs Surgery is the treatment of choice for recurrent (previously treated) basal cell carcinoma. J Dermatol Surg Oncol 15:424-432 (1989)
[19] Caccialanza M, Piccinno R, Kolesnikova L, Gnecchi L. Radiotherapy of skin carcinomas of the pinna: a study of 115 lesions in 108 patients. Int J Dermatol. 44, 513-7 (2005)
[20] Barnes EA, Breen D, Culleton S, et al. Palliative radiotherapy for non-melanoma skin cancer. Clin Oncol. 22, 844-849 (2010)
[21] Kohler-Brock A, Prager W, Pohlmann S, Kunze S. The indications for and results of HDR afterloading therapy in diseases of the skin and mucosa with standardized surface applicators (the Leipzig applicator). Strahlenther. Onkol. 175, 170-174 (1999)
[22] Gauden S, Egan C, Pracy M, HDR brachytherapy for the treatment of skin cancers using standard surface applicators. Brachytherapy 7, 159 (2008)
[23] Mebed AH, Soliman HO, Gad ZS, et al. Multimodality treatment for non melanoma skin cancer: a prospective study done on 120 Egyptian patients. J Egyp Nat Cancer Inst. 22, 49-55 (2010)

[24] Rivard MJ, Davis SD, DeWerd LA, Rusch TW, and Axelrod S, Calculated and measured brachytherapy dosimetry parameters in water for the Xoft Axxent X-Ray Source: An electronic brachytherapy source. Med. Phys. 33, 4020–4032 (2006)

[25] Mille MM, Xu XG, Rivard MJ. Comparison of organ doses for patients undergoing balloon brachytherapy of the breast with HDR 192Ir or electronic sources using monte carlo simulations in a heterogeneous human phantom. Med Phys. 37, 662-71 (2010)

[26] Dickler A, Kirk MC, Seif N, et al, A dosimetric comparison of MammoSite high dose-rate brachytherapy and Xoft Axxent electronic brachytherapy. Brachytherapy. 6, 164–168 (2007)

[27] Dickler A, Dowlatshahi K. Xoft Axxent electronic brachytherapy. Expert Rev Med Devices. 6, 27-31 (2009)

[28] Dickler A, Kirk MC, Coon A, et al, A dosimetric comparison of Xoft Axxent electronic brachytherapy and iridium-192 high-dose-rate brachytherapy in the treatment of endometrial cancer. Brachytherapy. 7, 351-354 (2008)

[29] Hiatt J, Cardarelli G, Hepel J, et al, A commissioning procedure for breast intracavitary electronic brachytherapy systems. J. App. Clin. Med. Phys. 9, 58-68 (2008)

[30] Rong Y, Welsh JS. Surface applicator calibration and commissioning of an electronic brachytherapy system for nonmelanoma skin cancer treatment. Med Phys. 37, 5509-5517 (2010)

[31] Liu D, Poon E, Bazalova M, Reniers B, Evans M, Rusch T, Verhaegen F. Spectroscopic characterization of a novel electronic brachytherapy system. Phys Med Biol. 53, 61-75 (2008)

[32] Ma CM, Coffey CW, DeWerd LA, et al. AAPM protocol for 40-300kV x-ray beam dosimetry in radiotherapy and radiobiology. Med. Phys. 28, 868-893 (2001)

[33] Bhatnagar A, Loper A, The initial experience of electronic brachytherapy for the treatment of non-melanoma skin cancer. Radiat Oncol. 28, 87 (2010)

[34] Brahme A, Dosimetric precision requirements in radiation therapy, Acta. Radiol. Oncol. 23, 379-391 (1984)

[35] Aldrich JE, Meng JS, and Andrew JW, The surface doses from orthovoltage x-ray treatment, Med. Dosim. 17, 69-72 (1992)

[36] Podgorsak MB, Schreiner LJ and Podgorsak EB, Surface dose in intracavitary orthovoltage radiotherapy, Med. Phys. 17, 635-640 (1990)

[37] Holt RW, Thomadsen BR, Orton CG. Miniature x-ray tubes will ultimately displace Ir-192 as the radiation sources of choice for high dose rate brachytherapy. Med Phys. 35, 815-817 (2008)

Part 3

Prevention

8

Chemoprevention of Skin Cancer with Dietary Phytochemicals

BuHyun Youn and Hee Jung Yang
Pusan National University
Republic of Korea

1. Introduction

Cancer is responsible for a major cause of death in human. It is calculated that more than 11 million people are diagnosed with cancer worldwide (Jemal et al., 2009). Cancer arises through accumulation of multiple genetic alterations. In skin, UV radiation-induced gene mutations have been considered as a driving force of the skin carcinogenesis. Over the past 30 years, ozone depletion has induced increase in the level of UV-B radiation at the earth's surface. As a result, incidence of the skin cancer has been significantly increased, and it is recognized as a serious public health issue. Many researchers have studied mechanisms of UV-B radiation-induced skin cancer and strategies for skin cancer prevention and treatment. Among the various cancer therapies, chemoprevention is a pharmacological approach using natural, synthetic or biological agents that can prevent, inhibit and reverse the carcinogenic progression. Especially, dietary natural products in chemoprevention have been appreciated as credible components for the management of cancer. Epidemiological studies including more than 250 populations indicated that people who take five different kinds of fruits and vegetables a day showed about 50% decrease in cancer incidence and development than not or less eating plant foods. Based on accumulated researches, dietary plants have been believed to outstanding sources of the cancer preventive substances, and received considerable attention due to their various biological effects – anti-oxidant, anti-inflammatory and anti-carcinogenic functions. Therefore, chemoprevention by dietary phytochemicals has been regarded as a new, safety and efficiency strategy for cancer treatment.

This chapter gives a useful overview of recent studies in chemoprevention of skin cancer with dietary phytochemicals, and especially, focuses on UV-B radiation as a major factor of skin cancer and summarizes the UV-B radiation-induced skin carcinogenic mechanism.

2. Ultraviolet (UV) radiation-induced skin cancer and chemoprevention with dietary phytochemicals

Currently, skin cancer occurs at a rate of one in every six Americans (18%), and constitutes more than 30% of all newly diagnosed cancer patients in the world (Gloster et al., 1996; Aziz et al., 2005). The incidence and mortality in the skin cancer have rapidly increased worldwide because of an increase in the level of UV radiation at the earth's surface due to ozone depletion. The new strategies for skin cancer prevention and treatment are demanded, and chemoprevention has come to the fore.

2.1 Skin cancer

Epidemiological researches on the relation between diseases and death have demonstrated a significant death rate decrease in stroke, heart and infectious diseases within the United States, however, cancer mortality rate has not been changed in last 50 years (Aggarwal & Shishodia, 2006). In spite of a better understanding of the cancer mechanism and improvement of medical and pharmacological technology, the efficiency of cancer treatment has not progressed. In various types of cancer, especially, skin cancer has recognized a serious public health issue because of rapid increase of incidence, morbidity and mortality (Katiyar, 2011). There are over one million patients per year diagnosed skin cancer in the United States, and these account for 40% of all new cases of cancer diagnosed (Gloster et al., 1996; Johnson et al., 1998). Magnitude of the skin cancer is closely associated with exposure to UV radiation. Indeed, the high incidence of skin cancer is reported in some countries of the world such as Australia (particularly in Queensland) indicating serious destruction of ozone layer (Diepgen & Mahler, 2002).

Depending on the cellular origin, skin cancer is divided into two major categories - melanomas (melanocytic) and non-melanoma (epithelial) skin cancers (NMSCs), and NMSCs are subdivided into basal cell carcinomas (BCCs) and squamous cell carcinomas (SCCs). Although both BCCs (the most common types of skin cancer, 80%) and SCCs are derived from the basal layer of the epidermis of the skin, BCCs and SCCs have a different feature - BCCs are characterized by slow growth and rare metastasis, whereas, SCCs have strong invasive and metastasis ability. Melanomas account for only 4% of skin cancer, but it is the main cause of death in patients with skin cancer (Marks, 1995).

2.1.1 UV radiation as a major risk factor for skin damages

Although various physical, chemical and environmental factors contribute to initiation and development of skin disorders - premature skin aging, wrinkling, scaling, dryness, mottled pigment abnormalities and skin cancer, UV radiation exerts the most detrimental effect in skin (Nichol & Katiyar, 2010; Katiyar, 2011).

Among invisible radiation emitted from the sun, UV radiation is classified into three categories according to its wavelength: UV-A (315-380 nm), UV-B (280-315 nm), and UV-C (190-280 nm) (Tyrrell, 1994). Because stratospheric ozone layer completely absorbs UV-C and mostly absorbs UV-B radiation, it has been considered that UV radiation reaching the surface of the earth is composed with 10% of the UV-B and 90% of the UV-A radiation. However, recently, the proportion of UV-B radiation at the surface of the earth has gradually increased due to depletion of the ozone layer (Latonen & Laiho, 2005). Although UV-B radiation accounts for a minor part of the sunlight arriving to the surface of the earth, previous studies have suggested that UV-B radiation could have the most cytotoxic and mutagenic effect to induce skin damage including skin cancer (Ichihashi et al., 2003).

2.2 UV-B radiation-induced cellular mechanisms in skin

UV-B radiation can cross the whole epidermis layer and portion of the dermis compartment in skin. UV-B radiation can induce both direct and indirect adverse biological effects including induction of DNA damage, oxidative stress, inflammation, immunosuppression, alterations in the extracellular matrix (ECM) and premature aging of the skin (Mukhtar & Elmets, 1996; Latonen & Laiho, 2005), which together perform critical functions in the generation and maintenance of UV-induced carcinogenesis (Hruza & Pentland, 1993). Actually, it is experimentally demonstrated that UV-B radiation can act as a strong carcinogen in mouse skin models, indicating that UV-B radiation can affect tumor initiation, promotion and progression in skin carcinogenesis (Aziz et al., 2004; Armstrong & Kricker, 2001).

Previous studies have suggested that the most important effect on UV-B radiation is DNA damage. UV-B radiation can provoke DNA single (or double) strand breaks and indirect DNA damage through reactive oxygen species (ROS) production. DNA damage activates (oxidative) stress signal transduction and DNA checkpoint signaling, and also induces cell cycle arrest, DNA repair and apoptosis. Although skin has an elaborate defense mechanism to protect the skin from the radiation-induced cellular damages, chronic exposure to UV-B radiation attenuates the cutaneous defense processes leading to initiation and development of skin cancer (Nichols & Katiyar, 2010). Especially, failure of DNA repair is regarded as a crucial factor of UV-B radiation-induced skin cancer.

2.2.1 Direct DNA damage by UV-B radiation

Cells include photosensitive molecules called chromophores, which, upon receiving photons in UV radiation, transfer electrons to a higher energy state. Moreover, the chromophore could transmit its excited energy to other molecules, therefore, chromophore can induce the chain reactions. The major cellular chromophore for UV-B radiation has been demonstrated to DNA. Due to the aromatic rings in DNA bases, DNA efficiently and directly absorbs UV-B radiation. On the other hands, although UV-A radiation is the most abundant (90%) light at the surface of the earth and has cytotoxic effects, UV-A radiation exhibits gentle extent of the DNA damage than UV-B radiation, because DNA is not a suitable chromophore for UV-A radiation (Tyrrell, 1994). The most typical types of UV-B radiation-induced DNA damage are production of abnormal DNA adducts - cyclobutane pyrimidine dimers (CPDs) and (6-4) photoproducts ((6-4) PPs), which cross-link adjacent DNA bases. Also, UV-B radiation could generate DNA double (or single) strand breaks and DNA-protein cross-links. CDPs and (6-4) PPs change the DNA structure through helix-distorting and induce mutations in the epidermal cells, causing to the tumor initiation and development (Ravanat et al., 2001). The occurrence of (6-4) PPs by UV-B radiation is 5-10 fold less than appearance of CPDs (Eveno et al., 1995). Part of CPDs, thymine-cytosine (TC) and cytosine-cytosine (CC) dimers are represented to be the most common mutation type, and TC→TT and CC→TT mutations in p53 tumor suppressor gene are repeatedly seen in the UV-B radiation-induced cancer cells (Ichihashi et al., 2003). Consequentially, distortions of the DNA helix due to UV-B radiation-induced abnormal DNA adducts can stop RNA polymerase (pol) and inhibit elongation along DNA during the transcription. Therefore, UV-B radiation could influence normal mammalian gene expression and function (Tornaletti & Hanawalt, 1999).

2.2.2 Indirect DNA damage by UV-B radiation

UV-B radiation-induced ROS induction results in oxidative damage to the DNA bases, lipid peroxidation and additional types of DNA damage (Kielbassa et al., 1997). Electron transfer and singlet molecular oxygen production induced by UV-B radiation mark guanine base and accelerate generation of 8-hydroxydeoxyguanosine (8-OHdG) in the DNA strand (Cadet et al., 2000). 8-OHdG has been represented to be a typical maker of oxidative stress because it is produced by ROS such as peroxynitrite, .OH radical and singlet oxygen. Also, 8-OHdG is a miscoding lesion inducing G to T transversion (de Gruijl et al., 2001).

UV-B radiation causes various types of DNA damage - protein-DNA cross-links, DNA double (single) strand breaks and thymine glycol (Ichihashi et al., 2003). Although skin cells possess the defense machinery against oxidative stresses by means of the cooperation of chemical and enzymatic anti-oxidant components, repeated exposure to UV-B radiation could induce crucial uncorrectable oxidative damage to DNA. Excessive amounts of UV-B radiation can cause the degeneration of inner and outer cell membranes and suppression of macromolecular synthesis (proteins and lipids) inducing abnormal cellular metabolism (Latonen & Laiho, 2005). Moreover, UV-B radiation is well known to up-regulate gene expression through many intracellular signal transduction pathways, which may contribute to initiation and development of skin cancer. UV-B radiation is proved to suppress immune reaction and to induce tolerance to antigens. These biological effects of UV-B radiation had been proven in experimental animal models (de Gruijl et al., 2001).

2.2.3 Repair mechanism of UV-B radiation-induced DNA damage

The repair process of UV-B radiation-induced DNA lesions occurs immediately after irradiation. Also, the cellular defensive events such as cell cycle arrest or apoptosis simultaneously proceed (Decraene et al., 2001). In skin, the UV-B radiation mediated–cellular photoprotective events are associated with paracrine regulation, ECM alteration, initiation of inflammation, and pigmentation (Clydesdale, 2001).

The predominant UV-B radiation-induced DNA damage is represented as pyrimidine dimers which induce helix-distorting lesion, and it is repaired by nucleotide excision repair (NER) process in mammalian cells (de Gruij et al., 2001). NER is a complicated process which is required 20-30 proteins (e.g., Xeroderma pigmentosum (XP): XPA - G) having specific functions such as recognition and incision of the DNA lesion (Friedberg, 2003). The NER repair complex is recruited to the DNA lesion and causes to regional unwinding around the damaged site by the DNA helicase activity of TFIIH (transcription factor II H). Then, the damaged DNA site is incised at almost 15 nucleotides from both sides of the bulge and is deleted. Incised DNA strand is sealed by new oligonucleotide synthesis and ligation through the reaction of DNA endonuclease, polymerase and ligase (Friedberg, 2001). NER pathways are divided into 2 subcategories – transcription-coupled repair (TCR) and global genomic repair (GGR). TCR is rapidly activated process in a gene-dependent manner, and it can repair the only template strand having transcriptional activity. While, GGR occurs more slowly than TCR and it can repair damaging sites from both non-transcribed genomic DNA and non-transcribed strand of expressed gene. Cell survival and proliferation are mainly regulated through TCR rather than GGR, however, genomic integrity and instability are controlled more by GGR (Hanawalt, 2002). Furthermore, GGR is initiated by the XPC-HR23B protein complex identifying the UV-B radiation-caused DNA lesion, and TCR is raised by pol II complex stopping at the DNA damage sites (Tornaletti & Hanawalt, 1999).

Although the DNA repair mechanisms are exquisitely regulated, deficiency in DNA repair often occurs, and unrepaired DNA damage could trigger in a mutations within the next cell division. Typical DNA polymerase cannot bypass the DNA lesion, however, a specific DNA polymerase can sometimes bypass the DNA lesion. Therefore mutations occasionally present, and the unrepaired DNA mutations are often misinterpreted during the DNA replication (Latonen & Laiho, 2005). Consequentially, failure of repair process in UV radiation-induced DNA damage could be regarded as a major cause one of the skin cancer.

2.3 UV-B radiation-induced skin carcinogenesis

The skin is the largest organ composing a body surface area, and it protects internal body organs as a first defense barrier against harmful influences of environmental and xenobiotic stimuli. Exposure to UV-B radiation could induce initiation of skin cancer and repeated exposure to UV-B radiation accelerates skin carcinogenesis through depleting cutaneous defense mechanisms (Nichols & Katiyar, 2010).

Photocarcinogenesis in skin is progressed through complex and multiple steps - tumor initiation, promotion and progression (Digiovanni, 1992). Tumor initiation is rapidly induced by exposure to carcinogenic agents (e.g., UV radiation, the best known carcinogenic agent in skin cancer) and associated with irreversible genetic alterations that modify the response of basal (stem) cells in the epidermis. Unlike initiation process within just few days, tumor promotion requires long time more than 10 years. And it is reversible event that relates clonal expansion of initiated cells under the repeated radiation exposure to induce a benign tumor. In tumor progression stage, the final step of carcinogenesis, transformation of the benign tumor to an invasive and metastatic malignant tumor is promoted through additional genotoxic UV-B radiation (Surh, 2003). In other words, the incidence of skin cancer is closely associated with sun exposure - total quantity and time exposed to sun, and type of sun light (de Gruijl et al., 2001). If radiation-induced abnormal DNA adducts are not repaired, the significant mutations could be accumulated through the replication of DNA including the abnormal DNA adducts. The initiation of skin carcinogenesis has some connection with pivotal gene mutations in proto-oncogenes or tumor suppressor genes, and the *TP53* tumor suppressor gene has been reported as representative example in repeated sun-exposed skin (Brash et al., 1991). UV-B radiation-mediated gene alteration events occur in the basal cells in the epidermis, and could induce initiated cells (Zhang et al., 2001). Then, repeated UV-B irradiation could accelerate the proliferation of the initiated cells and generate a benign tumor. The driving force in tumor promotion is regarded as modification in gene expression. Researches in various skin cell lines have established certain signal molecules that are activated by UV-B radiation. These signaling molecules contain epidermal growth factor receptors (EGFR), mitogen-activated protein kinases (MAPKs), phosphatidylinositol 3-kinase (PI3K), cyclooxygenase-2 (COX-2) and various transcription factors (AP-1, CREB and NF-κB) (Wan et al., 2001). In tumor progression stage, there are associated with further gene alterations, including changes of gene copy number, gene mutations and gene re-arrangements that take place in the progression of benign to malignant skin tumors (Zoumpourlis et al., 2003).

2.4 Chemoprevention of skin cancer

Skin cancer arises primarily from sun-exposed body site and is intimately associated with repeated sun exposure (Kwa et al., 1992). Thus, an approach aimed at preventing or protecting from UV-B radiation-induced cellular damages has considered as an effective strategy for the management of skin cancer (Aziz et al., 2005). Fundamental and primary prevention of skin cancer is an attempt to minimize the exposure to the sun through use of sunscreens or protective clothing, and these approaches could clearly be helpful at decreasing the risk of skin cancer. However, due to several causes, these primary prevention methods have shown limited success (Bode & Dong, 2000). Therefore, new strategies for skin cancer prevention and treatment are demanded, and chemoprevention has come to the fore. The term of 'chemoprevention' was first mentioned by Michael Sporn in the mid-1970's to depict the strategy of blocking or retarding the initiation of pre-malignant tumors with non-toxic chemical resources - natural, synthetic, or biological agents (Surh, 2003).

2.4.1 Chemoprevention with dietary phytochemicals

Since 1999, chemoprevention has been in spotlight as a new anti-cancer strategy, and various review articles focusing on the subjects, principles, mechanisms and prospects of chemoprevention have been pouring (Bode & Dong, 2000).

Chemopreventive agents have been reported to interfere with a multistep of the carcinogenesis such as tumor initiation, promotion and progression. Chemopreventive agents are classified into two major categories - blocking agents and suppressing agents. Blocking agents inhibit the carcinogens from interaction with target molecules, metabolic activation or subsequently interaction with important cellular molecules - DNA, RNA and proteins. Also, blocking agents suppress carcinogen activation and promote detoxification. Whereas, suppressing agents prevent the tumor promotion and progression. They are closely associated with apoptosis, cell-cycle, cell proliferation, differentiation, DNA repair, expression and activation of oncogenes (or tumor suppressor genes), angiogenesis and metastasis in initiated cells (Wattenberg, 1985).

Plants including vegetables, fruits, seeds, nuts, flowers, and bark, have been used as a source of traditional medicines throughout history and utilized as a basis for various pharmaceutical drugs today. Plants include macronutrients - protein, fat, carbohydrate, and micronutrients - dietary fiber, vitamins, and minerals. Also, they contain non-nutritive components like polyphenols, terpenes and alkaloids that could serve considerable health advantages beyond the basic nutrition (Aggarwal & Shishodia, 2006). These non-nutritive compounds in plants are named phytochemicals ('phyto' is derived from the Greek term signifying 'plant') and are reported to have substantial biological properties such as anti-carcinogenic and anti-mutagenic effects (Surh, 2003). The NCI (National Cancer Institute) identified approximately thirty five plant-based foods that show anti-cancer properties. These contain chilli peppers, grape, turmeric, green tea, soybean, ginger, cabbage, apple, onion, tomato and garlic etc. Hundreds of phytochemicals have been identified as potential chemopreventive agent: allicin, anethol, capsaicin, catechins, curcumin, diallyl sulfide, dietary fiber, diosgenin, ellagic acid, eugenol, evodiamine, genistein, gingerol, indole-3-carbinol, isoflavones, lutein, lycopene, phytosterols, resveratrol, S-allyl cysteine, saponins, selenium, silymarin, ursolic acid and β-carotene etc. (Nichols & Katiyar, 2010).

Actually, epidemiological studies have indicated that populations (206 human and 22 animals) that consume a great quantity of the vegetables and fruits, have lower risk of the colon, endometrium, esophagus, lung, oral cavity, pancreas, pharynx and stomach cancer (Steinmetz & Potter, 1996). Moreover, experimentally, numerous cell culture and animal model researches have been demonstrated that various phytochemicals can suppress the inflammatory processes that induce to transformation, hyperproliferation, and initiation of carcinogenesis. Their inhibitory effects could suppress the final steps of carcinogenesis such as angiogenesis and metastasis (Saunders & Wallace, 2010). In addition to their biological functions, especially, plant-based natural products are thought to be safe (having little or no toxicity) chemopreventive agents, because natural compounds are contained in generally consumed foods and beverages (Bode & Dong, 2000).

2.4.2 Biological properties of dietary phytochemicals

During the last several centuries, the intake of dietary phytochemicals through plant food has been related to health advantages such as a photoprotection of the skin. Previous studies have demonstrated that various dietary phytochemicals possess the sunscreen ability, anti-inflammatory, anti-cancer, anti-oxidant and anti-bacterial effects.

Sunscreen effects of phytochemicals - Most of the natural products have different colored pigments – typically yellow, red or purple, and can absorb UV radiation. Accordingly, the natural phytochemicals can block the penetration of the UV radiation into the skin. Actually, the entire UV-B radiation and part of the UV-C and UV-A radiation are absorbed by phytochemicals having the pigment. This sunscreen ability of natural products can reduce inflammation, oxidative stress and DNA damaging effects by UV-B radiation in the skin. However, sunscreen effects account for only a part of various photoprotective effects in dietary phytochemicals (Nichols & Katiyar, 2010).

Anti-inflammatory effects of phytochemicals - UV-B radiation-induced erythema, edema and hyperproliferattive epithelial responses are known to representative inflammatory markers, and play important functions in skin tumor promotion (Mukhtar & Elmets, 1996). UV-B radiation-induced COX-2 expression and prostaglandin (PG) generation are specific responses of keratinocytes (mainly localized in epidermis) in both acute and chronic irradiation. COX-2 is a rate-limiting inflammatory enzyme for the production of PG metabolites from arachidonic acid (Langenbach et al., 1999), and COX-2 expression has been related to the pathological inflammation and cancer. A number of researches have suggested that COX-2 overexpression is closely associated with UV-B radiation-induced skin cancer - premalignant lesions, BCCs and SCCs (Buckman et al., 1998). Curcumin, green tea extract, gingerol, resveratol and basil based-ulsoric acid are reported to have anti-inflammatory effects through inhibiting of the inflammatory COX-2 enzyme.

Anti-oxidant effects of phytochemicals - The skin has well-regulated anti-oxidant defense system against UV-B radiation-induced oxidative stresses. But, repeated and excessive exposure to UV-B radiation cannot handle cutaneous anti-oxidant capacity. UV-B radiation is reported to induce excessive production of ROS resulting in the oxidative stress and depletion of anti-oxidant defense enzymes (superoxide dismutase, catalase, thioredoxin reductase and glutathione reductase). The strategies targeted at counteracting ROS generation and anti-oxidant defense enzymes could be helpful for the skin cancer prevention (Afaq et al, 2002). Some botanical phytochemicals (e.g., Caffeic acid phenethyl ester (CAPE), curcumin, green tea extracts, genistein, gingerol, quercetin and resveratol) are suggested to carry out the role in protecting the anti-oxidant system of skin and preventing skin carcinogenesis (F'guyer et al., 2003).

Based on previous researches of biological properties of the natural products, there has been considerable attention in the use of various phytochemicals for prevention and treatment of skin cancer.

2.4.3 Molecular targets of dietary phytochemicals in skin

Extracellular stimuli (e.g., UV-B radiation)-induced signal transduction is transmitted from the plasma membrane (receptors) into the cell and then, an intracellular chain of signaling molecules stimulates complex cellular responses. Also, skin carcinogenesis is associated with many functional genes regulating important cellular functions (e.g., intracellular, cell-surface, or extracellular function). All signal transduction pathways relating skin carcinogenesis are prime targets for chemopreventive agents (Bode & Dong, 2000). However, although considerable research has been done in explaining the mechanisms of carcinogenesis, further investigations are demanded to verify molecular and cellular targets for effective use of chemopreventive agents. Exactly, identification of exact target molecules for phytochemicals in cellular reaction process is essential to apply dietary phytochemicals to safe and effective medical treatment.

Although chemoprevention with natural products has considerable advantages, the negative results obtained for phytochemicals on lung cancer prevention highlight the need for caution in application of the potential chemopreventive agents before their mechanism of action is entirely comprehended (Omenn et al., 1996). This example suggests the need to verify carcinogenic mechanisms and molecular and cellular targets for effective use of potential chemopreventive substances.

Skin carcinogenesis is a multistage process that can be activated by UV radiation (especially, UV-B radiation). The alteration of the signaling molecules regulating cell proliferation, differentiation and death are associated with UV-B radiation-induced skin cancer (Nichols et al., 2010). UV-B radiation are known to modulate the transcription factors (e.g., AP-1, NF-kB, STAT3), anti-apoptotic proteins (e.g., Akt, Bcl-2, Bcl-XL), pro-apoptotic proteins (e.g., caspases, PARP), numerous protein kinases (e.g., AKT, ERK, IKK, JNK, PI3K, p38), cell cycle proteins (e.g., cyclins, cyclin-dependent kinases), cell adhesion molecules, inflammatory enzymes (e.g., COX-2 and 5-LOX), and growth factor signaling pathways (e.g., EGFR, TNF, IGF).

There is summarization of the photoprotective effects and target molecules in some selected representative dietary phytochemicals, such as capsaicin, curcumin, resveratol, green tea polyphenol - (epigallocatechin-3-gallate (EGCG)), silymarin, quercetin and genistein, on external stimuli (e.g., UV-B radiation)-induced skin inflammation, oxidative stress and DNA damage condition. It is based on previous laboratory researches utilizing animal models and skin cell lines and indicating skin cancer chemopreventive activities of these phytochemicals.

Capsaicin - a pungent component of chilli peppers had been reported to work as a carcinogen in experimental animals due to its irritant effects. However, today, numerous studies have suggested that capsaicin has effects of chemoprevention and treatment in skin cancer through the regulation of the IκBα degradation, NF-κB activiation and translocation, AP-1 activation, pro-apoptosis proteins, generation of ROS and activation of JNK in dorsal skin of female ICR mice and mouse skin carcinogenesis model (Park et al.,1998; Han et al, 2001).

Curcumin - a yellow pigment that exists in the rhizome of turmeric is one of the most examined phytochemicals and owns powerful anti-inflammatory and anti-oxidant potential. Curcumin has been indicated to inhibit tumor promotion and progression in skin carcinogenesis through the regulation of the COX-2 expression, NF-κB and AP-1 activation, catalytic activity of ERK, caspase-mediated apoptosis and oxidative stresses in skin squamous carcinoma A431 cell line (Chan et al., 2003). Topical administration of the curcumin has been represented to enhance glutathione contents and glutathione-S-transferase (GST) activity, and suppresses lipid peroxidation and COX-2 activation in mouse skin and human IGR-39 melanoma cells (Iersel et al., 1996). Also, curcumin has been represented to attenuate the induction of ornithine decarboxylase (ODC) in mouse skin (Ishizaki et al, 1996) and to induce p53-associated apoptotic cell death through the blocking the NF-κB pathway and inhibiting the apoptotic inhibitor XIAP (X-linked inhibitor of apoptosis protein) in human basal carcinoma cells (Jee et al., 1998). These researches suggest that curcumin could be beneficial chemopreventive agent against the skin cancer (F'guyer et al., 2003).

Epigallocatechin-3-gallate (EGCG) - a polyphenol compound mainly contained in green tea has anti-oxidant properties. It has been demonstrated to suppress UV-B radiation-induced malignant transformation in skin through the regulation of the activation of AP-1, NF-κB and IKKα, phosphorylation and degradation of IκBα, activation of PI3K, STAT3, ERK, AKT and ERBB2 receptor, VEGF production, and cell cycle and apoptosis associating molecules (Afaq et al., 2003). As a potent anti-oxidant, EGCG can scavenge ROS, such as lipid free radicals, superoxide radical, hydroxyl radicals, hydrogen peroxide and singlet oxygen (Katiyar et al., 2000). Moreover, EGCG suppressed UV-B radiation-induced skin tumor initiation and development through inhibiting the AP-1 and NF-κB in SKH-1 hairless mouse skin (Mittal et al., 2003).

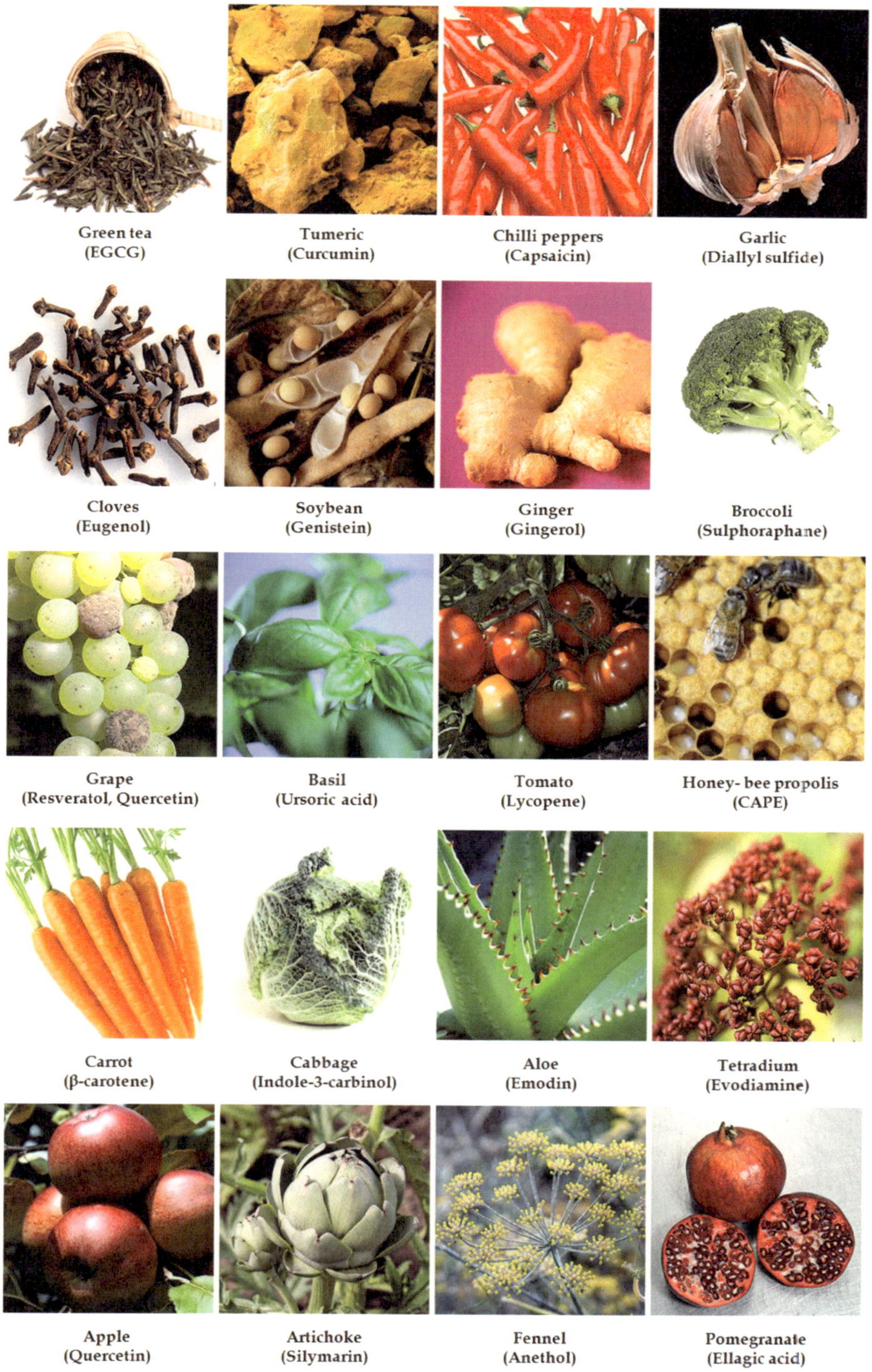

Fig. 1. Plant sources containing dietary chemopreventive phytochemicals

Genistein - a soy derived isoflavone has been mostly proven to contribute to the putative breast and prostate cancer preventive activity. In UV-B radiation-stimulated skin, it is reported that genistein suppresses NF-κB DNA binding and regulates to c-Jun and c-Fos in SENCAR mouse skin (Wang et al., 1998). Genistein has been known to have anti-oxidant and anti-carcinogenic properties in skin (Wei et al., 1998). Also, genistein downregulates the UV-B radiation-mediated phosphorylation of tyrosine protein kinase (TPK) and PGE_2 production in human epidermoid carcinoma A431 cells, and suppresses COX-2 expression in HaCaT keratinocytes (F'guyer et al., 2003).

Gingerol - a phenolic compound that takes charge of the spicy taste in ginger has been explained to prevent neoplastic transformation in skin carcinogenesis through the regulation of the ornithine decarboxylase (ODC) activity and TNF-α production and AP-1 activation in a two-stage mouse skin carcinogenesis model (Park et al., 1998).

Resveratol - a phytoalexin that is mainly contained in grapes has anti-oxidant, anti-inflammatory, anti-proliferative effects. Resveratol is an ingredient of red wine, colored grapes, peanuts and mulberries. Interest in red wine has been increased with so-called 'French paradox' - red wine has been presented to attenuate the mortality rates of cardiovascular diseases and some cancers (Kopp, 1998). The present study demonstrated that resveratrol conveys significant protection against UV-B radiation-induced skin carcinogenesis through modulation of the survivin and Smac/DIABLO in SKH-1 hairless mice (Aziz et al., 2005). Topical application of resveratrol inhibits UV-B radiation-induced skin tumor initiation, promotion and progression (Nichols & Katiyar, 2010). Resveratrol administration inhibits gene expression and catalytic activity of the COX-2, AP-1, MAPKs (ERK, JNK and p38), PKC and protein tyrosine kinases and activation of NF-κB through restriction of IKK phosphorylation. Resveratol presents effective chemoprevention properties based on anti-oxidant, anti-inflammatory in three major stages of skin carcinogenesis (Jang et al., 1997).

Quercetin - as the most abundant flavonol compound, quercetin is found plentifully in red wine, apples, tea and particularly onions (Gossé et al., 2005; Jeong et al., 2009; Murakami et al., 2008). Quercetin has anti-oxidant property as a free radical scavenger and metal ion chelator and is believed to prevent the harmful effects of UV radiation or reduce the damage (Aherne & O' Brien, 2002). Also, it has wide range of effects including anti-inflammatory and anti-cancer properties (Pan & Ho, 2008). The major functions of quercetin are regulation of the cell cycle arrest and induction of caspase-dependent cell death, and the major target molecules are indicated to p53, Wnt/β-catenin and ODC. Quercetin can protect skin anti-oxidant systems – glutathione peroxidase, glutathione reductase, catalase and superoxide dismutase activities, against UV radiation damage (Erden Inal et al., 2001). Oral administration of quercetin prevented UV-B radiation-mediated immunosuppression in SKH-1 hairless mice (Steerenberg et al., 1997; Svobodová et al., 2003)

Silymarin – a polyphenolic flavonoid isolated from milk thistle plant has anti-oxidant and anti-carcinogenic effects in mouse models (Berton et al., 1997). The exact molecular mechanism of the anti-carcinogenic effects of silymarin is still being examined. But, silymarin has been revealed to suppress UV radiation-induced NF-κB activation in human HaCaT keratinocytes. Also, treatment of the silymarin results in a significant downregulation of extracellular signalregulated protein kinase (ERK) and upregulation of stress-activated protein kinase/Jun NH(2)-terminal kinase (SAPK/JNK1/2) and p38 in human epidermoid carcinoma A431 cells (Singh et al., 2002). These results propose that silibinin could be possible underlying molecular events through inhibition of proliferation and induction of apoptosis in epidermoid A431 cancer cells. Silymarin is reported to protect skin against photocarcinogenesis in mice. Silymarin shows significant inhibition against UV-B-induced skin edema, skin sunburn, cell apoptosis, depletion of catalase activity, induction of COX-2 and ODC activities, and ODC mRNA expression (Katiyar et al., 1997). These results suggest that silymarin gives substantial protection against UV-B radiation-induced cellular damage in mouse skin. Moreover, recent investigation shows that silymarin suppresses endogenous tumor promoter, tumor necrosis factor-alpha (TNF-α) - a central mediator in skin tumor promotion in mouse skin (Singh & Agarwal, 2002; F'guyer et al., 2003).

Molecular targets of representative dietary phytochemicals in skin		
Plant name	**Active component**	**Molecular targets**
Honey bee propopolis	Caffeic acid phenethyl ester (CAPE) 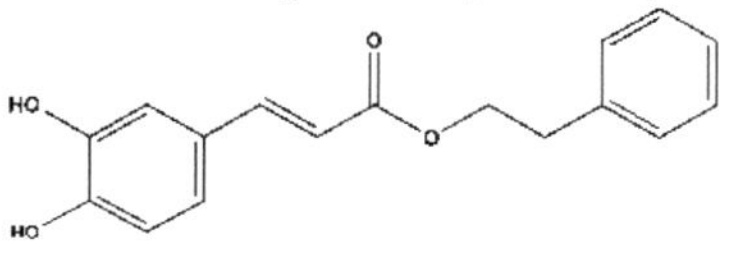	Bax↑, β-Catenin↓, Bcl-2↓, Bcl-xL↓, EGFR↓, PKC↓, ODC↓, Caspase-3↑ *↑: up-regulation *↓: down-regulation
Chilli peppers	Capsaicin 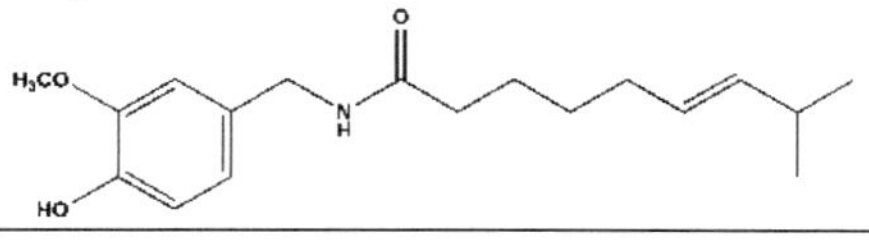	AP-1↓, Bcl-2↓, Bcl-xL↓, Cdc25↓, Cdk1↓, CIAP↓, NF-κB↓, Survivin ↓
Tumeric	Curcumin 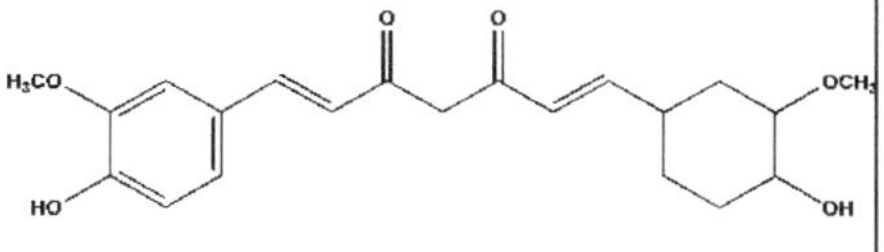	Akt↓, AP-1↓, Bcl-2↓, Bcl-xL↓, COX-2↓, c-Fos↓, c-Jun↓, c-Myc↓, CyclinD1↓, EGFR↓, ICAM1↓, Bcl-2↓, Bcl-xL↓, IL-6↓, iNOS↓, Jak2↓, JNK↓, MMP9↓, NF-κB↓, PKA↓, PKC↓, p53↓, Src↓, TNF↓, VCAM1↓, 5-LOX↓
Green tea	Epigallocatechin-3-gallate (EGCG) 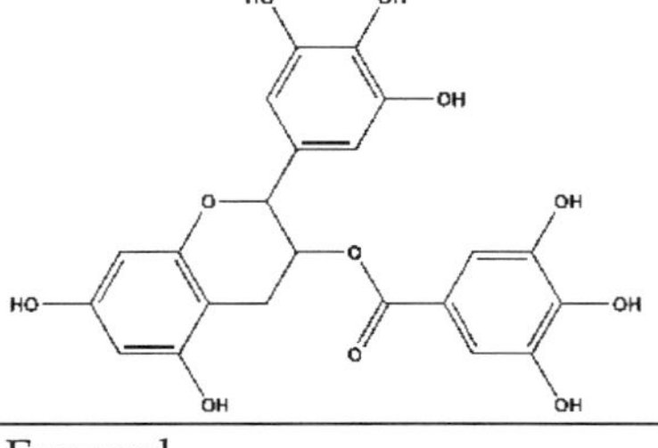	AP-1↓, Bcl-2↓, COX-2↓, c-Myc↓, IGF↓, IKKα↓, IL-6↓, iNOS↓, MAPKs↓, NF-κB↓, p21/WAF1↑, p53↑, VEGF↓, 5-LOX↓
Cloves	Eugenol 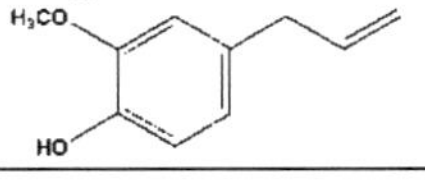	Caspase-3↓, NF-κB↓, PARP↓, p53↓

Molecular targets of representative dietary phytochemicals in skin		
Plant name	**Active component**	**Molecular targets**
Tetradium	Evodiamine 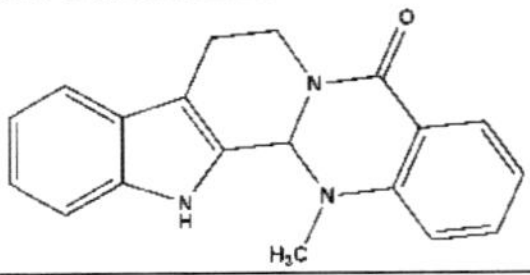	Caspase-3,-8,-9↓, Cdc25↓, Cdk 2↓, CyclinA ↓, CyclinB1↓
Soybean	Genistein 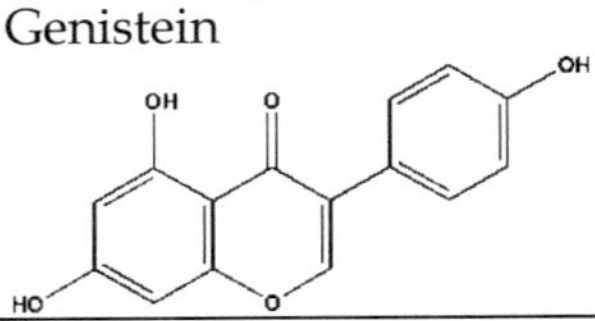	Caspase-12↓, Glutathione peroxidase↑, NF-κB↓, p21/WAF1↓
Ginger	Gingerol 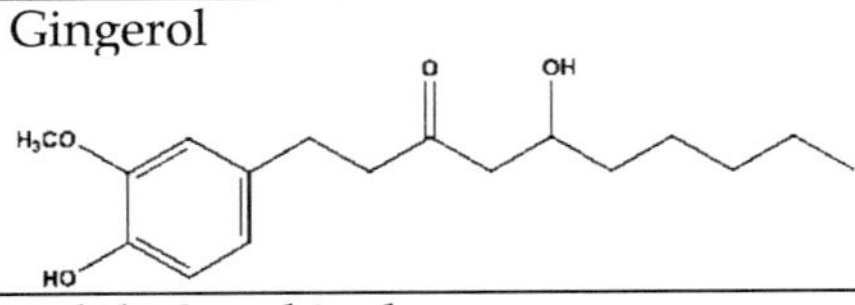	AP-1↓, COX-2↓, iNOS↓, NF-κB↓, ODC↓, TNF↓
Cabbage	Indole-3-carbinol 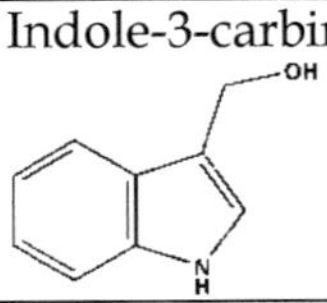	Bcl-2↓, Bcl-xL↓, Cdc25↓, Cdk1↓, CIAP↓
Apple	Quercetin 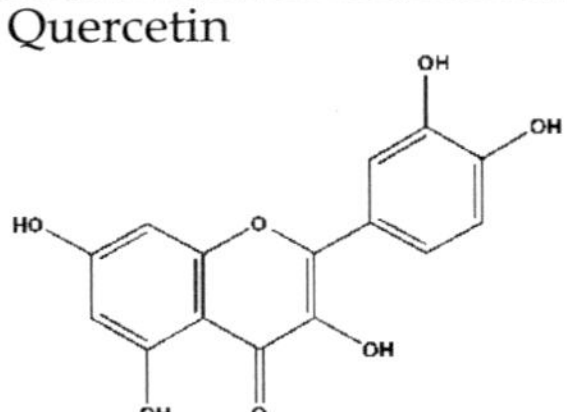	AP-1↓, IL-1,-6,-8↓, MAPKs↓, MMP-2,-3↓, NF-κB↓, PI3K↓, TNF↓, 5-LOX↓
Grape	Resveratol 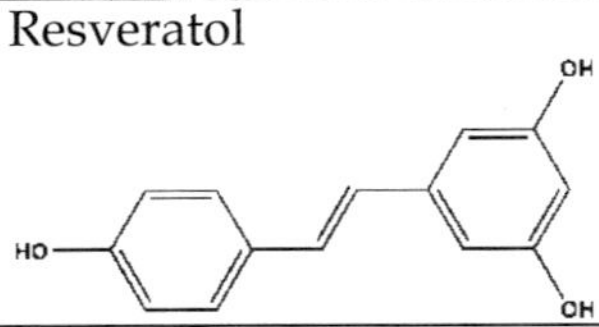	AP-1↓, COX-2↓, Cyclin D1↓, MAPKs ↓, 5-LOX↓, NF-κB↓, Survivin↓
Basil	Ursolic acid 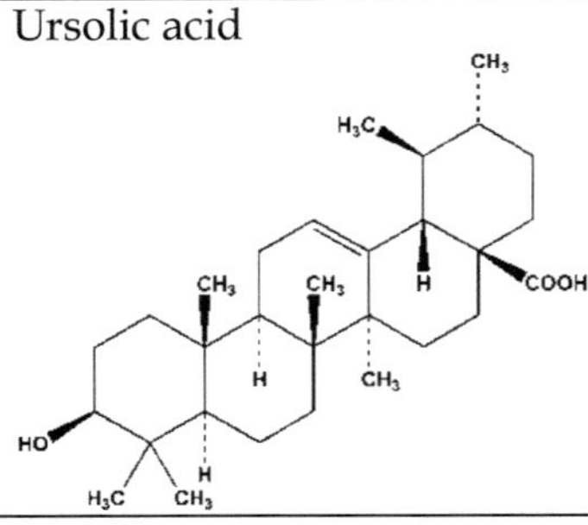	COX-2↓, Cyclin D1↓, NF-κB↓, MMP-9↓

Table 1. Molecular targets of representative dietary phytochemicals

3. Conclusion

The incidence of the skin cancer has recently accelerated worldwide because of an increase in the level of UV-B radiation at the earth's surface due to ozone depletion. Since it is very difficult to restore the once destroyed ozone layer to its original condition, incidence of the skin cancer will be significantly increased in future. Therefore, prevention and treatment of skin cancer will be the important problem. Among diverse strategies, chemoprevention by dietary phytochemicals has attracted considerable interest and it is now being studied in detail. Especially, chemoprevention using the natural products is considered to be an inexpensive, readily acceptable and accessible strategy to cancer management.

Dietary phytochemicals could directly interact with intracellular signaling molecule in prevention and treatment of skin cancer. Mostly dietary phytochemicals have been reported that they could have duplicity - a certain compound can 'switch on' the target molecules and sometimes 'switch off' the target molecules depend on various factors. Therefore, it is essential to identify the target molecules in the signaling network that can be influenced by individual chemopreventive compounds to allow medical application. In many cases, the chemopreventive effects of dietary phytochemicals confirmed in cultured cells or tissues are only achievable at supraphysiological concentrations - these concentrations would not be aquired when the phytochemicals are tried as food intake.

Moreover, phenolic compounds - the most widely used phytochemicals are frequently shown as glycosides or are conjugated to glucuronide, sulfate and methyl groups after administration, which might have a lower bioavailablity. Both pharmacokinetic properties and bioavailability are pivotal problems in investigating the prevention and treatment of the cancer and should be evaluated cautiously before attempting medical trials with dietary phytochemicals. From the viewpoint of the delivery of the phytochemicals, the penetration of phytochemicals into the skin is somewhat limited.

Although sufficient studies are demanded to apply dietary phytochemicals to clinic trials, chemoprevention by phytochemicals has been regarded as a safe strategy (having little or no genotoxicity) and a realistic method for controlling the risk of the cancers. Also, unlike the carcinogenic environmental factors that are difficult to control, individuals can modify their dietary habits and lifestyle in combination with a careful use of skin care products to prevent the photodamaging effects in the skin.

In this chapter, UV radiation (especially, UV-B radiation) is focused as a major factor of skin cancer, and mechanisms of the UV radiation-induced skin cancer and information of the chemoprevention of dietary phytochemicals are summarized. These contents will be useful to understand the 'chemoprevention of skin cancer with dietary phytochemicals'.

4. Acknowledgment

This work was supported by the Nuclear R&D Program through the National Research Foundation of Korea Grant funded by the Korean Government (Ministry of education science and technology, MEST) (grant code: 2010-0029553 and 2010-0021920).

5. References

Adhami, VM., Afaq, F., & Ahmad, N. (2003) Suppression of ultraviolet B exposure-mediated activation of NF-kappaB in normal human keratinocytes by resveratrol. *Neoplasia*, Vol. 5, No. 1, pp. 74-82, ISSN 1522-8002

Aggarwal, BB., & Shishodia, S. (2006) Molecular targets of dietary agents for prevention and therapy of cancer. *Biochemical Pharmacology*, Vol. 71, No. 10, pp.1397-1421, ISSN 0006-1421

Aherne, SA., & O' Brien, NM. (2002) Dietary flavonols: chemistry, food content, and metabolism. *Nutrition*, Vol. 18, No. 1, pp. 75-81, ISSN 0899-9007

Afaq, F., Adhami, VM., Ahmad, N., & Mukhtar, H. (2002) Botanical antioxidants for chemoprevention of photocarcinogenesis. *Frontiers in Bioscience*, Vol. 7, pp. d784-792, ISSN 1093-9946

Afaq, F., Adhami, VM., Ahmad, N., Mukhtar, H. (2003) Inhibition of ultraviolet B-mediated activation of nuclear factor kappaB in normal human epidermal keratinocytes by green tea Constituent (-)-epigallocatechin-3-gallate. *Oncogene*, Vol. 22, No. 7, pp. 1035-1044, ISSN 0950-9232

Ahmad, N., Gupta, S., & Mukhtar, H. (2000) Green tea polyphenol epigallocatechin-3-gallate differentially modulates nuclear factor kappaB in cancer cells versus normal cells. *Archives of Biochemistry and Biophysics*, Vol. 376, No. 2, pp. 338-346, ISSN 0003-9861

Anand, P., Kunnumakkara, AB., Newman, RA., & Aggarwal, BB. (2007) Bioavailability of curcumin: problems and promises. *Molecular Pharmacology*, Vol. 4, No. 6, pp. 807-818, ISSN 0026-895X

Armstrong, BK., & Kricker, A. (2001) The epidemiology of UV induced skin cancer. *Journal of Photochemistry and Photobiology B*, Vol. 63, No. 1-3, pp. 8-18, ISSN 1011-1344

Aziz, MH., Ghotra, AS., Shukla, Y., & Ahmad, N. (2004) Ultraviolet-B radiation causes an upregulation of survivin in human keratinocytes and mouse skin. *Photochemistry and Photobiology*, Vol. 80, No. 3, pp. 602-608, ISSN 0031-8655

Aziz, MH., Reagan-Shaw, S., Wu, J., Longley, BJ., & Ahmad, N. (2005) Chemoprevention of skin cancer by grape constituent resveratrol: relevance to human disease? *FASEB Journal*, Vol. 19, No. 9, pp. 1193-1195, ISSN 0892-6638

Berton, TR., Mitchell, DL., Fischer, SM., & Locniskar, MF. (1997) Epidermal proliferation but not quantity of DNA photodamage is correlated with UV-induced mouse skin carcinogenesis. *Journal of Investigative Dermatology*, Vol. 109, No. 3, pp. 340-347, ISSN 0022-202X

Bode, AM., & Dong, Z. (2000) Signal transduction pathways: targets for chemoprevention of skin cancer. *Lancet Oncology*, Vol. 1, pp. 181-188, ISSN 1470-2045

Bode, AM., Ma, WY., Surh, YJ., & Dong Z. (2001) Inhibition of epidermal growth factor-induced cell transformation and activator protein 1 activation by [6]-gingerol. *Cancer Research*, Vol. 61, No. 3, pp. 850-853, ISSN 0008-5472

Bowden, GT. (2004) Prevention of non-melanoma skin cancer by targeting ultraviolet-B-light signalling. *Nature Reviews Cancer*, Vol. 4, No. 1, pp. 23-35, ISSN 1474-175X

Brash, DE., Rudolph, JA., Simon, JA., Lin, A., McKenna, GJ., Baden, HP., Halperin, AJ., & Pontén, J. (1991) A role for sunlight in skin cancer: UV-induced p53 mutations in squamous cell carcinoma. *Proceedings of the National Academy of Sciences of the United States of America*, Vol. 88, No. 22, pp. 10124-10128, ISSN 0027-8424

Buckman, SY., Gresham, A., Hale, P., Hruza, G., Anast, J., Masferrer, J., & Pentland, AP. (1998) COX-2 expression is induced by UVB exposure in human skin: implications for the development of skin cancer. *Carcinogenesis*, Vol.19, No. 5, pp. 723-729, ISSN 0163-7258

Cadet, J., Douki, T., Pouget, JP., & Ravanat, JL. (2000) Singlet oxygen DNA damage products: formation and measurement. *Methods in Enzymology*, Vol. 319, pp. 143-153, ISSN 0076-6879

Chan, WH., Wu, CC., Yu, JS. (2003) Curcumin inhibits UV irradiation-induced oxidative stress and apoptotic biochemical changes in human epidermoid carcinoma A431 cells. *Journal of Cellular Biochemistry*, Vol. 90, No. 2, pp.327-338, ISSN 0730-2312

Clydesdale, GJ., Dandie, GW., & Muller, HK. (2001) Ultraviolet light induced injury: immunological and inflammatory effects. *Immunology and Cell Biology*, Vol. 79, No. 6, pp. 547-68, ISSN 0818-9641

Dampier, K., Hudson, EA., Howells, LM., Manson, MM., Walker, RA., & Gescher, A. (2001) Differences between human breast cell lines in susceptibility towards growth inhibition by genistein. *British Journal of Cancer*, Vol. 85, No. 4, pp. 618-624, ISSN 0007-0920

Decraene, D., Agostinis, P., Pupe, A., de Haes, P., & Garmyn, M. (2001) Acute response of human skin to solar radiation: regulation and function of the p53 protein. *Journal of Photochemistry and Photobiology B*, Vol. 63, No. 1-3, pp. 78-83, ISSN 1011-1344

de Gruijl, FR., van Kranen, HJ., & Mullenders, LH. (2001) UV-induced DNA damage, repair, mutations and oncogenic pathways in skin cancer. *Journal of Photochemistry and Photobiology B*, Vol. 63, No. 1-3, pp. 19-27, ISSN 1011-1344

Diepgen, TL., & Mahler, V. (2002) The epidemiology of skin cancer. *British Journal of Dermatology*, Vol. 146, No. Suppl 61, pp. 1-6, ISSN 0007-0963

Digiovanni, J. (1992) Multistage carcinogenesis in mouse skin. *Pharmacology & Therapeutics*, Vol.54, No. 1, pp. 63-128, ISSN 0163-7258

Erden Inal, M., Kahraman, A., & Köken, T. (2001) Beneficial effects of quercetin on oxidative stress induced by ultraviolet A. *Clinical and Experimental Dermatology*, Vol. 26, No. 6, pp. 536-539, ISSN 0307-6938

Eveno, E., Bourre, F., Quilliet, X., Chevallier-Lagente, O., Roza, L., Eker, AP., Kleijer, WJ., Nikaido, O., Stefanini, M., Hoeijmakers, JH., Dirk, B., James, EC., Alain, S., & Mauro, M. (1995) Different removal of ultraviolet photoproducts in genetically related xeroderma pigmentosum and trichothiodystrophy diseases. *Cancer Research*, Vol. 55, No. 19, pp. 4325-4332, ISSN 0008-5472

F'guyer, S., Afaq, F., & Mukhtar, H. (2003) Photochemoprevention of skin cancer by botanical agents. *Photodermatology, Photoimmunology & Photomedicine*, Vol. 19, No. 2, pp. 56-72, ISSN 0905-4383

Friedberg, EC. (2001) How nucleotide excision repair protects against cancer. *Nature Reviews Cancer*, Vol. 1, No. 1, pp. 22-33, ISSN 1474-175X

Friedberg, EC. (2003) DNA damage and repair. *Nature*, Vol. 421, No. 6921, pp. 436-40, ISSN 0028-0836

Gossé, F., Guyot, S., Roussi, S., Lobstein, A., Fischer, B., Seiler, N., & Raul, F. (2005) Chemopreventive properties of apple procyanidins on human colon cancer-derived metastatic SW620 cells and in a rat model of colon carcinogenesis. *Carcinogenesis*, Vol. 26, No. 7, pp. 1291-1295, ISSN 0143-3334

Gloster, HM Jr., & Brodland, DG. (1996) The epidemiology of skin cancer. *Dermatologic Surgery*, Vol. 22, No. 3, pp. 217-226, ISSN 1076-0512

Han, SS., Keum, YS., Seo, HJ., Chun, KS., Lee, SS., & Surh, YJ. (2001) Capsaicin suppresses phorbol ester-induced activation of NF-kappaB/Rel and AP-1 transcription factors in mouse epidermis. *Cancer Letters*, Vol. 164, No. 2, pp. 119-126, ISSN 0304-3835

Hanawalt, PC. (2002) Subpathways of nucleotide excision repair and their regulation. *Oncogene*, Vol. 21, No. 58, pp. 8949-8956, ISSN 0950-9232

Hruza, LL., & Pentland, AP. (1993) Mechanisms of UV-induced inflammation. *Journal of Investigative Dermatology*, Vol. 100, No. 1, pp. 35S-41S, ISSN 0022-202X

Ichihashi, M., Ueda, M., Budiyanto, A., Bito T., Oka, M., Fukunaga, M., Tsuru, K., & Horikawa, T. (2003) UV-induced skin damage. *Toxicology*, Vol. 189, No. 1-2, pp. 21-39, ISSN 0300-483X

Iersel, ML., Ploemen, JP., Struik, I., van Amersfoort, C., Keyzer, AE., Schefferlie, JG., & van Bladeren, PJ. (1996) Inhibition of glutathione S-transferase activity in human melanoma cells by alpha,beta-unsaturated carbonyl derivatives. Effects of acrolein, cinnamaldehyde, citral, crotonaldehyde, curcumin, ethacrynic acid, and trans-2-hexenal. *Chemico-biological Interactions*, Vol. 102, No. 2, pp. 117-132, ISSN 0009-2797

Ishizaki, C., Oguro, T., Yoshida, T., Wen, CQ., Sueki, H., & Iijima, M. (1996) Enhancing effect of ultraviolet A on ornithine decarboxylase induction and dermatitis evoked by 12-o-tetradecanoylphorbol-13-acetate and its inhibition by curcumin in mouse skin. *Dermatology*, Vol. 193, No. 4, pp. 311-317, ISSN 0190-9622

Jang, M., Cai, L., Udeani, GO., Slowing, KV., Thomas, CF., Beecher, CW., Fong, HH., Farnsworth, NR., Kinghorn, AD., Mehta, RG., Moon, RC., & Pezzuto, JM. (1997) Cancer chemopreventive activity of resveratrol, a natural product derived from grapes. *Science*, Vol. 275, No. 5297, pp. 218-220, ISSN 0036-8075

Jee, SH., Shen, SC., Tseng, CR., Chiu, HC., & Kuo, ML. (1998) Curcumin induces a p53-dependent apoptosis in human basal cell carcinoma cells. *Journal of Investigative Dermatology*, Vol. 111, No. 4, pp. 656-661, ISSN 0022-202X

Jemal, A., Siegel, R., Ward, E., Hao, Y., Xu, J., & Thun, MJ. (2009) Cancer statistics, 2009. *CA: A Cancer Journal for Clinicians*, Vol. 59, No. 4, pp. 225-249, ISSN 0007-9235

Jeong, JH., An, JY., Kwon, YT., Rhee, JG., & Lee, YJ. (2009) Effects of low dose quercetin: cancer cell-specific inhibition of cell cycle progression. *Journal of Cellular Biochemistry*, Vol. 106, No.1, pp. 73-82, ISSN 0730-2312

Johnson, TM., Dolan. OM., Hamilton, TA., Lu, MC., Swanson, NA., & Lowe, L. (1998) Clinical and histologic trends of melanoma. *Journal of the American Academy of Dermatology*, Vol. 38, No. 5 Pt 1, pp. 681-686, ISSN 0190-9622

Katiyar, SK., Korman, NJ., Mukhtar, H., & Agarwal, R. (1997) Protective effects of silymarin against photocarcinogenesis in a mouse skin model. *Journal of the National Cancer Institute*, Vol. 89, No. 8, pp. 556-566, ISSN 0027-8874

Katiyar, SK., Ahmad, N., & Mukhtar, H. (2000) Green tea and skin. *Archives of Dermatology*, Vol. 136, No. 8, pp. 989-994, ISSN 0003-987X

Katiyar, SK. (2011) Green tea prevents non-melanoma skin cancer by enhancing DNA repair. *Archives of Biochemistry and Biophysics*, Vol. 508, No. 2, pp. 152-158, ISSN 0003-9861

Kielbassa, C., Roza, L., & Epe, B. (1997) Wavelength dependence of oxidative DNA damage induced by UV and visible light. *Carcinogenesis*, Vol. 18, No. 4, pp. 811-816, ISSN 0143-3334

Kopp, P. (1998) Resveratrol, a phytoestrogen found in red wine. A possible explanation for the conundrum of the 'French paradox'? *European Journal of Endocrinology*, Vol. 138, No. 6, pp. 619-620, ISSN 0804-4643

Kwa, RE., Campana, K., & Moy, RL. (1992) Biology of cutaneous squamous cell carcinoma. *Journal of the American Academy of Dermatology*, Vol. 26, No. 1, pp. 1-26, ISSN 0190-9622

Langenbach, R., Loftin, CD., Lee, C., & Tiano, H. (1999) Cyclooxygenase-deficient mice. A summary of their characteristics and susceptibilities to inflammation and carcinogenesis. *Annals of the New York Academy of Sciences*, Vol. 889, pp. 52-61, ISSN 0077-8923

Latonen, L., & Laiho, M. (2005) Cellular UV damage responses-functions of tumor suppressor p53. *Biochimica et Biophysica Acta*, Vol. 1755, No. 2, pp. 71-89, ISSN 0304-419X

Marks, R. (1995) An overview of skin cancers. Incidence and causation. *Cancer*, Vol. 75, No. 2 Suppl, pp. 607-612, ISSN 0008-543X

Mittal, A., Piyathilake, C., Hara, Y., & Katiyar, SK. (2003) Exceptionally high protection of photocarcinogenesis by topical application of (-)-epigallocatechin-3-gallate in hydrophilic cream in SKH-1 hairless mouse model: relationship to inhibition of UVB-induced global DNA hypomethylation. *Neoplasia*, Vol. 5, No. 6, pp. 555-565, ISSN 1522-8002

Mukhtar, H., & Elmets, CA. (1996) Photocarcinogenesis: mechanisms, models and human health implications. *Photochemistry and Photobiology*, Vol. 63, pp. 355–447, ISSN 0031-8655

Murakami, A., Ashida, H., & Terao, J. (2008) Multitargeted cancer prevention by quercetin. *Cancer Letters*, Vol. 269, No. 2, pp. 315-325, ISSN 0304-3835

Nichols, JA., & Katiyar, SK. (2010) Skin photoprotection by natural polyphenols: anti-inflammatory, antioxidant and DNA repair mechanisms. Archives of *Dermatological Research*, Vol. 302, No. 2, pp. 71-83, ISSN 0340-3696

Nomura,M., Kaji, A., Ma, W., Miyamoto, K., & Dong, Z. (2001) Suppression of cell transformation and induction of apoptosis by caffeic acid phenethyl ester. *Molecular Carcinogenesis*, Vol. 31, No. 2, pp. 83-99, ISSN 0899-1987

Omenn, GS., Goodman, GE., Thornquist, MD., Balmes, J., Cullen, MR., Glass, A., Keogh, JP., Meyskens, FL., Valanis, B., Williams, JH., Barnhart, S., & Hammar, S. (1996) Effects of a combination of beta carotene and vitamin A on lung cancer and cardiovascular disease. *New England Journal of Medicine*, Vol. 334, No. 18, pp.1150-1155, ISSN 0028-4793

Pan, MH., & Ho, CT. (2008) Chemopreventive effects of natural dietary compounds on cancer development. *Chemical Society Reviews*, Vol. 37, No. 11, pp. 2558-2574, ISSN 0306-0012

Park, KK., Chun, KS., Lee, JM., Lee, SS., & Surh, YJ. (1998) Inhibitory effects of [6]-gingerol, a major pungent principle of ginger, on phorbol ester-induced inflammation, epidermal ornithine decarboxylase activity and skin tumor promotion in ICR mice. *Cancer Letters*, Vol. 129, No. 2, pp. 139-144, ISSN 0304-3835

Park, KK., Chun, KS., Yook, JI., & Surh, YJ. (1998) Lack of tumor promoting activity of capsaicin, a principal pungent ingredient of red pepper, in mouse skin carcinogenesis. *AntiCancer Research*, Vol. 18, No. 6A, pp. 4201-4205, ISSN 0250-7005

Patel, PS., Varney, ML., Dave, BJ., & Singh, RK. (2002) Regulation of constitutive and induced NF-kappaB activation in malignant melanoma cells by capsaicin modulates interleukin-8 production and cell proliferation. *Journal of Interferon and Cytokine Research*, Vol. 22, No. 4, pp. 427-435, ISSN 1079-9907

Pianetti, S., Guo, S., Kavanagh, KT., Sonenshein, GE. (2002) Green tea polyphenol epigallocatechin-3 gallate inhibits Her-2/neu signaling, proliferation, and transformed phenotype of breast cancer cells. *Cancer Research*, Vol.62, No. 3, pp. 652-655, ISSN 0008-5472

Ravanat, JL., Douki, T., & Cadet, J. (2001) Direct and indirect effects of UV radiation on DNA and its components. *Journal of Photochemistry and Photobiology B*, Vol. 63, No. 1-3, pp. 88-102, ISSN 1011-1344

Saunders, FR., & Wallace, HM. (2010) On the natural chemoprevention of cancer. *Plant Physiology and Biochemistry*, Vol. 48, No. 7, pp. 621-626, ISSN 0981-9428

Schmidt, B., Ribnicky, DM., Poulev, A., Logendra, S., Cefalu, WT., & Raskin, I. (2008) A natural history of botanical therapeutics. *Metabolism*, Vol.57, No. 7 Suppl 1, pp. S3-9, ISSN 0026-0495

Singh, RP., & Agarwal, R. (2002) Flavonoid antioxidant silymarin and skin cancer. *Antioxidants & Redox Signaling*, Vol. 4, No. 4, pp. 655-663, ISSN 1523-0864

Singh, RP., Tyagi, AK., Zhao, J., & Agarwal, R. (2002) Silymarin inhibits growth and causes regression of established skin tumors in SENCAR mice via modulation of mitogen-activated protein kinases and induction of apoptosis. *Carcinogenesis*, Vol. 23, No. 3, pp. 499-510, ISSN 0143-3334

Steinmetz, KA., & Potter, JD. (1996) Vegetables, fruit, and cancer prevention: a review. *Journal of the American Dietetic Association*, Vol. 96, No. 10, pp. 1027-1039, ISSN 0002-8223

Steerenberg, PA., Garssen, J., Dortant, PM., van der Vliet, H., Geerse, E., Verlaan, AP., Goettsch, WG., Sontag, Y., Bueno-de-Mesquita, HB., Van Loveren, H. (1997) The effect of oral quercetin on UVB-induced tumor growth and local immunosuppression in SKH-1. *Cancer Letters*, Vol. 114, No. 1-2, pp. 187-189, ISSN 0304-3835

Surh, YJ. (2003) Cancer chemoprevention with dietary phytochemicals. *Nature Reviews Cancer*, Vol. 3, No. 10, pp. 768-780, ISSN 1474-175X

Svobodová, A., Psotová, J., & Walterová, D. (2003) Natural phenolics in the prevention of UV-induced skin damage. A review. *Biomedical Papers-Olomouc*, Vol. 147, No. 2, pp. 137-145, ISSN 1213-8118

Tornaletti, S., & Hanawalt, PC. (1999) Effect of DNA lesions on transcription elongation. *Biochimie*, Vol. 81, No. 1-2, pp. 139-146, ISSN 0300-9084

Tyrrell, RM. (1994) The molecular and cellular pathology of solar ultraviolet radiation. *Molecular Aspects of Medicine*, Vol. 15, No. 1, pp. 1-77, ISSN 0098-2997

Wan, YS., Wang, ZQ., Shao, Y., Voorhees, JJ., & Fisher, GJ. (2001) Ultraviolet irradiation activates PI 3-kinase/AKT survival pathway via EGF receptors in human skin in vivo. *International Journal of Oncology*, Vol. 18, No. 3, pp. 461-466, ISSN 1019-6439

Wang, Y., Zhang, X., Lebwohl, M., DeLeo, V., & Wei, H. (1998) Inhibition of ultraviolet B (UVB)-induced c-fos and c-jun expression in vivo by a tyrosine kinase inhibitor genistein. *Carcinogenesis*, Vol. 19, No. 4, pp. 649-654, ISSN 0143-3334

Wattenberg, LW. (1985) Chemoprevention of cancer. *Cancer Research*, Vol. 45, No. 1, pp. 1-8, ISSN 0008-5472

Wei, H., Bowen, R., Zhang, X., Lebwohl, M. (1998) Isoflavone genistein inhibits the initiation and promotion of two-stage skin carcinogenesis in mice. *Carcinogenesis*, Vol. 19, No. 8, pp. 1509-1514, ISSN 0143-3334

Yu, R., Hebbar, V., Kim, DW., Mandlekar, S., Pezzuto, JM., Kong, AN. (2001) Resveratrol inhibits phorbol ester and UV-induced activator protein 1 activation by interfering with mitogen-activated protein kinase pathways. *Molecular Pharmacology*, Vol. 60, No. 1, pp. 217-224, ISSN ISSN 0026-895X

Zhang, W., Remenyik, E., Zelterman, D., Brash, DE., & Wikonkal, NM. (2001) Escaping the stem cell compartment: sustained UVB exposure allows p53-mutant keratinocytes to colonize adjacent epidermal proliferating units without incurring additional mutations. *Proceedings of the National Academy of Sciences of the United States of America*, Vol. 98, No. 24, pp. 13948-13953, ISSN 0027-8424

Zoumpourlis, V., Solakidi, S., Papathoma, A., & Papaevangeliou, D. (2003) Alterations in signal transduction pathways implicated in tumour progression during multistage mouse skin carcinogenesis. *Carcinogenesis*, Vol. 24, No. 7, pp. 1159-1165, ISSN 0143-3334

9

Bioactive Food Components for Melanoma: An Overview

Imtiaz A. Siddiqui[1], Rohinton S. Tarapore[2], Jean Christopher Chamcheu[1] and Hasan Mukhtar[1]
[1]*Department of Dermatology, School of Medicine and Public Health, University of Wisconsin, Madison, WI*
[2]*Gastroenterology Division, University of Pennsylvania School of Medicine, Philadelphia, PA*
USA

1. Introduction

The skin being the largest organ in the body accounts for the most common cancer in humans. Skin cancer is typically of three types, basal cell carcinoma (BCC), squamous cell carcinoma (SCC) and melanoma. Despite accounting for only 4% of all cases, melanoma is the most deadly skin cancer, resulting in over 79% of skin cancer related deaths [1, 2]. In the year 2011 in the United States melanoma is thought to cause 70,230 cases (40,010 in men and 30,220 in women) with 8,790 deaths (5,750 in men and 3,040 in women) associated with the disease [3]. The median age at diagnosis is between 45 and 55, although 25% of cases occur in individuals before age 40. It is the second most common cancer in women between the ages of 20 and 35, and the leading cause of cancer death in women ages 25 to 30.

There are multiple risk factors that contribute to the escalating incidences of melanomas in humans (Table 1). Among all, ultraviolet (UV)-radiation emitted from the sun is the main contributing factor towards the development of melanomas. It is well documented that UV-radiation is absorbed by the chromophores such as DNA, RNA, protein and melanin in the skin [4]. This UV absorption in the skin results in different photochemical reactions and the secondary interactions involving ROS (reactive oxygen species) result in damaging effects. UV irradiation of the skin causes erythema, edema, hyperplasia, hyperpigmentation, sunburn cells, immunosuppression, photoaging and photocarcinogenesis [5, 6]. UV irradiation to skin also has direct effects on biomolecules such as formation of cyclobutane pyrimidine dimers (CPDs), 8-hydroxy-2'-deoxyguanosine (8-OHdG), protein oxidation and generation of ROS [4, 7, 8].

Over the years, changes in lifestyle patterns have led to a significant increase in the amount of UV radiation that people receive, leading to a surge in the incidence of skin cancer and photoaging. Since these trends are likely to continue in the foreseeable future, the adverse effects of ultraviolet radiation have become a major human concern. One way of combating against the melanomas is through "chemoprevention" which is defined as the use of natural or synthetic agents to reverse, suppress or prevent premalignant lesions from progressing to invasive cancers. Chemoprevention broadly is divided into 3 categories: (i) *primary-* preventing initial cancer in high risk individuals; (ii) *secondary-* preventing cancers in those with premalignant conditions; and (iii) *tertiary-* preventing second cancers in patients cured or an initial cancer [9, 10].

Ultraviolet (UV) radiation	
	UVA
	UVB
Genetic syndromes	
	Xeroderma pigmentosum
	Oculocutaneous albinism
	Basal cell nevus syndrome
Ionizing radiation	
	X-rays
Other risk factors	
	Artificial UV radiation (tanning)
	Skin color (having fair skin, especially with blue or hazel eyes)
	History of lesions
	Chronically injured or non-healing wounds
	Working outdoors
	Increasing age

Table 1. Risk factors for melanomas [Reviewed in [136-142]]

In recent years, natural agents have gained considerable attention because of their skin photoprotective effects [11, 12]. Nutritional agents with potential antioxidant, anti-inflammatory, anti-mutagenic and anti-carcinogenic properties, and that have the ability to exert striking inhibitory effects on diverse cellular and molecular events are gaining considerable attention for the prevention of UV-induced skin damage [11-13]. Botanical anti-oxidants have also been shown to reduce the incidence of ROS-mediated photocarcinogenic and photoaging. This has generated a great interest in using botanical supplements rich in anti-oxidants to delay photocarcinogenesis and prevent photoaging. This chapter presents an overview of selected few botanical agents and their protective properties of the skin against melanoma.

2. Tea polyphenols

Tea, derived from the plant *Camellia sinensis*, is the most popular beverage consumed by two-thirds of the world's population. It is processed in different ways in different parts of the world to give green, black or oolong tea. "Black tea" is fully fermented, "oolong tea" is partially fermented and "green tea" is strained and not fermented. For the preparation of green tea, the young leaves are steamed to inactivate the enzymes thereby preserving as much as 90% of the polyphenols contained in fresh leaves from being degraded [14].

The most studied formulation of tea is the green tea. Green tea contains characteristic polyphenolic conpounds, (-)-epigallocatechin-3-gallate (EGCG), (-)-epicatechin-3-gallate (ECG) and (-)-epicatechin (EC). A typical tea beverage (1 g leaf per 200 mL water in a 3 minute brew) usually contains 250-300 mg tea solids comprised of 30-40% catechins and 3-

6% caffeine [14]. Green tea is considered a dietary source of anti-oxidants nutrients like polyphenols (catechin and gallic acid), carotenoids, tocopherols, ascorbic acid and certain phytochemical compounds. They may also function indirectly as anti-oxidants through inhibition of the redox-sensitive transcription factors, inhibition of pro-oxidant enzymes, such as inducible nitric oxide synthase, lipoxygenases, cyclooxygenases, and xanthine oxidase and induction of anti-oxidant enzymes, such as glutathione-S-transferases and superoxide dismutases [15].

The activity of tea polyphenols on the inhibition of skin tumorigenesis has been studied in depth. Studies have shown that green tea polyphenols (GTP) have a significant inhibitory effect on tumor induction in a chemically induced initiation-promotion mouse model [16]. EGCG significantly inhibited the binding of ^{3}H-labelled polycyclic aromatic hydrocarbons to epidermal DNA. Topical application of EGCG resulted in significant inhibition in TPA-mediated induction of epidermal ornithine decarboxylase (ODC) activity. The application of EGCG before challenge with DMBA also resulted in significant inhibition both in percentage of mice with tumors and the number of tumors per mouse compared with non-EGCG-pretreated mice [17].

Oral consumption or topical application of brewed green tea or green tea extracts showed meaningful protection against ultraviolet or chemically induced carcinogenesis in mice. Oral consumption of brewed green tea at concentrations similar to human consumption (1.5-2.5%) significantly inhibited UVB or TPA-induced tumorigenesis [18, 19]. Mechanistically, oral consumption of GTP resulted in decreased UVB-induced ODC and carboxylase (COX) activities [20]. Oral administration or intra-peritoneal injection of GTP achieved similar effects to inhibit the growth of UV-induced skin papillomas [18] or TPA-induced COX2 in rodent models [21]. EGCG treatment was found to result in a dose-dependent decrease in the viability and growth of A-375 amelanotic malignant melanoma and Hs-294T metastatic melanoma cell lines [22]. Oral administration of GTP was found to reduce UVB-induced tumor incidence, tumor multiplicity and growth in SKH-1 mice. Reduced expression of matrix metalloproteinase (MMP)-2 and MMP-9, vascular endothelial growth factor (VEGF) and proliferating cell nuclear antigen (PCNA) was also observed [23]. Furthermore, oral administration of green tea to UV-pretreated high risk mice for 23 weeks inhibited skin tumorigenesis [24]. Pretreatment of SKH-1 hairless mice with green tea for 2 weeks enhances UV-induced increase in epidermal p53, p21 (WAF1/CIP1) and apoptotic sunburns in the epidermis [25]. Furthermore, mice treated with green tea during chronic UVB irradiation changed the mutation profile of the p53 gene in early mutant p53 positive epidermal patches [26].

3. Curcumin

Curcumin (diferuloylmethane) is a yellow substance extracted from the root of the turmeric plant *Curcuma longa* which belongs to the *Zingiberaceae* family. Curcumin has been used for centuries in indigenous medicine for the treatment of a variety of inflammatory and other diseases, and was shown for the first time in 1988, to have antimutagenic activity using the Ames *Salmonella* test [27]. It has a wide range of pharmacological activities including anti-inflammatory, anti-cancer, anti-oxidant, wound healing and anti-microbial effects [28], as well as several documented clinical applications referenced to its anti-inflammatory and anti-oxidant properties. Curcumin is also a potent scavenger of a variety of reactive oxygen species (ROS) such as superoxide anion radicals, hydroxyl radicals, and nitrogen dioxide

radicals. The molecular basis of anti-carcinogenic and chemopreventive effects of curcumin is attributed to its effect on several targets including transcription factors, growth regulators, adhesion molecules, apoptotic genes, angiogenesis regulators and other cellular signaling molecules [29]. Curcumin is able to block multiple targets conferring protective effects against oxidative stress and inflammation and has proven useful in photoaging skin and photocarcinogenesis [30]. It was shown to induce apoptosis and cell cycle arrest in melanoma cells, associated with down-regulation of iNOS, the catalytic subunit of DNA-dependent protein kinase, and up-regulation of p53, p21(CIP1), p27(KIP1) and Chk-2 [31] and its apoptosis inducible ability has also been associated to the Fas receptor/caspase-8 pathway, independent of p53. It has been shown to down regulate the production of pro-inflammatory cytokines such as tumor necrosis factor-α (TNF-α) and IL-1β, and to inhibit the activation of transcription factors NF-κB, and activator protein-1 (AP-1), which regulate the genes for pro-inflammatory mediators and protective anti-oxidant genes [32].
Curcumin also suppresses the apoptotic inhibitor XIAP, decreases NF-κB downstream target genes such as COX-2 and cyclin D1 expression and blocks it cell survival pathway and selectively induced apoptosis in melanoma cells but not in normal melanocytes [33, 34]. It was shown to inhibit proteasomal activity, inhibit Ca^{2+}-adenosine triphosphatase (ATP) pump leading to accumulation of cytosolic calcium which then activates caspases, cleave p23 and downregulate the antiapoptotic Mcl-1 protein and thus inducing ER stress in melanoma cells [35]. The antiproliferative and proapoptotic effects induced by curcumin are shown to be independent of the B-Raf/ERK MAPK and the AKT pathway [36]. In spite the proapoptotic effects, curcumin has reportedly been associated with the inhibition of the ability of IFN-alpha, IFN-gamma, and IL-2 to phosphorylate STAT1 and STAT5 proteins [37], suggesting the possibility of it to adversely affect immune effector cells responses to clinically relevant cytokines with antitumor properties [36].
Moreover, curcumin was also reported to cause cell death in 8 melanoma cell lines, four with wild type and four with mutant p53. In highly metastatic murine melanoma cells B16F10 as well as other cells, it significantly inhibited the activity of MMP2 , collagenase and focal adhesion kinase (FAK), important components of the intracellular signaling pathway, meanwhile it enhanced the expression of anti-metastatic proteins such as tissue inhibitor metalloproteinase-2, nonmetastatic gene 23, and E-cadherin [38, 39]. Curcumin-treated B16F10 cells formed eight fold fewer lung metastasis in C57Black 6 mice [39], and showed a dose dependent reduction in their binding affinity to extracellular matrix (ECM) protein including fibronectin, vitronectin and collage IV and a reduced α5β1 and α5β3 integrin receptors expression in the cell adhesion assays. In stimulated melanoma cells, curcumin has been shown to suppress melanogenesis by down regulating melanogenesis related proteins such as MITF, tyrosinase and tyrosinase-related proteins 1 and 2 [40]. Interestingly, its antimetastatic effects has been linked to the modulation of the expression of integrin receptors, collagenase activity, tissue inhibitor metalloproteinase (TIMP)-2, nonmetastatic gene 23 (Nm23) and E-cadherin [38], [39].
In resistant cases, a two hit combination of curcumin and other factors has been shown to enhance curcumin induced effects on melanoma cells in cell culture models. Small inhibitory RNA silencing of ABCA1 gene was shown to sensitize melanoma cells to the apoptotic effect of curcumin most likely due to a reduced basal levels of active NFκB as well as a reduction of P65 expression [41]. Moreover, C6 ceramide was shown to sensitize melanoma cells to curcumin-induced cell death and apoptosis by partially increasing the

intrinsic apoptotic pathway [42]. More recently, it has been shown that a combination of curcumin and tamoxifen concomitantly induced apoptosis and autophagy in melanoma cells without affecting non-cancerous cells [43].

Recent advances in view of selecting new antitumor agents with more potent and selective growth inhibitory activity has revolutionized the synthesis and testing of several analogous "curcumin-like" compounds. For instance the compound α,β-unsaturated ketone D6 was shown to be more effective in inhibiting melanoma growth when compared to curcumin [44]. Synthetic curcuminoid derivatives have been analyzed *in vivo* to test their inhibitory role to tumor-specific angiogenesis such that in mice injected with melanoma cells an intraperitoneal administration of tetrahydro curcumin, salicyl curcumin and curcumin III reduced the number of induced tumor-directed capillaries. Moreover, these curcuminoids have been shown to reduce serum Nitric Oxide (NO) and tumor-necrosis factor (TNF)-α levels in treated animals, perhaps by decreasing the production by activated macrophages [45]. A small molecule FLLL32, an analog of curcumin and STAT3-specific inhibitor for melanoma therapy was shown to induce caspase-dependent apoptosis in cells through reduced STAT3 phosphorylation and retained the cellular response to cytokines with antitumor activity, and most remarkably did not reduce the function or viability of normal donor immune cells. FLLL32 has also been shown to inhibit IL-6-induced STAT3 phosphorylation without reducing signaling due to IFN-γ and IL-2 [37, 46].

Despite the highly recognized chemotherapeutic potential of curcumin, its poor solubility to water and fast degradation has significantly hindered its clinical application. However, amphiphilic block copolymer micelles of poly(ethylene oxide)-b-poly(epsilon-caprolactone) used as solubilization and stabilization vehicles, were able to effectively solubilize curcumin, protect the degradation of encapsulated curcumin and control it release over several days [47]. A combination of curcumin and catechin was shown to inhibit the melanoma cell invasion by inhibiting MMPs, thus inhibiting lung metastasis [48]. Curcumin also was shown to inhibit the phosphorylation of Src kinase and STAT3 partly by downregulating PRL-3 and preventing melanoma cells from invading the draining lymph nodes [49]. In Mice, curcumin was reported to decrease the induction of epidermal ODC activity, epidermal cyclooxygenase and lipoxygenase enzyme levels, epidermal glutathione content, oxidation of DNA bases, and the number of tumors per mouse and tumor volume per mouse. Topical application of curcumin together with TPA was shown to induce epidermal hyperplasia and *c-Jun* and *c-Fos* expression in CD-1 mice [50]. Curcumin treatment successfully reduced the number and volume of tumors when given in diet to animals in which skin tumors had been inhibited with DMBA and promoted with TPA. The dietary consumption of curcumin resulted in decreased expression of proto-oncogenes, *ras* and *fos*, in the skin tissue [51, 52]. Topical application of curcumin together with TPA twice weekly for 18 weeks markedly inhibited TPA-induced tumor promotion [53]. Topical application on the dorsal side of the skin with curcumin before TPA exposure inhibited TPA-induced expression of c-fos, c-jun and c-myc [54]. Currently, several clinical trials are investigating the effect of curcumin in diverse cancerous and non-cancerous conditions but without any of them evaluating its effects against melanoma in human populations.

4. Genistein

Genistein (4', 5, 7-trihydroxyisoflavone) is a widely distributed isoflavone primarily present in soy, *Ginkgo biloba* extract, oregano and sage [55, 56]. It was first isolated from soybean in

1931 [57]. Increasing incidence has accumulated that genistein shows preventive and therapeutic use for cancers, osteoporosis and cardiovascular disease in both humans and animals. Genistein is a potent inhibitor of cytochrome P450-medicated activation of benz-a-pyrene [58]. In an *in vitro* setting, genistein inhibits the activities of tyrosine protein kinase, topoisomerase II and ribosomal S6 kinase [59, 60]. Genistein has been reported to inhibit the growth of ras-transfected NIH3T3 cells without affecting the growth of normal cells [61]. Genistein can modulate the inflammatory responses that are commonly involved in the promotional stage of carcinogenesis [62]. It displays many anticancer properties which includes suppressing the growth of a variety of human gastrointestinal cancer cell lines, induction of differentiation of leukemia cells, and inhibition of endothelial cell angiogenesis relevant to tumor metastasis [63].

Genistein treatment in human NCTC 2544 keratinocytes prevented UV-induced enhancement of STAT1 (signal transducer and activator 1) thereby limiting lipid peroxidation [64]. Genistein inhibited UV-induced DNA damage as evaluated with the formation of pyrimidine dimers [65]. A dose-dependent inhibition of UVB-induced pyrimidine dimer formation was observed relative to increasing genistein concentrations [65]. Genistein substantially inhibits skin carcinogenesis and cutaneous aging induced by UV in mice and photodamage in humans [66]. Topical application of genistein before UVB radiation reduced the expression of c-fos and c-jun in the SENCAR mouse skin in a dose dependent manner [67]. Two promotion studies using DMBA and TPA protocol were conducted using CD-1 and SENCAR mice. Both these studies consistently showed that genistein substantially inhibited TPA-promoted skin tumorigenesis by reducing the tumor multiplicity. Genistein also inhibited DMBA-induced bulky DNA adduct formation and substantially suppressed TPA-stimulated H_2O_2 inflammatory responses and ODC activity in mouse skin [68].

5. Fisetin

Fisetin (3,7,3′,4′-tetrahydroxyflavone) is a flavonol, a structurally distinct chemical substance that belongs to the flavonoid group of polyphenols together with quercetin, myricetin and kaempferol with a chemical formula described earlier by the Austrian chemist Josef Herzig in 1891. It can be found in various plants, fruits and vegetables including apples, onions, persimmons and strawberries, where it functions as coloring agent [69], and was originally identified as an oxidative stress-induced nerve cell death inhibiting compound [70]. It has also been shown to possess neurotropic effects, promoting nerve cell differentiation and to enhance learning and memory in mice upon oral administration [71, 72]. In addition to its direct antioxidant and anti-inflammatory activities, fisetin can increase the intracellular levels of glutathione, and can as well reduce the production of lipid peroxides and their pro-inflammatory by products [73]. In addition to its neuroprotective and anti-ageing effects, recent data suggests that fisetin possess anticancer properties, and have been shown to induce apoptosis in diverse cancer cell lines [73]. A more recent report showed that fisetin treatment of human melanoma cells resulted in decreased cell viability and disruption of Wnt/β-catenin signaling associated with reduction of Wnt protein and its co-receptors expression, parallel by an increase expression of two endogenous Wnt inhibitor proteins, increased cytosolic levels of Axin and β-TrCP and decreased phosphorylation of GSK3-β [74]. An intraperitoneal administration of fisetin to mice was shown to significantly inhibit human melanoma tumor development and suggested that this "nontargeted therapies" is promising to be effectively developed as a therapy armamater against melanoma since targeted therapies do not targ*et all* of the pathways required for melanoma growth [74].

6. Resveratrol

Resveratrol (3,5,4'-trihydroxystilbene), a polyphenolic flavonoid belonging to the stilbene family of phytoalexins, is found in grapes, nuts, berries and red wine. Resveratrol has been reported to exhibit a wide range of biological and pharmacological properties. Several plants including grapevine synthesize resveratrol when attacked by fungal pathogens [75]. Epidemiological studies indicate that the French have relatively lower risk of cardiovascular disease despite consuming a diet rich in fat. In reality, the high concentration of resveratrol in red wine consumed by the French is frequently cited to account for the "French Paradox" [5]. There have been extensive studies demonstrating that resveratrol possesses an ability to intervene in multistep carcinogenesis. In addition, resveratrol may be beneficial in the control of artherosclerosis, heart disease, arthritis or autoimmune disease. According to a study by Pezzerto *et al.* [76] resveratrol significantly reduced the number of tumors per mouse in a two-stage skin carcinogenesis model. In the *in vivo* assay, resveratrol offered a 60% reduction in DMBA and TPA-induced skin papillomas in mouse at 20 weeks [77]. Single topical application of resveratrol to SKH-1 hairless mice resulted in significant inhibition of UVB-mediated increase in skin edema. Resveratrol treatment to mouse skin also resulted in significant inhibition of UVB-mediated induction of COX and decreased ODC activity. It was also observed that resveratrol inhibited UVB-mediated increased level of lipid peroxidation which is a biomarker of oxidative stress [78]. Further, topical application of resveratrol to SKH-1 hairless mouse skin prior to UVB-radiation resulted in the inhibition of UVB-induced cellular proliferation, phosphorylation of surviving and upregulation of apoptotic factors (Smac and Diablo). The anti-proliferative effects of resveratrol might be mediated via modulation in the expression and function of cell cycle regulatory proteins like cyclin D1 and D2, cdk 2, 4, 6 and p21 and maybe associated with the inhibition of the MAPK pathway [79]. In normal human epidermal keratinocytes, resveratrol blocked UVB-mediated activation of NF-κB in a dose- and time- dependent fashion. Resveratrol treatment in these cells also inhibited UVB-mediated phosphorylation and degradation of IKBα and activation of IKKα [80]. Studies have demonstrated that topical application of resveratrol resulted in the inhibition of UVB-induced tumor incidence and a delay in the onset of skin tumorigenesis [81].

7. Pomegranate

The pomegranate (*Punica granatum*) fruit has been used for centuries in ancient cultures for its medicinal purposes. Pomegranate is a rich source of two types of phenolic compounds: anthocyanins (delphinidn-3-glycoside, delphinidin-3,5-diglycoside, pelargonidin-3-glycoside, pelargonidin-3,5-diglycoside, cyanidin-3-glycoside, cyanidin-3,5-diglycoside) and hydrolysable tannins. The other flavonoids present in pomegranate are quercetin, kaempherol and luteolin glycosides [82]. Pomegranate possesses strong anti-oxidant, anti-inflammatory and anti-cancer properties [58, 83]. Pomegranate juice shows potent anti-oxidant propterties that can be attributed to its high content of polyphenols (ellagic acid, EA), anthocyanins and other flavonoids [83].

Studies have demonstrated that treatment of NHEK with pomegranate fruit extract (PFE) prior to UVB-exposure inhibited UVB-mediated phosphorylation of ERK1/2, JNK1/2 and p38 proteins in a dose- and time- dependent manner [84]. The treatment also resulted in inhibition of UVB-mediated degradation and phosphorylation of IκBα, activation of IKK, nuclear translocation and phosphorylation of NF-κB/p65 at Ser 536 [84]. Another study has reported that PFE treatment of NHEK inhibited UVA-mediated phosphorylation of STAT-3, AKT and ERK1/2 [85]. Topical application of PFE resulted in inhibition of TPA-induced tumor promotion in DMBA-initiated CD-1 mice. Mice pretreated with PFE showed reduced tumor incidence and lower tumor burden when compared to mice that did not receive PFE [86]. Treatment of HaCaT cells with PFE prior to UVB-exposure protected cells from UVB mediated decrease in cell viability, inhibited UVB-mediated decrease in endogenous glutathione levels, lipid peroxidation and expression of MMP-2 & MMP-9 [87].

Delphinidin, a major anthocyanin present in pomegranate, protected NHEK from UVB-mediated decrease in cell death [88]. The study reported an induction of apoptosis, a decrease in PCNA, activation of caspases and an increase in PARP expression [88]. Topical application of delphinidin to SKH-1 hairless mice inhibited UVB-mediated apoptosis and markers of DNA damage such as CPDs and 8-OHdG. Oral feeding of PFE to SKH-1 mice inhibited single UVB exposure mediated epidermal hyperplasia, infiltration of leucocytes, generation of hydrogen peroxide and lipid peroxidation [89]. PFE consumption further protects mouse skin against the adverse effects of UVB radiation by modulating UVB-induced signaling pathways such as NF-κB, MAPKs, c-Jun [86]. Topical and oral administration of pomegranate to humans was shown to augment the protective effects of sunscreens and afforded protection from UVB. A double blind, placebo-controlled clinical trial indicated that oral intake of PFE inhibited UV-induced pigmentation in the human skin [90].

8. Lupeol

Lupeol, a triterpene found in fruits such as olives, mango, strawberry, grapes, figs and in medicinal plants like ginseng, shea butter plant, *Tamarindus indica, Bombax ceiba* [91] and has been used by native people in North America, Latin America, Japan, China, Africa and the Caribbean islands [92-97]. Lupeol has been demonstrated to inhibit various pharmacological activities under *in vitro* and *in vivo* conditions. These include its beneficial activity against inflammation, cancer, arthritis, diabetes, heart disease, renal- and hepatic toxicity [94, 98-107]. Topical application of lupeol alleviated TPA-induced inflammation in the ear mouse model [98] and decreased the expression of myeloperoxidase, a neutrophil specific marker, resulting in reduced infiltration into inflamed tissues [98]. Lupeol was found to reduce infiltration in mouse model of arthritis, an inflammation associated disease [108]. This beneficial effect was shown to be associated with the potential of lupeol to modulate the immune system. Lupeol was reported to suppress CD4+ and CD8+ T cell counts resulting in reduced cytokine expression (IL-2, IL-4,IFN-gamma) [109].

Epidemiological data suggests that the content of phytosterols (like lupeol) in the diet is associated with a reduction in common cancers including cancer of breast, prostate and colon [110, 111]. Tumorigenic animal models suggest that phytosterols modulate host systems potentially enabling more robust anti-tumor responses such as enhancing immune recognition of tumor cells, altering hormone-dependent growth of endocrine tumors, and modulating sterol biosynthesis [91, 111]. Mutation that occurs through DNA strand breaks have been shown to form the precursor of cancer development [112-115]. An accumulation of these mutations transform neoplastic cells into malignant carcinomas. Lupeol was reported to exhibit strong anti-mutagenic activity under *in vitro* and *in vivo* systems [102, 116]. A study demonstrated that topical application of lupeol prevents DMBA-induced DNA strand breaks in murine skin [102]. Recently, lupeol was shown to inhibit benz-a-pyrene induced genotoxicity in mouse models [117].

There is increasing evidence that lupel inhibits tumor promotion in two stage skin carcinogenesis in mouse model [103]. Topical application of lupeol for 28 weeks was shown to significantly decrease tumor burden and tumor multiplicity [103]. The anti-tumor effects were observed to be associated with the potential of lupeol to modulate signaling pathways like NF-κB and phosphatidylinositol-3-kinase (PI3K)/Akt, that play an important role in tumorigenesis [103]. Lupeol was shown to significantly inhibit NF-ΚB translocation to the nucleus and its DNA-binding activity in a mouse model of skin tumorigenesis [103]. Lupeol was also observed to inhibit ODC activity, an important biomarker of tumor promotion [103, 118]. Lupeol was also shown to inhibit growth of highly metastatic tumors of human melanoma origin by modulating the expression of BCl-2 and Bax proteins [104]. A recent study demonstrated that lupeol significantly inhibits the growth of metastatic melanoma cells that harbor constitutive activation of Wnt/β-catenin signaling [119].

9. Silymarin

Silymarin refers to three mixtures of flavonoids including silybin, silydianin and silychristin, a flavanolignan, isolated from the fruits and seeds of the plant milk thistle (*Silybum marianum* L. Gaertn.) which are protective against photocarcinogenesis. Mouse models studies elucidated that silymarin possess antioxidant, anti-inflammatory and immunomodulatory properties responsible for its efficacy against photocarcinogenesis [120, 121]. Using UV-irradiated human melanoma cells silymarin was shown to protect against UV-induced apoptosis as well as modulation of the cell cycle with increase in the G2/M phase [120]. Silymarin's potential to reduce UV-induced apoptosis is partially through activation of human deacetylase SIRT1 as well as by activation of the AKT and MAPK pathways [122]. An unclear knowledge of whether the protective effects of silymarin in melanoma cells is beneficial to melanoma prevention still lingers, but it was shown to enhanced the cytotoxic effect of anti-Fas agonistic antibody on human melanoma cells [123]. A more recent report showed that silybinin, a major active constituent of silymarin, prevented mitomycin C-induced apoptosis in human melanoma cells through suppression of the mitochondria-mediated intrinsic but not the extrinsic apoptosis pathway [124]. However, further studies are required to delineate the role of silymarin in the prevention of melanoma carcinogenesis.

10. Other multifaceted food bioactive agents

It has become clear that plants and phytosynthetic agents possess a broad spectrum of targeted and non-targeted potential drug compounds for cancer prevention and therapy. The anticancer properties of other fruits and vegetables are partly related to their isoprenoid constituents. A report showed that isoprenoids extracted from different plants possesses variable degrees of potency in suppressing the growth and proliferation of melanoma and other cancer cells [125]. Perillyl alcohol, derived from essential oils of lavendin, peppermint and other diverse plants, is known to inhibit melanoma cell growth [125], but only few reports examined their efficacy in melanoma in situ. In a recent report topical perillyl alcohol was demonstrated to delay melanoma tumors appearance in TPras transgenic mice [126]. However, only a modest protective effect was detected in sun-burned skin subjects in a double-blind, randomized, phase II trial of topical perillyl alcohol possibly as a result of inadequate delivery through the epidermis [127].

Other bioactive agents such as garlic extract [128], exo-biopolymer from rice bran [129], and isothiocyanates extract of wasabi [130], as well as flavonoids such as hesperitin, naringenin [131] and chrysin derived from acacia honey [132] have been evaluated for their cytotoxic effect on melanoma cells. A limited number of studies have been effectuated on these compounds with several of them appearing as potential agents against melanoma, but the exact knowledge regarding their active excipient as well as their mechanistic potentials requires extensive *in vitro* cell culture and *in vivo* animal model studies to elucidate.

11. Nanotechnology for melanoma

There are several issues in the effective prevention and therapy of melanoma which include development of novel agents, determination of optimal therapeutic combinations and effective delivery of agents to the tumor. The optimal agent delivery, which is the most important issue, is essential to improve drug concentrations, reduce side effects, and lower effective doses for better efficacy of the agents. We recently employed the use of nanotechnology to improve the outcome of chemopreventive intervention and coined the term 'nanochemoprevention' [119]. Utilization of nanotechnology for the development of efficient anticancer drug delivery system is one of the most recent advancement in medical science. The structure and tunable surface functionality of nanoparticulate system allows it to encapsulate/conjugate single or multiple entities either in the core or on the surface, rendering them ideal carriers for various anticancer drugs. Further, most drugs have poor solubility and low bioavailability, and are formulated with undesirable solvents, and, the use of nanocarriers, allows for the preparation of low water soluble cancer medications as solid or liquid formulations.

For melanoma research, utilization of nanotechnology is a relatively new and rapidly developing field with constant research going on all around the world. So far no natural agents have been nanoformulated but constant work is going on and nanotechnology is being actively utilized in melanoma research. In one of the first study in the field, Banciu *et al.* [133] evaluated the inhibitory effects of glucocorticoids (GC) encapsulated in long-circulating liposomes (LCL-PLP) (LCL-GC). The effects of all LCL-GC on the production of angiogenic/inflammatory factors *in vivo* in the B16.F10 murine melanoma model as well as on the viability and proliferation of tumor cells and endothelial cells *in vitro* were investigated. The results showed that all four selected LCL-GC formulations inhibit tumor growth, albeit to different degrees. The differences in antitumor activity of LCL-GC correlate with their efficacy to suppress tumor angiogenesis and inflammation. The *in vitro* results presented suggested that LCL-BUP has strong cytotoxic effects on B16.F10 melanoma cells and the anti-proliferative effects of all LCL-GC towards angiogenic endothelial cells play a role in their antitumor activity.

Tran *et al.* [134] discussed some promising new nanotechnology based therapies under development for the treatment of melanoma. This article summarized the utilization of liposomes for effective therapy of melanoma. A recent study demonstrated that the delivery of doxorubicin using a nanotechnology-based platform significantly reduces the systemic toxicity of the drug, keeping unchanged its therapeutic efficacy in a mouse melanoma tumor model. Single-walled carbon nanotubes were used to conjugate a doxorubicin prodrug. The CNT-doxorubicin conjugate (CNT-Dox) induced time-dependent cell death in B16-F10 melanoma cells *in vitro*. The nanoparticle was rapidly internalized into the lysosome of melanoma cells and was retained in the subcellular compartment for over 24 h. In an *in vivo* melanoma model, treatment with the nanotube-doxorubicin conjugate abrogated tumor growth without the systemic side-effects associated with free doxorubicin. High-resolution photoacoustic tomography (PAT) with extraordinarily optical absorbing gold nanocages (AuNCs) was utilized in a study [135]. When bioconjugated with [Nle(4),D-Phe(7)]-alpha-melanocyte-stimulating hormone, the AuNCs served as a novel contrast agent for *in vivo* molecular PAT of melanomas with both exquisite sensitivity and high specificity. The bioconjugated AuNCs enhanced contrast approximately 300% more than the control, PEGylated AuNCs. A study optimized the antitumoral effects of direct electric current (DC) with poly(ε-caprolactone) (PCL) nanoparticles loaded with the amino acid tyrosine. The authors observed that the *in vitro* cytotoxicity of DC was significantly increased when associated with L-tyrosine-loaded NPs, using a murine multidrug-resistant melanoma cell line model. More studies involving nanotechnology are certainly required to be utilized in melanoma research that will open new avenues for prevention and therapy of melanoma. Studies involving nanoformulation of bioactive food components will be a welcome addition where nanotechnology could be involved to improve pharmacokinetics and reduce side effects associated with drugs.

12. Conclusions

With incessant efforts by the researchers worldwide, the prospect for the therapy of advanced melanoma has improved considerably and currently the future of this avenue is considered very optimistic. As described throughout this manuscript bioactive food components have great potential for melanoma therapy with each agent demonstrating multidimensional effects and targets as summarized under table 3. Although the preclinical data with these and other natural agents is encouraging, data from epidemiological studies is still needed to indicate a definite efficacy. Also, further understanding of the molecular and immunologic mechanisms that promote survival of melanoma tumor cells is needed. Several gene and protein modulation as depicted in table 2 could be targeted for better regulation of melanoma progression. Such information will undeniably lead to the development of better, more specific and less toxic agents. With careful planning and rational design of future human intervention trials and cohort studies natural agents could be easily exploited for betterment of patients with melanoma.

Another approach that seems promising is utilizing a combination of two or more bioactive food components. In contrast to the single agent approach, researchers should direct their attention upon different natural and synthetic products as a complex mixture, a cocktail approach, which together may have synergistic anti-cancer benefits. This approach could be exploited both *in vitro* and *in vivo* as well as in clinical and epidemiological studies. Since utilization of these bioactive food agents is relatively inexpensive, simple to use and possibly non-toxic, studies to assess its role in clinical melanoma is accessible and will be of interest. As many *in vitro* and *in vivo* studies assessing the role of dietary agents on melanoma have shown significant effects against multiple targets, an in-depth analysis of our approach with the chemopreventive cocktail is warranted.

Gene	Protein	References
Gene amplification		
MITF	Mitf	[142, 143]
BRAF	Braf	[143, 144]
c-MYC	c-Myc	[144-147]
HRAS	H-Ras	[148, 149]
CCND1	Cyclin D1	[150]
CDK4	Cdk4	[150]
CDH2	N-cadherin	[145, 151]
Gene losses		
ITGB3BP	beta 3 endonexin	[152]
CDKN2A	P16Ink4a/ p14Arf	[144, 150]
PTEN	Pten	[145, 150]

Table 2. Alterations involving known genes found in melanomas

Agent	Effects observed	References
Tea polyphenols	Inhibition of skin tumorigenesis	[16-19]
	Decreased UVB induced ODC, COX and tumorigenesis;	[20, 21, 23-25]
Curcumin	Inhibition of photoaging and photocarcinogenesis;	[30, 31]
	Modulation of multiple signaling pathways	[29, 32-34, 39, 48, 50, 54]
	Increase of intrinsic apoptotic pathway and/or autophagy	[42, 43]
Genistein	Inhibition of UV-induced effects *in vitro* Inhibition of inflammation and ODC activity	[64-66] [68]
Fisetin	Decreased cell viability and disruption of Wnt/β-catenin pathway	[74]
Resveratrol	Inhibition of skin tumorigenesis	[76, 77, 81]
	Decreased oxidative stress	[78]
Pomegranate	Modulation of multiple signaling pathways	[84-87]
	Inhibit UV-mediated apoptosis and DNA damage, photoprotection	[88, 89]
	Inhibit UV-induced pigmentation	[90]
Lupeol	Inhibit DMBA-induced DNA strand breaks and B(a)P induced genotoxicity	[102, 117]
	Inhibit tumor promotion, ODC activity etc.	[103, 104, 118]
Silymarin	Exhibit antioxidant, anti-inflammatory and immunomodulatory properties	[120, 121]

Table 3. Observed effects of various bioactive food components in skin cancer

13. Glossary

UVB	Ultraviolet B
ROS	reactive oxygen species
CPD	cyclobutane pyrimidine dimers
8-OHdG	8-hydroxy-2'-deoxyguanosine
EGCG	epigallocatechin-3-gallate
ECG	epicatechin-3-gallate
EC	Epicatechin
GTP	green tea polyphenols
TPA	12-O-tetradecanoyl-phorbol-13-acetate
ODC	ornithine decarboxylase
DMBA	7,12-dimethylbenz-a-anthracene
NF-ƘB	Nuclear factor-kappa B
TNF-α	tumor necrosis factor-alpha
XIAP	X-linked inhibitor of apoptosis
MMP	matrix metalloproteinase
TIMP	tissue inhibitor metalloproteinase
MT1-MMP	membrane type 1-matrix metalloproteinase
FAK	Focal Adhesion Kinase
Nm23	Non-metastatic 23
STAT1	signal transducer activator 1
NHEK	Normal Human Epidermal Keratinocyte

14. References

[1] A. Jemal, R. Siegel, J. Xu, E. Ward, Cancer statistics, 2010, CA Cancer J Clin 60 (2010) 277-300.

[2] A. Jemal, F. Bray, M.M. Center, J. Ferlay, E. Ward, D. Forman, Global cancer statistics, CA Cancer J Clin 61 (2011) 69-90.

[3] R. Siegel, E. Ward, O. Brawley, A. Jemal, Cancer statistics, 2011: The impact of eliminating socioeconomic and racial disparities on premature cancer deaths, CA Cancer J Clin (2011).

[4] V.M. Adhami, D.N. Syed, N. Khan, F. Afaq, Phytochemicals for prevention of solar ultraviolet radiation-induced damages, Photochem Photobiol 84 (2008) 489-500.

[5] F. Afaq, H. Mukhtar, Botanical antioxidants in the prevention of photocarcinogenesis and photoaging, Exp Dermatol 15 (2006) 678-684.

[6] G.T. Bowden, Prevention of non-melanoma skin cancer by targeting ultraviolet-B-light signalling, Nat Rev Cancer 4 (2004) 23-35.

[7] Y.P. Lu, Y.R. Lou, P. Yen, D. Mitchell, M.T. Huang, A.H. Conney, Time course for early adaptive responses to ultraviolet B light in the epidermis of SKH-1 mice, Cancer Res 59 (1999) 4591-4602.

[8] P. McLoone, E. Simics, A. Barton, M. Norval, N.K. Gibbs, An action spectrum for the production of cis-urocanic acid in human skin *in vivo*, J Invest Dermatol 124 (2005) 1071-1074.

[9] S.M. Lippman, J.J. Lee, A.L. Sabichi, Cancer chemoprevention: progress and promise, J Natl Cancer Inst 90 (1998) 1514-1528.

[10] M.F. Demierre, L. Nathanson, Chemoprevention of melanoma: an unexplored strategy, J Clin Oncol 21 (2003) 158-165.

[11] F. Afaq, V.M. Adhami, H. Mukhtar, Photochemoprevention of ultraviolet B signaling and photocarcinogenesis, Mutat Res 571 (2005) 153-173.

[12] Y.J. Surh, Cancer chemoprevention with dietary phytochemicals, Nat Rev Cancer 3 (2003) 768-780.

[13] J.A. Nichols, S.K. Katiyar, Skin photoprotection by natural polyphenols: anti-inflammatory, antioxidant and DNA repair mechanisms, Arch Dermatol Res 302 (2010) 71-83.

[14] D.A. Balentine, S.A. Wiseman, L.C. Bouwens, The chemistry of tea flavonoids, Crit Rev Food Sci Nutr 37 (1997) 693-704.

[15] C. Cabrera, R. Artacho, R. Gimenez, Beneficial effects of green tea--a review, J Am Coll Nutr 25 (2006) 79-99.

[16] W.A. Khan, Z.Y. Wang, M. Athar, D.R. Bickers, H. Mukhtar, Inhibition of the skin tumorigenicity of (+/-)-7 beta,8 alpha-dihydroxy-9 alpha,10 alpha-epoxy-7,8,9,10-tetrahydrobenzo[a]pyrene by tannic acid, green tea polyphenols and quercetin in Sencar mice, Cancer Lett 42 (1988) 7-12.

[17] S.K. Katiyar, R. Agarwal, Z.Y. Wang, A.K. Bhatia, H. Mukhtar, (-)-Epigallocatechin-3-gallate in Camellia sinensis leaves from Himalayan region of Sikkim: inhibitory effects against biochemical events and tumor initiation in Sencar mouse skin, Nutr Cancer 18 (1992) 73-83.

[18] Z.Y. Wang, M.T. Huang, C.T. Ho, R. Chang, W. Ma, T. Ferraro, K.R. Reuhl, C.S. Yang, A.H. Conney, Inhibitory effect of green tea on the growth of established skin papillomas in mice, Cancer Res 52 (1992) 6657-6665.

[19] Z.Y. Wang, M.T. Huang, T. Ferraro, C.Q. Wong, Y.R. Lou, K. Reuhl, M. Iatropoulos, C.S. Yang, A.H. Conney, Inhibitory effect of green tea in the drinking water on tumorigenesis by ultraviolet light and 12-O-tetradecanoylphorbol-13-acetate in the skin of SKH-1 mice, Cancer Res 52 (1992) 1162-1170.

[20] R. Agarwal, S.K. Katiyar, S.G. Khan, H. Mukhtar, Protection against ultraviolet B radiation-induced effects in the skin of SKH-1 hairless mice by a polyphenolic fraction isolated from green tea, Photochem Photobiol 58 (1993) 695-700.

[21] J.K. Kundu, H.K. Na, K.S. Chun, Y.K. Kim, S.J. Lee, S.S. Lee, O.S. Lee, Y.C. Sim, Y.J. Surh, Inhibition of phorbol ester-induced COX-2 expression by epigallocatechin gallate in mouse skin and cultured human mammary epithelial cells, J Nutr 133 (2003) 3805S-3810S.

[22] M. Nihal, N. Ahmad, H. Mukhtar, G.S. Wood, Anti-proliferative and proapoptotic effects of (-)-epigallocatechin-3-gallate on human melanoma: possible implications for the chemoprevention of melanoma, Int J Cancer 114 (2005) 513-521.

[23] S.K. Mantena, S.M. Meeran, C.A. Elmets, S.K. Katiyar, Orally administered green tea polyphenols prevent ultraviolet radiation-induced skin cancer in mice through activation of cytotoxic T cells and inhibition of angiogenesis in tumors, J Nutr 135 (2005) 2871-2877.

[24] A.H. Conney, Y.P. Lu, Y.R. Lou, M.T. Huang, Inhibitory effects of tea and caffeine on UV-induced carcinogenesis: relationship to enhanced apoptosis and decreased tissue fat, Eur J Cancer Prev 11 Suppl 2 (2002) S28-36.
[25] Y.P. Lu, Y.R. Lou, X.H. Li, J.G. Xie, D. Brash, M.T. Huang, A.H. Conney, Stimulatory effect of oral administration of green tea or caffeine on ultraviolet light-induced increases in epidermal wild-type p53, p21(WAF1/CIP1), and apoptotic sunburn cells in SKH-1 mice, Cancer Res 60 (2000) 4785-4791.
[26] P. Kramata, Y.P. Lu, Y.R. Lou, J.L. Cohen, M. Olcha, S. Liu, A.H. Conney, Effect of administration of caffeine or green tea on the mutation profile in the p53 gene in early mutant p53-positive patches of epidermal cells induced by chronic UVB-irradiation of hairless SKH-1 mice, Carcinogenesis 26 (2005) 1965-1974.
[27] R.G. Shah, M.S. Netrawali, Evaluation of mutagenic activity of turmeric extract containing curcumin, before and after activation with mammalian cecal microbial extract of liver microsomal fraction, in the Ames Salmonella test, Bull Environ Contam Toxicol 40 (1988) 350-357.
[28] R.K. Maheshwari, A.K. Singh, J. Gaddipati, R.C. Srimal, Multiple biological activities of curcumin: a short review, Life Sci 78 (2006) 2081-2087.
[29] B.B. Aggarwal, A. Kumar, A.C. Bharti, Anticancer potential of curcumin: preclinical and clinical studies, Anticancer Res 23 (2003) 363-398.
[30] M.C. Heng, Curcumin targeted signaling pathways: basis for anti-photoaging and anti-carcinogenic therapy, Int J Dermatol 49 (2010) 608-622.
[31] M. Zheng, S. Ekmekcioglu, E.T. Walch, C.H. Tang, E.A. Grimm, Inhibition of nuclear factor-kappaB and nitric oxide by curcumin induces G2/M cell cycle arrest and apoptosis in human melanoma cells, Melanoma Res 14 (2004) 165-171.
[32] Y.J. Surh, S.S. Han, Y.S. Keum, H.J. Seo, S.S. Lee, Inhibitory effects of curcumin and capsaicin on phorbol ester-induced activation of eukaryotic transcription factors, NF-kappaB and AP-1, Biofactors 12 (2000) 107-112.
[33] Y.E. Marin, B.A. Wall, S. Wang, J. Namkoong, J.J. Martino, J. Suh, H.J. Lee, A.B. Rabson, C.S. Yang, S. Chen, J.H. Ryu, Curcumin downregulates the constitutive activity of NF-kappaB and induces apoptosis in novel mouse melanoma cells, Melanoma Res 17 (2007) 274-283.
[34] J.A. Bush, K.J. Cheung, Jr., G. Li, Curcumin induces apoptosis in human melanoma cells through a Fas receptor/caspase-8 pathway independent of p53, Exp Cell Res 271 (2001) 305-314.
[35] J. Bakhshi, L. Weinstein, K.S. Poksay, B. Nishinaga, D.E. Bredesen, R.V. Rao, Coupling endoplasmic reticulum stress to the cell death program in mouse melanoma cells: effect of curcumin, Apoptosis 13 (2008) 904-914.
[36] D.R. Siwak, S. Shishodia, B.B. Aggarwal, R. Kurzrock, Curcumin-induced antiproliferative and proapoptotic effects in melanoma cells are associated with suppression of IkappaB kinase and nuclear factor kappaB activity and are independent of the B-Raf/mitogen-activated/extracellular signal-regulated protein kinase pathway and the Akt pathway, Cancer 104 (2005) 879-890.
[37] M.A. Bill, C. Bakan, D.M. Benson, Jr., J. Fuchs, G. Young, G.B. Lesinski, Curcumin induces proapoptotic effects against human melanoma cells and modulates the

cellular response to immunotherapeutic cytokines, Mol Cancer Ther 8 (2009) 2726-2735.

[38] A. Banerji, J. Chakrabarti, A. Mitra, A. Chatterjee, Effect of curcumin on gelatinase A (MMP-2) activity in B16F10 melanoma cells, Cancer Lett 211 (2004) 235-242.

[39] S. Ray, N. Chattopadhyay, A. Mitra, M. Siddiqi, A. Chatterjee, Curcumin exhibits antimetastatic properties by modulating integrin receptors, collagenase activity, and expression of Nm23 and E-cadherin, J Environ Pathol Toxicol Oncol 22 (2003) 49-58.

[40] J.H. Lee, J.Y. Jang, C. Park, B.W. Kim, Y.H. Choi, B.T. Choi, Curcumin suppresses alpha-melanocyte stimulating hormone-stimulated melanogenesis in B16F10 cells, Int J Mol Med 26 (2010) 101-106.

[41] B.E. Bachmeier, C.M. Iancu, P.H. Killian, E. Kronski, V. Mirisola, G. Angelini, M. Jochum, A.G. Nerlich, U. Pfeffer, Overexpression of the ATP binding cassette gene ABCA1 determines resistance to Curcumin in M14 melanoma cells, Mol Cancer 8 (2009) 129.

[42] T. Yu, J. Li, H. Sun, C6 ceramide potentiates curcumin-induced cell death and apoptosis in melanoma cell lines *in vitro*, Cancer Chemother Pharmacol 66 (2010) 999-1003.

[43] S.J. Chatterjee, S. Pandey, Chemo-resistant melanoma sensitized by tamoxifen to low dose curcumin treatment through induction of apoptosis and autophagy, Cancer Biol Ther 11 (2011) 216-228.

[44] M. Pisano, G. Pagnan, M.A. Dettori, S. Cossu, I. Caffa, I. Sassu, L. Emionite, D. Fabbri, M. Cilli, F. Pastorino, G. Palmieri, G. Delogu, M. Ponzoni, C. Rozzo, Enhanced anti-tumor activity of a new curcumin-related compound against melanoma and neuroblastoma cells, Mol Cancer 9 (2010) 137.

[45] P.V. Leyon, G. Kuttan, Studies on the role of some synthetic curcuminoid derivatives in the inhibition of tumour specific angiogenesis, J Exp Clin Cancer Res 22 (2003) 77-83.

[46] M.A. Bill, J.R. Fuchs, C. Li, J. Yui, C. Bakan, D.M. Benson, Jr., E.B. Schwartz, D. Abdelhamid, J. Lin, D.G. Hoyt, S.L. Fossey, G.S. Young, W.E. Carson, 3rd, P.K. Li, G.B. Lesinski, The small molecule curcumin analog FLLL32 induces apoptosis in melanoma cells via STAT3 inhibition and retains the cellular response to cytokines with anti-tumor activity, Mol Cancer 9 (2010) 165.

[47] Z. Ma, A. Haddadi, O. Molavi, A. Lavasanifar, R. Lai, J. Samuel, Micelles of poly(ethylene oxide)-b-poly(epsilon-caprolactone) as vehicles for the solubilization, stabilization, and controlled delivery of curcumin, J Biomed Mater Res A 86 (2008) 300-310.

[48] L.G. Menon, R. Kuttan, G. Kuttan, Anti-metastatic activity of curcumin and catechin, Cancer Lett 141 (1999) 159-165.

[49] L. Wang, Y. Shen, R. Song, Y. Sun, J. Xu, Q. Xu, An anticancer effect of curcumin mediated by down-regulating phosphatase of regenerating liver-3 expression on highly metastatic melanoma cells, Mol Pharmacol 76 (2009) 1238-1245.

[50] Y.P. Lu, R.L. Chang, Y.R. Lou, M.T. Huang, H.L. Newmark, K.R. Reuhl, A.H. Conney, Effect of curcumin on 12-O-tetradecanoylphorbol-13-acetate- and ultraviolet B

light-induced expression of c-Jun and c-Fos in JB6 cells and in mouse epidermis, Carcinogenesis 15 (1994) 2363-2370.

[51] P. Limtrakul, S. Anuchapreeda, S. Lipigorngoson, F.W. Dunn, Inhibition of carcinogen induced c-Ha-ras and c-fos proto-oncogenes expression by dietary curcumin, BMC Cancer 1 (2001) 1.

[52] P. Limtrakul, S. Lipigorngoson, O. Namwong, A. Apisariyakul, F.W. Dunn, Inhibitory effect of dietary curcumin on skin carcinogenesis in mice, Cancer Lett 116 (1997) 197-203.

[53] M.T. Huang, W. Ma, P. Yen, J.G. Xie, J. Han, K. Frenkel, D. Grunberger, A.H. Conney, Inhibitory effects of topical application of low doses of curcumin on 12-O-tetradecanoylphorbol-13-acetate-induced tumor promotion and oxidized DNA bases in mouse epidermis, Carcinogenesis 18 (1997) 83-88.

[54] S.S. Kakar, D. Roy, Curcumin inhibits TPA induced expression of c-fos, c-jun and c-myc proto-oncogenes messenger RNAs in mouse skin, Cancer Lett 87 (1994) 85-89.

[55] Y. Cao, Q. Chu, Y. Fang, J. Ye, Analysis of flavonoids in Ginkgo biloba L. and its phytopharmaceuticals by capillary electrophoresis with electrochemical detection, Anal Bioanal Chem 374 (2002) 294-299.

[56] V. Exarchou, N. Nenadis, M. Tsimidou, I.P. Gerothanassis, A. Troganis, D. Boskou, Antioxidant activities and phenolic composition of extracts from Greek oregano, Greek sage, and summer savory, J Agric Food Chem 50 (2002) 5294-5299.

[57] T. Whitsett, M. Carpenter, C.A. Lamartiniere, Resveratrol, but not EGCG, in the diet suppresses DMBA-induced mammary cancer in rats, J Carcinog 5 (2006) 15.

[58] N. Khan, F. Afaq, H. Mukhtar, Cancer chemoprevention through dietary antioxidants: progress and promise, Antioxid Redox Signal 10 (2008) 475-510.

[59] C. Linassier, M. Pierre, J.B. Le Pecq, J. Pierre, Mechanisms of action in NIH-3T3 cells of genistein, an inhibitor of EGF receptor tyrosine kinase activity, Biochem Pharmacol 39 (1990) 187-193.

[60] E.B. Yang, D.F. Wang, P. Mack, L.Y. Cheng, Genistein, a tyrosine kinase inhibitor, reduces EGF-induced EGF receptor internalization and degradation in human hepatoma HepG2 cells, Biochem Biophys Res Commun 224 (1996) 309-317.

[61] A. Okura, H. Arakawa, H. Oka, T. Yoshinari, Y. Monden, Effect of genistein on topoisomerase activity and on the growth of [Val 12]Ha-ras-transformed NIH 3T3 cells, Biochem Biophys Res Commun 157 (1988) 183-189.

[62] J. Wang, I.E. Eltoum, C.A. Lamartiniere, Genistein alters growth factor signaling in transgenic prostate model (TRAMP), Mol Cell Endocrinol 219 (2004) 171-180.

[63] T. Fotsis, M. Pepper, H. Adlercreutz, G. Fleischmann, T. Hase, R. Montesano, L. Schweigerer, Genistein, a dietary-derived inhibitor of *in vitro* angiogenesis, Proc Natl Acad Sci U S A 90 (1993) 2690-2694.

[64] C. Maziere, F. Dantin, F. Dubois, R. Santus, J. Maziere, Biphasic effect of UVA radiation on STAT1 activity and tyrosine phosphorylation in cultured human keratinocytes, Free Radic Biol Med 28 (2000) 1430-1437.

[65] J.O. Moore, Y. Wang, W.G. Stebbins, D. Gao, X. Zhou, R. Phelps, M. Lebwohl, H. Wei, Photoprotective effect of isoflavone genistein on ultraviolet B-induced pyrimidine

dimer formation and PCNA expression in human reconstituted skin and its implications in dermatology and prevention of cutaneous carcinogenesis, Carcinogenesis 27 (2006) 1627-1635.

[66] H. Wei, R. Saladi, Y. Lu, Y. Wang, S.R. Palep, J. Moore, R. Phelps, E. Shyong, M.G. Lebwohl, Isoflavone genistein: photoprotection and clinical implications in dermatology, J Nutr 133 (2003) 3811S-3819S.

[67] Y. Wang, X. Zhang, M. Lebwohl, V. DeLeo, H. Wei, Inhibition of ultraviolet B (UVB)-induced c-fos and c-jun expression *in vivo* by a tyrosine kinase inhibitor genistein, Carcinogenesis 19 (1998) 649-654.

[68] H. Wei, R. Bowen, X. Zhang, M. Lebwohl, Isoflavone genistein inhibits the initiation and promotion of two-stage skin carcinogenesis in mice, Carcinogenesis 19 (1998) 1509-1514.

[69] M. Kimira, Y. Arai, K. Shimoi, S. Watanabe, Japanese intake of flavonoids and isoflavonoids from foods, J Epidemiol 8 (1998) 168-175.

[70] K. Ishige, D. Schubert, Y. Sagara, Flavonoids protect neuronal cells from oxidative stress by three distinct mechanisms, Free Radic Biol Med 30 (2001) 433-446.

[71] P. Maher, T. Akaishi, K. Abe, Flavonoid fisetin promotes ERK-dependent long-term potentiation and enhances memory, Proc Natl Acad Sci U S A 103 (2006) 16568-16573.

[72] Y. Sagara, J. Vanhnasy, P. Maher, Induction of PC12 cell differentiation by flavonoids is dependent upon extracellular signal-regulated kinase activation, J Neurochem 90 (2004) 1144-1155.

[73] D.N. Syed, Y. Suh, F. Afaq, H. Mukhtar, Dietary agents for chemoprevention of prostate cancer, Cancer Lett 265 (2008) 167-176.

[74] D.N. Syed, F. Afaq, N. Maddodi, J.J. Johnson, S. Sarfaraz, A. Ahmad, V. Setaluri, H. Mukhtar, Inhibition of Human Melanoma Cell Growth by the Dietary Flavonoid Fisetin Is Associated with Disruption of Wnt/beta-Catenin Signaling and Decreased Mitf Levels, J Invest Dermatol 131 (2011) 1291-1299.

[75] R. Hain, H.J. Reif, E. Krause, R. Langebartels, H. Kindl, B. Vornam, W. Wiese, E. Schmelzer, P.H. Schreier, R.H. Stocker, *et al.*, Disease resistance results from foreign phytoalexin expression in a novel plant, Nature 361 (1993) 153-156.

[76] M. Jang, L. Cai, G.O. Udeani, K.V. Slowing, C.F. Thomas, C.W. Beecher, H.H. Fong, N.R. Farnsworth, A.D. Kinghorn, R.G. Mehta, R.C. Moon, J.M. Pezzuto, Cancer chemopreventive activity of resveratrol, a natural product derived from grapes, Science 275 (1997) 218-220.

[77] G.J. Kapadia, M.A. Azuine, H. Tokuda, M. Takasaki, T. Mukainaka, T. Konoshima, H. Nishino, Chemopreventive effect of resveratrol, sesamol, sesame oil and sunflower oil in the Epstein-Barr virus early antigen activation assay and the mouse skin two-stage carcinogenesis, Pharmacol Res 45 (2002) 499-505.

[78] F. Afaq, V.M. Adhami, N. Ahmad, Prevention of short-term ultraviolet B radiation-mediated damages by resveratrol in SKH-1 hairless mice, Toxicol Appl Pharmacol 186 (2003) 28-37.

[79] S. Reagan-Shaw, F. Afaq, M.H. Aziz, N. Ahmad, Modulations of critical cell cycle regulatory events during chemoprevention of ultraviolet B-mediated responses by resveratrol in SKH-1 hairless mouse skin, Oncogene 23 (2004) 5151-5160.

[80] V.M. Adhami, F. Afaq, N. Ahmad, Suppression of ultraviolet B exposure-mediated activation of NF-kappaB in normal human keratinocytes by resveratrol, Neoplasia 5 (2003) 74-82.

[81] S.H. Jee, S.C. Shen, C.R. Tseng, H.C. Chiu, M.L. Kuo, Curcumin induces a p53-dependent apoptosis in human basal cell carcinoma cells, J Invest Dermatol 111 (1998) 656-661.

[82] M.I. Gil, F.A. Tomas-Barberan, B. Hess-Pierce, D.M. Holcroft, A.A. Kader, Antioxidant activity of pomegranate juice and its relationship with phenolic composition and processing, J Agric Food Chem 48 (2000) 4581-4589.

[83] N.P. Seeram, L.S. Adams, S.M. Henning, Y. Niu, Y. Zhang, M.G. Nair, D. Heber, *In vitro* antiproliferative, apoptotic and antioxidant activities of punicalagin, ellagic acid and a total pomegranate tannin extract are enhanced in combination with other polyphenols as found in pomegranate juice, J Nutr Biochem 16 (2005) 360-367.

[84] F. Afaq, N. Ahmad, H. Mukhtar, Suppression of UVB-induced phosphorylation of mitogen-activated protein kinases and nuclear factor kappa B by green tea polyphenol in SKH-1 hairless mice, Oncogene 22 (2003) 9254-9264.

[85] D.N. Syed, A. Malik, N. Hadi, S. Sarfaraz, F. Afaq, H. Mukhtar, Photochemopreventive effect of pomegranate fruit extract on UVA-mediated activation of cellular pathways in normal human epidermal keratinocytes, Photochem Photobiol 82 (2006) 398-405.

[86] F. Afaq, M. Saleem, C.G. Krueger, J.D. Reed, H. Mukhtar, Anthocyanin- and hydrolyzable tannin-rich pomegranate fruit extract modulates MAPK and NF-kappaB pathways and inhibits skin tumorigenesis in CD-1 mice, Int J Cancer 113 (2005) 423-433.

[87] M.A. Zaid, F. Afaq, D.N. Syed, M. Dreher, H. Mukhtar, Inhibition of UVB-mediated oxidative stress and markers of photoaging in immortalized HaCaT keratinocytes by pomegranate polyphenol extract POMx, Photochem Photobiol 83 (2007) 882-888.

[88] F. Afaq, D.N. Syed, A. Malik, N. Hadi, S. Sarfaraz, M.H. Kweon, N. Khan, M.A. Zaid, H. Mukhtar, Delphinidin, an anthocyanidin in pigmented fruits and vegetables, protects human HaCaT keratinocytes and mouse skin against UVB-mediated oxidative stress and apoptosis, J Invest Dermatol 127 (2007) 222-232.

[89] F. Afaq, N. Khan, D.N. Syed, H. Mukhtar, Oral feeding of pomegranate fruit extract inhibits early biomarkers of UVB radiation-induced carcinogenesis in SKH-1 hairless mouse epidermis, Photochem Photobiol 86 (2010) 1318-1326.

[90] K. Kasai, M. Yoshimura, T. Koga, M. Arii, S. Kawasaki, Effects of oral administration of ellagic acid-rich pomegranate extract on ultraviolet-induced pigmentation in the human skin, J Nutr Sci Vitaminol (Tokyo) 52 (2006) 383-388.

[91] M. Saleem, Lupeol, a novel anti-inflammatory and anti-cancer dietary triterpene, Cancer Lett 285 (2009) 109-115.

[92] T.H. Beveridge, T.S. Li, J.C. Drover, Phytosterol content in American ginseng seed oil, J Agric Food Chem 50 (2002) 744-750.

[93] S. Imam, I. Azhar, M.M. Hasan, M.S. Ali, S.W. Ahmed, Two triterpenes lupanone and lupeol isolated and identified from Tamarindus indica linn, Pak J Pharm Sci 20 (2007) 125-127.

[94] B.G. Harish, V. Krishna, H.S. Santosh Kumar, B.M. Khadeer Ahamed, R. Sharath, H.M. Kumara Swamy, Wound healing activity and docking of glycogen-synthase-kinase-3-beta-protein with isolated triterpenoid lupeol in rats, Phytomedicine 15 (2008) 763-767.

[95] T. Geetha, P. Varalakshmi, R.M. Latha, Effect of triterpenes from Crataeva nurvala stem bark on lipid peroxidation in adjuvant induced arthritis in rats, Pharmacol Res 37 (1998) 191-195.

[96] Y.J. You, N.H. Nam, Y. Kim, K.H. Bae, B.Z. Ahn, Antiangiogenic activity of lupeol from Bombax ceiba, Phytother Res 17 (2003) 341-344.

[97] M.L. Macias-Rubalcava, B.E. Hernandez-Bautista, M. Jimenez-Estrada, R. Cruz-Ortega, A.L. Anaya, Pentacyclic triterpenes with selective bioactivity from Sebastiania adenophora leaves, Euphorbiaceae, J Chem Ecol 33 (2007) 147-156.

[98] M.A. Fernandez, B. de las Heras, M.D. Garcia, M.T. Saenz, A. Villar, New insights into the mechanism of action of the anti-inflammatory triterpene lupeol, J Pharm Pharmacol 53 (2001) 1533-1539.

[99] V. Sudhahar, S. Ashok Kumar, P. Varalakshmi, V. Sujatha, Protective effect of lupeol and lupeol linoleate in hypercholesterolemia associated renal damage, Mol Cell Biochem 317 (2008) 11-20.

[100] T. Akihisa, K. Yasukawa, H. Oinuma, Y. Kasahara, S. Yamanouchi, M. Takido, K. Kumaki, T. Tamura, Triterpene alcohols from the flowers of compositae and their anti-inflammatory effects, Phytochemistry 43 (1996) 1255-1260.

[101] L. Novotny, A. Vachalkova, D. Biggs, Ursolic acid: an anti-tumorigenic and chemopreventive activity. Minireview, Neoplasma 48 (2001) 241-246.

[102] N. Nigam, S. Prasad, Y. Shukla, Preventive effects of lupeol on DMBA induced DNA alkylation damage in mouse skin, Food Chem Toxicol 45 (2007) 2331-2335.

[103] M. Saleem, F. Afaq, V.M. Adhami, H. Mukhtar, Lupeol modulates NF-kappaB and PI3K/Akt pathways and inhibits skin cancer in CD-1 mice, Oncogene 23 (2004) 5203-5214.

[104] M. Saleem, N. Maddodi, M. Abu Zaid, N. Khan, B. bin Hafeez, M. Asim, Y. Suh, J.M. Yun, V. Setaluri, H. Mukhtar, Lupeol inhibits growth of highly aggressive human metastatic melanoma cells *in vitro* and *in vivo* by inducing apoptosis, Clin Cancer Res 14 (2008) 2119-2127.

[105] M. Saleem, S. Kaur, M.H. Kweon, V.M. Adhami, F. Afaq, H. Mukhtar, Lupeol, a fruit and vegetable based triterpene, induces apoptotic death of human pancreatic adenocarcinoma cells via inhibition of Ras signaling pathway, Carcinogenesis 26 (2005) 1956-1964.

[106] T.K. Lee, R.T. Poon, J.Y. Wo, S. Ma, X.Y. Guan, J.N. Myers, P. Altevogt, A.P. Yuen, Lupeol suppresses cisplatin-induced nuclear factor-kappaB activation in head and

neck squamous cell carcinoma and inhibits local invasion and nodal metastasis in an orthotopic nude mouse model, Cancer Res 67 (2007) 8800-8809.
[107] M. Saleem, I. Murtaza, R.S. Tarapore, Y. Suh, V.M. Adhami, J.J. Johnson, I.A. Siddiqui, N. Khan, M. Asim, B.B. Hafeez, M.T. Shekhani, B. Li, H. Mukhtar, Lupeol inhibits proliferation of human prostate cancer cells by targeting beta-catenin signaling, Carcinogenesis 30 (2009) 808-817.
[108] T. Geetha, P. Varalakshmi, Anticomplement activity of triterpenes from Crataeva nurvala stem bark in adjuvant arthritis in rats, Gen Pharmacol 32 (1999) 495-497.
[109] S. Bani, A. Kaul, B. Khan, S.F. Ahmad, K.A. Suri, B.D. Gupta, N.K. Satti, G.N. Qazi, Suppression of T lymphocyte activity by lupeol isolated from Crataeva religiosa, Phytother Res 20 (2006) 279-287.
[110] W.N. Setzer, M.C. Setzer, Plant-derived triterpenoids as potential antineoplastic agents, Mini Rev Med Chem 3 (2003) 540-556.
[111] P.G. Bradford, A.B. Awad, Phytosterols as anticancer compounds, Mol Nutr Food Res 51 (2007) 161-170.
[112] T.R. Devereux, J.I. Risinger, J.C. Barrett, Mutations and altered expression of the human cancer genes: what they tell us about causes, IARC Sci Publ (1999) 19-42.
[113] W.B. Coleman, G.J. Tsongalis, The role of genomic instability in human carcinogenesis, Anticancer Res 19 (1999) 4645-4664.
[114] R.A. DePinho, The age of cancer, Nature 408 (2000) 248-254.
[115] B.A. Ponder, Cancer genetics, Nature 411 (2001) 336-341.
[116] M. Lira Wde, F.V. dos Santos, M. Sannomiya, C.M. Rodrigues, W. Vilegas, E.A. Varanda, Modulatory effect of Byrsonima basiloba extracts on the mutagenicity of certain direct and indirect-acting mutagens in Salmonella typhimurium assays, J Med Food 11 (2008) 111-119.
[117] S. Prasad, V. Kumar Yadav, S. Srivastava, Y. Shukla, Protective effects of lupeol against benzo[a]pyrene induced clastogenicity in mouse bone marrow cells, Mol Nutr Food Res 52 (2008) 1117-1120.
[118] U.K. Basuroy, E.W. Gerner, Emerging concepts in targeting the polyamine metabolic pathway in epithelial cancer chemoprevention and chemotherapy, J Biochem 139 (2006) 27-33.
[119] I.A. Siddiqui, V.M. Adhami, D.J. Bharali, B.B. Hafeez, M. Asim, S.I. Khwaja, N. Ahmad, H. Cui, S.A. Mousa, H. Mukhtar, Introducing nanochemoprevention as a novel approach for cancer control: proof of principle with green tea polyphenol epigallocatechin-3-gallate, Cancer Res 69 (2009) 1712-1716.
[120] M. Vaid, S.K. Katiyar, Molecular mechanisms of inhibition of photocarcinogenesis by silymarin, a phytochemical from milk thistle (Silybum marianum L. Gaertn.) (Review), Int J Oncol 36 (2010) 1053-1060.
[121] S.K. Katiyar, Silymarin and skin cancer prevention: anti-inflammatory, antioxidant and immunomodulatory effects (Review), Int J Oncol 26 (2005) 169-176.
[122] L.H. Li, L.J. Wu, S.I. Tashiro, S. Onodera, F. Uchiumi, T. Ikejima, The roles of Akt and MAPK family members in silymarin's protection against UV-induced A375-S2 cell apoptosis, Int Immunopharmacol 6 (2006) 190-197.

[123] L.H. Li, L.J. Wu, Y.Y. Jiang, S. Tashiro, S. Onodera, F. Uchiumi, T. Ikejima, Silymarin enhanced cytotoxic effect of anti-Fas agonistic antibody CH11 on A375-S2 cells, J Asian Nat Prod Res 9 (2007) 593-602.

[124] Y.Y. Jiang, H.J. Wang, J. Wang, S. Tashiro, S. Onodera, T. Ikejima, The protective effect of silibinin against mitomycin C-induced intrinsic apoptosis in human melanoma A375-S2 cells, J Pharmacol Sci 111 (2009) 137-146.

[125] D. Tatman, H. Mo, Volatile isoprenoid constituents of fruits, vegetables and herbs cumulatively suppress the proliferation of murine B16 melanoma and human HL-60 leukemia cells, Cancer Lett 175 (2002) 129-139.

[126] M. Lluria-Prevatt, J. Morreale, J. Gregus, D.S. Alberts, F. Kaper, A. Giaccia, M.B. Powell, Effects of perillyl alcohol on melanoma in the TPras mouse model, Cancer Epidemiol Biomarkers Prev 11 (2002) 573-579.

[127] S.P. Stratton, D.S. Alberts, J.G. Einspahr, P.M. Sagerman, J.A. Warneke, C. Curiel-Lewandrowski, P.B. Myrdal, K.L. Karlage, B.J. Nickoloff, C. Brooks, K. Saboda, M.L. Yozwiak, M.F. Krutzsch, C. Hu, M. Lluria-Prevatt, Z. Dong, G.T. Bowden, P.H. Bartels, A phase 2a study of topical perillyl alcohol cream for chemoprevention of skin cancer, Cancer Prev Res (Phila) 3 (2010) 160-169.

[128] H. Hakimzadeh, T. Ghazanfari, B. Rahmati, H. Naderimanesh, Cytotoxic effect of garlic extract and its fractions on Sk-mel3 melanoma cell line, Immunopharmacol Immunotoxicol 32 (2010) 371-375.

[129] H.Y. Kim, J.H. Kim, S.B. Yang, S.G. Hong, S.A. Lee, S.J. Hwang, K.S. Shin, H.J. Suh, M.H. Park, A polysaccharide extracted from rice bran fermented with Lentinus edodes enhances natural killer cell activity and exhibits anticancer effects, J Med Food 10 (2007) 25-31.

[130] Y. Fuke, S. Shinoda, I. Nagata, S. Sawaki, M. Murata, K. Ryoyama, K. Koizumi, I. Saiki, T. Nomura, Preventive effect of oral administration of 6-(methylsulfinyl)hexyl isothiocyanate derived from wasabi (Wasabia japonica Matsum) against pulmonary metastasis of B16-BL6 mouse melanoma cells, Cancer Detect Prev 30 (2006) 174-179.

[131] A. Lentini, C. Forni, B. Provenzano, S. Beninati, Enhancement of transglutaminase activity and polyamine depletion in B16-F10 melanoma cells by flavonoids naringenin and hesperitin correlate to reduction of the *in vivo* metastatic potential, Amino Acids 32 (2007) 95-100.

[132] E. Pichichero, R. Cicconi, M. Mattei, A. Canini, Chrysin-induced apoptosis is mediated through p38 and Bax activation in B16-F1 and A375 melanoma cells, Int J Oncol 38 (2011) 473-483.

[133] M. Banciu, J.M. Metselaar, R.M. Schiffelers, G. Storm, Liposomal glucocorticoids as tumor-targeted anti-angiogenic nanomedicine in B16 melanoma-bearing mice, J Steroid Biochem Mol Biol 111 (2008) 101-110.

[134] M.A. Tran, R.J. Watts, G.P. Robertson, Use of liposomes as drug delivery vehicles for treatment of melanoma, Pigment Cell Melanoma Res 22 (2009) 388-399.

[135] C. Kim, E.C. Cho, J. Chen, K.H. Song, L. Au, C. Favazza, Q. Zhang, C.M. Cobley, F. Gao, Y. Xia, L.V. Wang, *in vivo* molecular photoacoustic tomography of melanomas targeted by bioconjugated gold nanocages, ACS Nano 4 (2010) 4559-4564.

[136] D.L. Narayanan, R.N. Saladi, J.L. Fox, Ultraviolet radiation and skin cancer, Int J Dermatol 49 (2010) 978-986.

[137] D.S. Preston, R.S. Stern, Nonmelanoma cancers of the skin, N Engl J Med 327 (1992) 1649-1662.

[138] H.M. Gloster, Jr., K. Neal, Skin cancer in skin of color, J Am Acad Dermatol 55 (2006) 741-760; quiz 761-744.

[139] K. Glanz, D.B. Buller, M. Saraiya, Reducing ultraviolet radiation exposure among outdoor workers: state of the evidence and recommendations, Environ Health 6 (2007) 22.

[140] K. Glanz, A.L. Yaroch, M. Dancel, M. Saraiya, L.A. Crane, D.B. Buller, S. Manne, D.L. O'Riordan, C.J. Heckman, J. Hay, J.K. Robinson, Measures of sun exposure and sun protection practices for behavioral and epidemiologic research, Arch Dermatol 144 (2008) 217-222.

[141] A.J. Swerdlow, M.A. Weinstock, Do tanning lamps cause melanoma? An epidemiologic assessment, J Am Acad Dermatol 38 (1998) 89-98.

[142] D.C. Whiteman, C.A. Whiteman, A.C. Green, Childhood sun exposure as a risk factor for melanoma: a systematic review of epidemiologic studies, Cancer Causes Control 12 (2001) 69-82.

[143] G. Jonsson, C. Dahl, J. Staaf, T. Sandberg, P.O. Bendahl, M. Ringner, P. Guldberg, A. Borg, Genomic profiling of malignant melanoma using tiling-resolution arrayCGH, Oncogene 26 (2007) 4738-4748.

[144] B.C. Bastian, P.E. LeBoit, H. Hamm, E.B. Brocker, D. Pinkel, Chromosomal gains and losses in primary cutaneous melanomas detected by comparative genomic hybridization, Cancer Res 58 (1998) 2170-2175.

[145] M. Balazs, Z. Adam, A. Treszl, A. Begany, J. Hunyadi, R. Adany, Chromosomal imbalances in primary and metastatic melanomas revealed by comparative genomic hybridization, Cytometry 46 (2001) 222-232.

[146] M.R. Speicher, G. Prescher, S. du Manoir, A. Jauch, B. Horsthemke, N. Bornfeld, R. Becher, T. Cremer, Chromosomal gains and losses in uveal melanomas detected by comparative genomic hybridization, Cancer Res 54 (1994) 3817-3823.

[147] C.M. Vajdic, A.M. Hutchins, A. Kricker, J.F. Aitken, B.K. Armstrong, N.K. Hayward, J.E. Armes, Chromosomal gains and losses in ocular melanoma detected by comparative genomic hybridization in an Australian population-based study, Cancer Genet Cytogenet 144 (2003) 12-17.

[148] B.C. Bastian, U. Wesselmann, D. Pinkel, P.E. Leboit, Molecular cytogenetic analysis of Spitz nevi shows clear differences to melanoma, J Invest Dermatol 113 (1999) 1065-1069.

[149] J. Bauer, B.C. Bastian, Distinguishing melanocytic nevi from melanoma by DNA copy number changes: comparative genomic hybridization as a research and diagnostic tool, Dermatol Ther 19 (2006) 40-49.

[150] J.A. Curtin, J. Fridlyand, T. Kageshita, H.N. Patel, K.J. Busam, H. Kutzner, K.H. Cho, S. Aiba, E.B. Brocker, P.E. LeBoit, D. Pinkel, B.C. Bastian, Distinct sets of genetic alterations in melanoma, N Engl J Med 353 (2005) 2135-2147.

[151] J.S. White, I.W. McLean, R.L. Becker, A.E. Director-Myska, J. Nath, Correlation of comparative genomic hybridization results of 100 archival uveal melanomas with patient survival, Cancer Genet Cytogenet 170 (2006) 29-39.

[152] T. Hausler, A. Stang, G. Anastassiou, K.H. Jockel, S. Mrzyk, B. Horsthemke, D.R. Lohmann, M. Zeschnigk, Loss of heterozygosity of 1p in uveal melanomas with monosomy 3, Int J Cancer 116 (2005) 909-913.